THE
SAVVY PATIENT

THE
SAVVY PATIENT

The Ultimate Advocate for
Quality Health Care

Mark C. Pettus, M.D.

A CAPITAL CARES BOOK

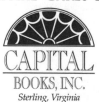

CAPITAL
BOOKS, INC.
Sterling, Virginia

Capital Books, Inc.
P.O. Box 605
Herndon, Virginia 20172-0605

ISBN 1-931868-80-8 (alk. paper)

The following illustrations in chapter two were provided with permission from Philips Medical Systems: A typical AED device; Attending to an unresponsive person and finding an AED device; Placing the defibrillator pads; On command, pressing the button to defibrillate.

Library of Congress Cataloging-in-Publication Data

Pettus, Mark C.
The savvy patient : the ultimate advocate for quality health care /
  Mark C. Pettus.
     p. cm.—(A Capital cares book)
  Includes bibliographical references and index.
  ISBN 1-931868-80-8 (alk. paper)
    1. Patient education—United States.   2. Medical care—United States.
  I. Title. II. Series.
  R727.4.P48 2004
  615.5'071—dc22
                                         2004005357

Printed in the United States of America on acid-free paper that meets the American National Standards Institute Z39-48 Standard.

Book design and composition by Susan Mark
Coghill Composition Company
Richmond, Virginia

First Edition

10 9 8 7 6 5 4 3 2 1

To my wife LeeAnn, my sister Nancy, and my children Anna and Alex. Words cannot express my love for you. This book is largely about what I do when I am not at home. I am grateful for your patience, love, and understanding.

To my courageous friend and colleague Jordan. Thank you for sharing your strength, faith, and wisdom.

ACKNOWLEDGMENTS

I AM very grateful to the many individuals who supported this effort. Special thanks to Helen Austin for her many hours of work in the preparation of *The Savvy Patient*. I also wish to thank the individuals who reviewed the manuscript and whose feedback was most valuable. Thanks to Brian Andrews, President of Berkshire County Ambulance, for his assistance with the chapter on pre-hospital care; Ken Tabor, Pharm.D., for his assistance with the chapter on taking medications; and Michelle Franklin and John Gottung for their assistance in the chapter on ICU/CCU care. I also wish to thank Gray Ellrodt, M.D., Burgess Record, M.D., and John St. Laurent for their valuable feedback.

DISCLAIMER

OPEN ANY publication that provides medical information and you will see, up front, a disclaimer. One important reason for the disclaimer is to make clear that any medical information must be interpreted on an individualized basis and discussed with your own physician (assuming you have one—many people do not) prior to the application of this newfound knowledge. As there is no one-size-fits all approach to health, wellness, and disease management, I have tried to focus on generalizations that I believe most people will find extremely beneficial when applied to their lives and to their health-care encounters. The second reason for the disclaimer is to protect the author from possible litigation if an adverse or negative event occurs as a consequence of the advice given.

We live in a litigious society (see the Epilogue for further thoughts on this). Many decisions are made, enormous sums of money are spent, and much energy is invested with the explicit purpose of minimizing medical legal risk; that is, avoiding a lawsuit. This has gotten way out of control in health care and in every other aspect of our social enterprise. With that said, the author (that would be me) will not assume responsibility for any adverse events that may occur as a consequence of your application of the advice to follow. I would be glad to assume, however, at least partial responsibility for any meaningful and positive outcomes that occur.

Stated more succinctly:

> *"Be careful about reading health books. You may die of a misprint."*
>
> —MARK TWAIN

"There is a strong feeling abroad among people . . . you see it in the newspapers—that we doctors are given over nowadays to science; That we care much more for the disease and its scientific aspects than for the individual patient . . . you have to keep your heart soft and tender lest you have too great a contempt for your fellow creatures."

—WILLIAM OSLER, M.D., 1915

CONTENTS

HOW TO USE THIS BOOK

THIS IS a book that you may not necessarily want to read from beginning to end. It's really more of a personalized reference text than a book to be read cover to cover. The chapters focus on specific health care scenarios that may or may not be relevant to your particular circumstances. These scenarios were chosen because of their common occurrence and because of their difficult and challenging nature. The overwhelming majority of questions and concerns shared with me and experienced by me over the last twenty years fall into one or more of these scenarios. You may, for example, already have a primary care physician. You may be struggling with the situation of a loved one who is critically ill, or a health care provider whose attitude leaves you angry and frustrated. I view *The Savvy Patient* as more of a reference companion that you can use as your individual circumstances require. Some chapters, for example on coping with illness or on spirituality and health, may have broader interest as they speak to general dimensions of the health care encounter.

A lot of technical information is integrated into the book. I apologize in advance if some of the material seems overwhelming. I strongly feel that some proficiency on the technical side can serve you well. If it seems confusing, it may serve as a good starting point for discussing the issue with your own physician.

Feel free to skip around among chapters, to find the information you want. As this is my first book, I anticipate much response, both positive and constructive. My ability to explain complicated problems to patients and families in person may be more effective than my ability to write about such problems. I am open to learning from your responses and shared experiences. This will not only allow me to refine the book for future consideration but also to add your feedback to a growing "library" of health care experiences that will allow me to be more effective as a physician and educator. Feel free to contact me with your thoughts and ideas.

I have tried to keep the chapters concise and focused. Each chapter opens with objectives for the chapter. There are many bullet points to emphasize key concepts. Each chapter ends with "Do Not Miss Take Home Points" that summarize and reinforce the most important messages and conclusions.

Mark C. Pettus, M.D.
(*markpettus@savvy*patient.com)
www.savvypatient.com

INTRODUCTION

THERE'S AN old joke. Two people are sitting in a Catskill mountain resort restaurant. As the food is served one person takes a bite and says, "My, the food here is terrible." The other responds, "Yeah . . . and in such small portions." This is how many people I meet characterize their health-care encounters. They can be impersonal, confusing, and unsatisfactory. And they are over much too quickly. Have you ever been really frustrated by a health-care encounter? Have you recently had a health-care experience where you were left with more questions than answers? If your answer is a resounding yes, you are a member of a large and growing club.

Our health-care system is a remarkable enterprise. It has become incredibly sophisticated. We are all witnesses to the unprecedented pace of advances and breakthroughs. Our health-care system is also becoming increasingly difficult and challenging for patients or "consumers" to navigate. Health-care encounters encompass many dimensions, not always visible to the naked eye or obvious in the spoken word. The most well-intentioned people, provider and patient alike, sometimes fall short of meeting mutual expectations.

It is my purpose in *The Savvy Patient* to demystify the average health care encounter. I wish to make your experiences more informed and more effective. It is my objective to inspire and empower you with a greater understanding of how our complex health-care system works and how you can make it work better for you. It is my objective to provide you with as much insight as possible as you contemplate the relevance of the health-care system in your life. While confronting health and health-care issues can be daunting and frustrating at times, I hope some or all of the content in *The Savvy Patient* will resonate with your interests and serve to compassionately satisfy an appetite too often left dissatisfied and with a bitter aftertaste.

Health-care consumption has skyrocketed in America. With an aging baby boomer population, longer life expectancy, and growing complexity with respect to health-care organization and delivery, there has never been a greater need to be empowered as a savvy health-care consumer and self-advocate. If the health-care system were a chemical reaction, it would look something like this:

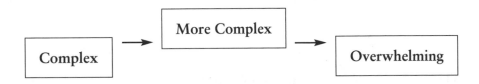

I hope to help you appreciate the lens through which health-care providers see their complex worlds. I hope to help you understand the emotions and feelings of health-care providers and how to derive opportunities for better service from that understanding. It is indeed my purpose to help you be the best advocate possible for you and for your loved ones. I hope to help you see and understand how you can have greater *influence* over the quality of your health and health-care experiences.

Encounters for health-care professionals and patients alike can be quite challenging. The stakes are sometimes very high. The pace of activity is brisk. Circumstances may overwhelm. You may feel like you are riding on a fragile, unsafe, and emotionally consuming roller coaster. Patience—the virtue, not the person—will be pushed to the limit. Information will sometimes be conflicting and will come from many sources. You may hear different perspectives from your care providers, and you most certainly will hear many unsolicited opinions. People like talking about their health-care experiences as much as they like talking about the weather. It is hard at times to know what to believe. Health-care professionals may use unintelligible medical jargon, without realizing that you do not have a clue to its meaning. You may be reluctant to ask for clarification for fear of appearing stupid or taking up too much time. These are ripe conditions for quality shortfalls. Why is this? The awareness, skills, and systems necessary for effective navigation are often lacking or are compromised by virtue of challenging and stressful interpersonal circumstances for everyone involved.

Not all health-care professionals, caring and committed though they may be, possess the skills necessary to excel interpersonally. Not all patients and families can cope and function at their best under the burden of illness. It is impossible for you as a patient or family member to take full advantage of a system you do not clearly understand. What information is of the highest value or quality? How do you feel about your role in the process of receiving medical information and making medical decisions? How can your needs, preferences, and values best be expressed to serve your health? How much information do you need to satisfy your values? This is critical in examining your health care. It is necessary now more than ever before to be savvy about your health. My goal in this book is to get you moving in the right direction. This is hard work! It is also well worth it.

I graduated from medical school over twenty years ago. Afterward I completed a three-year internship and residency in internal medicine, the study of adult diseases. From there I went on to complete a fellowship (specialty training after residency) in nephrology. Nephrology is the study of kidney diseases and high blood pressure in its more complex forms. I have now been practicing medicine for over fifteen years in the beautiful Berkshires in western Massachusetts. *The Savvy Patient* was inspired and made possible by the many relationships I have had with patients and their families over the last twenty years. It is by way of these relationships that my awareness, interest, and understanding of the common questions and concerns raised in *The Savvy Patient* have been sharpened. Over the last twenty years, as a physician, a family care provider, and as a healthcare consumer, I have been to some pretty interesting places. Not exotic locations, but up close and personal with the human condition via many encounters across the spectrum of health care.

I have applied the most sophisticated science, technology, and pharmaceuticals. I have looked into the eyes and held the hands of many people like you, your parents, and your grandparents. I have observed and shared with patients and families all that can be shared in the context of a healthcare encounter. I have had countless discussions with patients and families about their wishes regarding CPR, being placed on a breathing machine, needing to be in a nursing home, confronting terminal illness, starting dialysis, discontinuing dialysis, organ donation, and other subjects. I have shared the sanctity of end-of-life care with many, many people. Difficult and challenging though these circumstances can be, as a physician-patient advocate, I have viewed this opportunity with reverence. I see these remarkable encounters as a picture window to the soul. I have entered this "secret garden" with eyes, mind, spirit, and heart wide open. *The Savvy Patient* is an attempt to describe what I have seen and experienced in this secret garden over the last twenty years. It is my hope to transform these experiences into insights and advice that will leave you feeling more clear, connected, and comfortable with whatever circumstance you and your family may be confronting.

I have tried, in writing *The Savvy Patient*, to reach out in a personal way, as I have tried to do in practice (with variable success). I can speak personally and empathetically. I know what it is like to care for sick family members. Both my parents had numerous medical problems, probably similar to what you or a loved one may be confronting—diabetes, high blood pressure, high cholesterol, heart disease. Both my parents were smokers. And in a painfully ironic way, both my parents had kidney failure and required dialysis treatments to stay alive. I am, after all, a kidney specialist, a career decision made long before their medical problems developed. I suspect there are not many nephrologists who have experienced the enormous irony of witnessing irreversible kidney failure in both parents! My parents died at much too young an age. I was angry and saddened by their unfair plight. Their pain was my pain. Their uncertainty was at times my uncertainty. Their frustration was my frustration. I knew too much, and at the same time, not enough. I have experienced many of the needs and concerns that countless patients and families have shared with me over the years. I have seen remarkable outcomes of modern science. I have marveled at the resilient strength and courage of the human spirit. I have seen the potent combination of science and spirit transcend the most trying of circumstances.

If there is a principle or core value that resonates in the stories and information to follow, it is this:

Relationships rule. Relationships are the basis for trusting partnerships. Any health-care encounter should be defined as a partnership between you and your care providers.

I am convinced that the quality of the relationship between patient and care provider ultimately defines the quality of the encounter. Of course we always want our medical outcomes to be excellent. Medical outcomes, however, are only part of the equation. The process of how we got to the outcome, in addition to the outcome itself, is of vital importance to patients and families I have cared for. The interpersonal dimension of these experiences is what people carry in their hearts and minds at the end of the day. People crave quality face-time. People are much more likely to be "moved" by the quality of the human exchange than they are by the experience of sophisticated technology. The desire, of course, is to have both!

Physicians and patients alike often cite time constraints as obstacles to achieving quality encounters in health care. Surely, the demands on health-care professionals have never been greater. Individuals also bring more complex issues to the average health-care encounter. Without question, more time shared between physicians and patients would benefit all involved. Interestingly, the average clinical encounter for an internist has not changed significantly over the last fifteen years. It has decreased, on average, from seventeen minutes to approximately fifteen minutes. *Face-time is at a premium!* We are moving forward at high speed in the health-care express lane. The very nature of the health-care encounter has shifted, to a large extent unintentionally, from a patient-provider covenant to a more scientifically and technologically sophisticated and automated endeavor. The once time-honored personal space between patient and provider has become an overcrowded dance floor full of third-party personnel.

While the average time per outpatient primary care encounter has not changed considerably (a fact that surprises many clinicians), the nature of our encounters has changed a lot. The nature and complexity of the circumstances you and your physicians confront are much greater now than in the past. Options once limited to a patient-physician conversation and a handful of testing/treatment considerations have become much more complicated. With a vast array of tests, treatment options, and complex information to share and comprehend, we have unintentionally undermined our capacity to "cash in" on the people dividend. We all struggle with a growing awareness that quality face-time is slipping away. We all struggle with the frustration of experiences that fall short of our needs and expectations. The health-care encounter is more fragmented, specialized, and compartmentalized. For physicians, the fifteen-minute encounter has become more challenging, with many issues to address, necessitating a rapid process of prioritization. For the patient, it is more common for important issues to seem rushed or minimized.

As an indirect consequence, the depth of the physician-patient encounter has become more "diluted" from a humanistic perspective. With growing constraints on the *quantity* of shared time, we need to reinvest our shared energy in areas we can more effectively influence, such as the *quality* of shared time.

It is a myth that a quality health-care encounter is purely time dependent.

In a very short time, minutes or even instantaneously, I have experienced with patients and families an "in-the-moment" sharing that is experienced mutually as meaningful and of high quality. The effectiveness of any complex health-care encounter goes only as far as the quality of sharing of the people involved. Clear communication of needs, concerns, and expectations can be very challenging and is often missing in the average health-care encounter. This is a *shared* responsibility between the physician and the patient. What allows health-care providers to best apply their knowledge and skills? The answer is in the telling of your story. Your story is everything! Prepare to reveal anything that may shed light on your circumstances, physical, emotional, mental, and spiritual. Focus on what concerns you most. Try to resist the temptation to hold back. Time constraints may dictate which concerns need most to be addressed. Any important burden you bear, however, should eventually have time for discussion.

Which brings me to another important principal:

> *No one will ever have the potential to influence your health as much as you will. You also have much greater potential than you think to influence the quality of your health-care experiences.*

As marvelous as the scientific and technologic innovations in health care have been, there is simply no role more meaningful or important than that which you play in your life each day. Health maintenance, disease prevention, and treatment are serious responsibilities shared among you, your family, and your care providers. Consider your response to these questions very carefully and honestly:

- Are you doing all you can to promote your health and wellness?
- Do you see yourself as an active contributor to your health-care experiences and how your needs are met?
- Do you feel you can have greater influence on those caring for you?
- Do you see your relationship with your doctor as a partnership?
- What is the difference between *real* and *ideal* as it relates to your commitment to health and your health-care encounters?

If you are anything like me, the answer is that the difference between real and ideal is a *big* difference. How important is it for you to examine successful ways to transform that big difference to minimal or *no* difference? Helping you to attain greater awareness, understanding, and commitment to your role in the health-care partnership and how you can be more successful in this partnership is the goal of *The Savvy Patient*.

It is my impression that many people become frustrated by a lack of clarity with "what's going on" in the midst of a health-care encounter. These can be challenging encounters to sort out. Ours is a difficult system to understand! It is hard even for those who work in the system. Another important objective of *The Savvy Patient* is to empower you by giving you an "insider's" perspective on our health-care system. It is my hope that this book will allow you to more effectively anticipate, recognize, and manage health-care scenarios that are critically important and that all too often meet with frustration.

Emotions have the deceptive potential to undermine our effectiveness, despite our best intentions and analytical skills. When I examine poor health-care encounters, skills such as listening, communication, negotiation, influence, conflict resolution, and empathetic expression are conspicuously deficient or totally absent. The final common pathway for these shortcomings is the creation of an *expectation-reality gap*. When our experiences are miles apart from our expectations, the results are erosion of trust and perpetuation of frustration and anger.

Despite this, you can play a vital role in working with your health-care providers to close these gaps in understanding that lead to quality shortcomings. For you and your family, the "system" may seem impossible to budge or figure out. And though our system may not easily lend itself to change or understanding, individuals always have the potential and power to examine all available options present within the context of our health-care encounters. *The Savvy Patient* is more oriented to the interpersonal dimensions of the health-care encounter. While providing timely and practical state-of-the-art information on disease prevention and health promotion, it is more tailored to assist you in the *systems and processes* within which care is received. Chapters on medical decision making, conflict resolution, communication, and the power of the family meeting are unique perspectives, not found in most reference texts. If I could reduce the contents of *The Savvy Patient* to a simple picture, it would look something like the figure on page xxiv.

Now it would be reasonable for you to be saying, "C'mon Pettus . . . this is your responsibility . . . not mine!" And I would not disagree. Health-care professionals and the sophisticated resources available to them must be integrated in ways that allow basic human values such as respect, compassion, communication, and understanding to be nurtured and sustained. What you know and how you relate to individuals responsible for your care have the greatest potential to influence your health-care encounter positively. We are after all, people treating people. I will attempt to help you appreciate the perspective of the health-care professional. Is it possible for you to influence health-care professionals to make satisfaction of your needs and values more likely? The answer is a resounding yes! Physicians and patients need to rally together to reclaim center stage in the moment of health care.

Transforming the Health-Care Experience

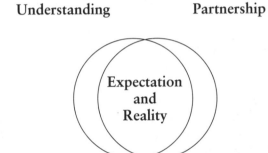

Our local health-care system, like many, is investing resources to make the patient encounter a more effective one. With greater understanding of our system, more meaningful insight into the perspective of health-care providers, and with an awareness of your contribution to the encounter, the health-care experience can be taken to a higher level. Many patients and families feel "out of control" when they encounter the health-care system. Patients and families relinquish considerable control over their circumstances, particularly when ill. This can be frightening and unsettling. A theme woven throughout this book is that of ongoing potential for more positive and effective self-control, regardless of the circumstances.

The health-care system in America is remarkable *and* far from perfect. I have attempted to integrate stories from patients and families I have cared for with practical and personal advice that will allow you to better leverage your health-care encounters and your health in general. The medical information I have incorporated is a combination of the best available current medical evidence, time-proven principles, and sincere heartfelt common sense. While this is a book that examines some challenging realities about our health-care encounters and about our lives, this is more a book about hope, faith, and transformation in the vast potential of the human encounter.

I hope health-care professionals and consumers alike will benefit from *The Savvy Patient*. I am very interested in your thoughts, experiences, and feedback.

CHAPTER 1

FINDING A PRIMARY CARE PROVIDER
What to Look For

"Don't live in a town where there are no doctors."

—Jewish Proverb

THE OBJECTIVES of this chapter are:

- To review the evolving role that primary care providers play in your health care
- To review why it is essential to have an excellent primary care provider
- To highlight the ingredients of a good primary care provider and practice
- To provide sample questions you can use to gauge the quality of the physican-practice

A logical place to start a book on navigating our health-care system is with finding a good doctor who can provide primary care—*a primary care provider*, or PCP. Though it seems self-evident that finding a primary care provider is of utmost importance, many people I meet either do not have one or if they do, cannot tell me who the doctor is. I know a lot of people who have barbers or hairdressers, auto mechanics, travel agents, financial advisers, accountants, realtors, and repairmen. These are among the many people we often need in our lives to serve our values and needs, and who, ideally, we can trust and count on to provide quality and reliable service.

Why isn't everyone connected with a doctor or a physicians' practice? Shouldn't everyone have one? Yes—but finding a primary care provider is not always an easy process. I have observed that the absence of a physician-practice in many peoples' lives speaks to a very large systemic problem in American health care. What I mean is that the problem has more to do with health-care finance, organization, and delivery, than it has to do with individuals. However, many people, and you may be one, have insurance (employer based, private, or government funded), have access to excellent physicians, and yet have not made the connection. You could have a doctor-practice available to meet your needs but for many reasons, some beyond your control, you do not.

It is important to keep in mind that when you find a primary care provider, you are in fact becoming attached to a practice. Although the ideal is to see the same person as much as possible, circumstances such as emergencies, after-hours needs, turnover, and practice organization and activity will often result in your interacting with other members of the practice. They may include other physicians, physician assistants, nurse practitioners, registered nurses, and medical assistants.

The challenge is twofold. You want to find a physician who is first, available and second, a good fit. The office staff, in any physician practice, plays a key role in determining the quality of the encounter. The staff should be professional, interested, and caring. The attitudes and behaviors of an office staff are a reflection of the attitudes and philosophies of the physician leadership within the practice. For example, are receptionists clear, engaging, and polite? Are attitudes professional and caring? They should be, always. During a health-care encounter, observe how the staff relates to you and to each other. How does your physician relate to staff and vice versa? Is there a "team" feeling? Is there an esprit de corps? Does the staff seem pleasant? Are they a cohesive crew? They should be.

How important is it to have a primary care provider? At the turn of the twentieth century, all physicians did all things. Surgery as a specialty soon followed. In the 1950s the general practitioner began to give way to specialized care, reflecting the growth and sophistication of biomedical and clinical capacity. Significant growth of specialization followed, diminishing to some extent the spectrum of care provided by primary care clinicians. The decentralization of care shifted back in the HMO era of the eighties. In this unproven model of health-care management, the primary care provider resumed center stage as the "gatekeeper." Flow of care, by necessity, went through the primary care provider in an effort to enhance efficiency, and to improve resource use and outcomes, with greater emphasis on health maintenance and disease prevention.

Worthy though the philosophy of care may have been, it created a wedge between physicians and patients with onerous paperwork, referrals, pre-approvals, and the precarious conflict between controlling costs and providing care. This model of care is becoming, for the most part, history. The role of the primary care provider continues to evolve. The following points are clear to me:

- People desire choice of care providers, with as few restrictions as possible.
- People are willing to make reasonable choices when provided with reasonable information.
- Specialists do not want to provide primary care.
- As we age, have more medical problems, take more medications, and tell a more complex story, the need for someone to pull it together, as the primary caring historian, will never be greater.
- Primary care physicians such as family practitioners and internists need to be compensated more equitably, commensurate with the value they contribute to patients' overall care.

Why is it so common for people to be without a primary care provider? One common reason is lack of health-care insurance.

No Insurance = No Doctor

Maybe you have had a change in insurance requiring a change in your provider. You may have moved to a new location or your physician may have left the area. Perhaps you are uncertain about how to find a doctor. Other sentiments I hear frequently include:

- "I'm in good health. I really don't need a doctor."
- "I've gone this long without a doctor and nothing has happened to me."
- "Doctors I've had in the past have changed just as I'm getting to know them."
- "I hate doctors. All they do is order a lot of tests."
- "I am afraid of what they might find. What I don't know can't hurt me."
- "My father never saw a doctor and lived to be eighty-five!"
- "It's hard for me to find a doctor I really like."

Perhaps some of this sounds familiar.

Some areas in our country are experiencing shortages of primary care providers. My own community has that problem. There are many reasons for this.

- Physicians, like people working in other industries, tend to be migratory because of personal factors such as family needs, quality of life, and opportunity.
- External factors such as malpractice insurance premiums, potential for practice growth, and market forces influence the decision to stay in a particular area for a long period of time. Massachusetts, where I live, has a growing reputation for very high practice costs, low rates of reimbursement, and a high cost of living. For a growing number of physicians this is not a suitable practice environment. While no one's empathy tank for physician income will be on full, many physicians confront enormous overhead, malpractice premium costs, and capital investment expenditures; for example, for new information technology systems. It can simply be too expensive to practice in some areas.
- Physicians who historically have provided primary care in addition to specialty care (e.g. cardiology, gastroenterology, and rheumatology) now often limit their practices to specialty-consulting care.
- There has also been a decline nationally in medical students' interest in pursuing careers in primary care (e.g. pediatrics, internal medicine, and family practice). Issues pertaining to quality of life, such as income (enormous educational debt, often exceeding $150,000 upon graduating from medical school) and on-call responsibility are important considerations in the minds of medical students, strongly influencing career choice.

A diminished provider pool, however, does not fully explain the disproportionate number of people without a primary care provider. The disparity of provider supply and increasing health care demand has placed greater burdens on our emergency departments and urgent care facilities. Many people feel they have no choice but to receive their care in these clinical settings. Excellent though that care may be, primary care is most effective when the emphasis is on health maintenance and disease prevention. Accessing the system only when you feel sick misses the fundamental point of health care.

As you will see repeatedly in the pages to follow, many of the most dangerous medical problems are silent and often preventable. Waiting until you feel sick to "open the door" makes less possible the identification and potential treatment of problems that routine preventive care would otherwise allow more promptly. Recognition and treatment of diabetes, high blood pressure, and high lipid levels (cholesterol) are common examples. I will elaborate on this in chapter 20, "Parting Wisdom."

Ideally, health care is about establishing long-term relationships between those who provide care and those in need of care. Having a sporadic and random sequence of encounters with clinicians with whom you have no meaningful relationship is far from the ideal of repeated encounters with providers who know you and with whom you feel comfortable and trusting.

Trust is at the core of any meaningful relationship.

Trust, in and of itself, is therapeutic and can only be strengthened over time and with commitment and sharing between you and your primary care provider. The ultimate goal is to find a physician who feels more like a trusted friend than a randomly assigned professional stranger. You may be saying: "Sure, Pettus, I'll go out and find a great doctor tomorrow. There aren't that many out there." I sometimes hear this from people who have had an unsatisfactory experience with a previous physician or physicians and lose faith in the possibility of finding a good one. Don't give up! They are out there and you can find them. The purpose of this chapter is to show you how.

If you do not have a physician, write this down and post it on your refrigerator:

Today I am going to start the process of finding my physician-practice. Four weeks from today and no later, I will have an appointment set up!

Be patient (no pun intended). Finding a physician-practice takes time and can be frustrating. Surely, the effort of finding individuals to whom you can comfortably entrust your life is worth it. Here the responsibility is largely on you. In the immortal (and modified) words of Woody from *Toy Story*, as he rallied his fellow toys to get a "buddy" in anticipation of a big move, "If you don't have a primary care provider . . . get one!"

The types of providers available in our system include the following.

M.D.—Medical Doctor

M.D.s are graduates of medical school, licensed to practice in their particular states, usually after completing a residency training program and if necessary, specialty fellowship training. I say usually because in some states it may be possible to get a license after only successful completion of an internship year after medical school. While this is uncommon, confirm that your physician has completed an accredited residency-training program. This can be done by asking the provider directly, inquiring through your state's Board of Registration in Medicine, or checking through your health insurance provider. There should be documented evidence of successful training for a minimum of three years after medical school. It would be extremely unlikely for any physician serving on a panel of providers for an insurer, or who receives Medicare or Medicaid payments, not to have this confirmed and documented. You should, however, appreciate that not all M.D.s are created equal.

D.O.—Doctor of Osteopathy

D.O.s train in much the same way as M.D.s. It is increasingly difficult to distinguish an osteopathic from an allopathic, or "traditional" M.D. curriculum in medical school. In addition to traditional allopathic techniques, osteopathic teaching places more emphasis on hands-on manipulation of the musculoskeletal system, such as the backbone, head, neck, and extremities. One of my roles as a teacher is to oversee the training of medical students and medical residents. Medical residents are graduates from both allopathic and osteopathic schools. In my experience there are few distinguishable differences, and in practice I do not even recognize a significant distinction between a D.O. and an M.D. The important issues are level of training, board eligibility and certification, state licensure, ethics of the highest standards, and the caring quality of the individual. Successful completion of a residency program, as for an M.D., should be the expectation.

P.A.—Physician Assistant

P.A.s usually require two years of intensive clinical training after four years of college. In 2002 it was estimated that 46,000 P.A.s were in clinical practice. Most P.A.s work in primary care practices such as family practice, general internal medicine, and pediatrics. A growing number are working in obstetrics, as well as some medical and surgical subspecialties such as cardiology and orthopedics. You will encounter P.A.s in clinics and in hospital settings. Their responsibilities vary based on their experience and the practice needs of the supervising physician. They can conduct physical exams, diagnose and treat illnesses, counsel patients on preventive care, prescribe medications, and order and interpret tests. They are always under the supervision of a physician. Currently I supervise a P.A. who is essential as a member of the treatment team.

N.P.—NURSE PRACTITIONER

An N.P. is a registered nurse who is qualified, through advanced training, to assume some of the duties and responsibilities formerly assumed only by a physician. A nurse practitioner may provide comprehensive primary care evaluation and treatment. In addition, they may write prescriptions. They work under the supervision of a physician. Physician assistants and nurse practitioners are particularly important in the evaluation and management of less complex and non-emergency medical problems. If you call your physician-practice with a concern, who handles it and how it is handled will depend on the urgency and complexity of the concern.

Regardless of the training background of the provider, a relationship with a primary care provider is like a marriage. It requires mutual give and take, shared commitment to health and wellness, and like a marriage, should be nurtured "in sickness and in health." Which of the following scenarios do you find yourself confronting?

I have a primary care provider whom I like.

You're there! There is no substitute for having a physician you know, like, and trust. If you are aware of anyone who needs a physician, ask your doctor if he or she is accepting new patients. Congratulations, you are a member of a special club and can go on to the next chapter.

I have a primary care provider, but I do not feel satisfied with the quality of the encounters.

This is not an uncommon scenario. In my experience, the dissatisfaction a patient or client may feel has more to do with interpersonal issues than with competency issues. Most individuals assume that a standard of competence exists in a licensed professional. Most people are not able to distinguish gaps in clinical competency as they could an imperfection on an appliance, television screen, or sound system. Interpersonal skills are extremely important and readily accessible to the average observer.

However, they should not be equated with medical knowledge, technical expertise, or clinical reasoning skill.

Let me give you two examples. First, I was asked to do a consult in our hospital on a patient having some kidney problems. Her primary care provider asked me to see her to assist in this aspect of her hospital care. Her doctor had been a friend and colleague of mine for many years. I knew that he was an incredibly competent fellow, but also somewhat reserved and at times awkwardly shy. He had had only one or two previous encounters with this patient and I was very confident he would let nothing slip through the cracks. When I met his patient she said, "I would like to change my primary care provider." Naturally (and curiously) I asked why. She responded, "My doctor doesn't look at me directly when he talks to me. He seems to be more focused on my chart than on me. He seems quiet and I'm uncomfortable he may be hiding something from me and is uncertain." I reassured her about his clinical competence and explained his shy nature. Though this might be a significant issue, understanding her doctor better very much changed the patient's perspective.

As a second example, I once asked my mother, "Do you like your nephrologist?"

"Oh yes," she replied, "Dr. Owen is a real peach."

Now I am as savvy a judge as anyone when it comes to nephrology and I was interested in learning more about her perception of his quality. "What else do you like about him?"

She responded, "Oh, he's a great doctor. He calls me Agnes. I feel comfortable whenever he comes around the dialysis unit. He sits down when he talks to me during his rounds."

Sitting face-to-face and looking eye-to-eye are very powerful body language behaviors when a physician is interacting with a patient during hospital rounds.

"He asks me how you're doing (referring to me). He's always in a pleasant mood."

You get the picture. Of course, I knew Dr. Owens to be a very well-trained and skilled clinician. My mother's perception of his skills had little to do with where he trained or if he had published in a major medical journal (which he had). She, like most people, assumed that his training and competence were sufficient. Her perceptions were shaped more by his interpersonal skills than by his analytical skills. Ahhh . . . to find a physician who has both.

If you have a primary care provider and do not feel satisfied with the quality of the relationship, try the following: Generate and write down a list of reasons you feel dissatisfied or uncomfortable. Attempt to separate "style" or "interpersonal" issues from competency/care issues. Common examples of each include:

Interpersonal Characteristics

- Communication style
- Bedside manner
- Empathy—relates to and understands your individual circumstances
- Caring disposition
- Professionalism
- Respect for you, the patient
- Active listening—engaged, in the moment, and tuned in to nonverbal messages
- Sense of humor
- Responsiveness—anticipates what is on your mind

Competence Concerns

- Inability to explain circumstances satisfactorily
- Repeatedly making decisions with adverse or bad consequences
- Frequent pattern of uncertainty
- Frequently missed, delayed, or wrong diagnosis and treatment
- Inappropriate behavior
- Lack of professionalism
- Failure to respond to or return important phone calls
- Tendency to order a lot of tests

It is possible you can avoid the challenge of finding another primary care provider by explicitly addressing interpersonal concerns, particularly if you feel your physician is smart enough. If you invest in a greater understanding of the circumstances, you may be surprised at the outcome. In the process you may learn something about yourself and help your provider to care more effectively for you and others. Physicians are people, too. Though most are quite intelligent, it is not necessarily true that acquiring an M.D. means having great people skills.

As Bernie Siegel says, "the physician is the tourist. The patient is the native." This is such a poignant metaphor for the relationship. Creating and sustaining relationships is very hard work. A good physician understands the opportunity and value of discovering as much about your landscape as possible. The emphasis is as much on the experience as it is the diagnosis.

As Anatole Broyard, a writer for the *New York Times* and author of

Intoxicated By My Illness, wrote: "A doctor's job would be so much more interesting and satisfying if he would occasionally let himself plunge into the patient, if he could lose his own fear of falling."

If the effort of strengthening this connection seems much greater than the effort of finding another provider, then it's time to move on.

I need a doctor and I'm starting from scratch.

Here are a few tips to consider: First, examine your health plan and determine whether you must choose from a list of providers. Finding someone you like only to learn they are not a provider in your plan is unfortunate and frustrating. If you are unfamiliar with the choices available, ask friends, family, or fellow workers for their opinions. It always makes sense to consider a physician who is already caring for someone you know and trust. In my experience, even the provider with a full practice may be willing to make an exception for a family member or a close friend of a current patient. There is no better advertisement, in my opinion, than the endorsement of someone you trust who can speak to the quality of care a physician provides. Find out what the person's experiences have been like. Why does he or she like this provider? Would the individual recommend a family member to the physician? If you are seen in your local emergency department and need primary care follow-up, ask your treating provider for some recommendations.

If you are unable to come up with a personal reference, you might try contacting a local hospital. Many have physician referral services. Is there a patient relations person (or ombudsman) at your local hospital? He or she may have the "inside information" on local physicians and be able to guide you in a positive way. If all else fails, a random choice may turn out to be a good fit. Set up an introductory appointment (perhaps for a routine physical). The time to do this is when you are well, so that the encounter will be less urgent and distracting. As you undoubtedly know, the wait may be weeks to months. If you're well, the wait will matter less. If the physician, as Anatole Broyard observed, "has no fear of falling" the wait will be well worth it!

Availability: Patient-Centered Access

A pervasive frustration for patients and physicians alike is the challenge of matching need with availability. Some needs result in visits that could have been managed over the telephone or, in a few practices, over the Internet. Needs best served by a prompt visit cannot always be seen to quickly.

Health-care needs in a large, busy office practice are numerous and diverse. Our conventional office appointment model contributes to inefficient use of health-care resources. The challenge of our health-care delivery system is matching an individual's needs to the most appropriate resource, in the timeliest fashion. For example, your specific needs and concerns may require only a brief telephone conversation with an R.N., N.P., or M.D. On the other hand, you may have a problem that requires you to be seen on the day of the call. People who need to be seen should not have to wait, and people who need timely advice, available by telephone or e-mail, should not have to come in to the office. Some problems are appropriate for a physician extender such as a P.A. or N.P., and others are more complicated and best evaluated by a physician. Many physician practices are attempting to reconfigure their office practice to better serve their patients. So as you attempt to find the right physician-practice for you, ask these questions:

- Do you always keep appointments open each day for more time-sensitive needs and urgent problems?
- Does the practice have evening or Saturday hours?
- Does the practice have a process for handling telephone calls?
- Who usually triages—screens and prioritizes—telephone calls to the office?
- Can I communicate with your providers directly by telephone or e-mail?
- Does the practice use a Web site for appointments, education, or advice?
- How does the practice handle urgent needs?

The Initial Encounter

The first appointment is an opportunity for you to interview the provider as much as for the provider to interview and get to know you. This is an important point. The flow of information is often unidirectional or "one-way" between a patient and a physician, particularly during an initial encounter. Necessary though this is at times, you should feel comfortable asking questions to allow you to determine whether the fit between you and the provider is right.

It is also important to ensure that your needs and concerns are adequately addressed. Before your initial meeting, take a moment to list the attributes you find most important in a physician. These might include a personable demeanor, a caring quality, a sense of humor, an ability to communicate clearly, a willingness to be a good listener, good eye contact, and open-ended questions, for example. Ethnic and cultural background or gender may be important to you. Some people might care only about quality of training and credentials with less emphasis on personality. Some might put more emphasis on personality and interpersonal skills. In any event, the fit should feel comfortable.

Here are some revealing, non-threatening questions to ask your provider. You can minimize the risk of putting a physician on the defensive by framing your questions in the context of gaining more insight into the doctor's views on patient care. For example: "Dr. Smith, I know these questions may seem personal. As a physician, I know you understand how important your role is in my care. It is important to me that this be a comfortable fit for both of us."

1. **What do you love most about what you do?**
   See if the doctor's eyes open wide and if his or her face lights up.
2. **What do you suppose other patients say about you?**
   Look for the virtues you wish to find in an M.D.
3. **If you don't mind my asking, what do you like most about yourself?**
   Humility should rule the day.
4. **What do you think is most important in your therapeutic relationships with patients?**
   Does the response feel more like a covenant or more like a business partnership?
5. **What is your policy/philosophy for handling phone messages? Do patients ever e-mail the office?**
   Well-defined policies for screening and prioritizing return of phone calls should be in place.
6. **Are you Board Certified? In what specialty/specialties?**
   Board certification is recognition by a certifying medical specialty society that attests to an excellent and reasonable standard of competency—attained by passing a challenging examination. It is important to appreciate that Board certification measures the individual's analytical skills more than it does interpersonal competency.
7. **Are you a member of your specialty's medical society?**
8. **Do you care for your patients in the hospital or do you have hospitalist colleagues who do this?**

9. **Do you think spiritual wellness is an important aspect of one's health?**
   This may be an important need and value for you and your health.
10. **How long have you been in practice?**
11. **Do you foresee any significant changes in your practice in the near future?** This might include addition or departure of some staff, changes in health insurer contractual agreements, change of location, etc.
12. **How long have you been in the community?**
13. **What would nurses at the hospital say about you?**
14. **Are you open-minded to feedback?**
   A solid physician understands that ego should never interfere with acceptance of feedback. The ability to say "I'm sorry" and to learn from patients, families, and colleagues are hallmarks of humility. A physician who is not a responsive listener will not allow good advice to penetrate the filter of ego protection. There is little hope of personal and professional development—not a good choice.
15. **Do you like it here?**
   Physicians who have practiced for long periods of time, for example longer than five or ten years in one community, are perhaps more rooted and less likely to leave. However, physicians who are starting out offer many advantages, as their batteries are fresh and their practices sometimes less busy. They are more likely to be in a position of accepting new patients.
16. **Do you have children?**
   This gives the interaction a more personal quality. I have always loved it when patients ask me about my children or other interests.

This is just a sampling of questions to consider. You may, of course, think of other specific questions. The point here is to participate. This is an enormously important relationship! I believe most people, after one encounter, will have a sense of whether the fit is right based on the physician's response to these or some of these questions.

After the encounter, consider these self-awareness issues: Did the physician and staff make you feel comfortable? Did they look you in the eye or were they more focused on your chart and paperwork? Were you asked how you wanted to be addressed; for example, as "Mrs. Jones" or as "Virginia"? A hot button for my wife was being in our pediatrician's office when our children were very young and being asked, "How is mom and baby?" This seemed rather generic and impersonal, well-intentioned though we knew the staff to be. Do you feel that you can trust the physician? Is his or her style a good fit? Listen to your gut feeling—our deeper instincts are telling. If it feels positive, you are there. If there is uncertainty, see how it goes in future encounters. It may be worth the time and effort to work with a physician on improving things that do not feel right rather than to find another provider. The truth is that many excellent health-care providers may not be aware of behaviors, communication styles, or body language that affect others they see and care for. Awkward though it may feel, feedback regarding your observations will probably help you, your provider, and others in future encounters. If the vibes are bad, however, consider another choice. I feel it would even be fair, difficult though it would be, to ask the individual for a recommendation for someone who might provide a better fit.

Trusting Reassurance

The majority of information in *The Savvy Patient* examines the *art* of the health-care encounter more than the science. Good encounters always require some mutual awareness and effectiveness of the "art" piece. If science is the body upon which medicine rests, the interpersonal art of communication, listening, humility, and empathy are the wings upon which it soars. As an aside, I firmly believe that all people, providers and recipients of care alike, can cultivate listening, communicating, and empathetic expression—the important interpersonal attributes. Innate though these skills are for some people, they are not automatically attached to the health-care professional. Your ability to cultivate these skills is also essential to your satisfaction in health-care encounters and in all life encounters

A good marker of an effective health-care provider is the ability to succeed at delivering trusting reassurance. When I say "trusting reassurance," I mean the kind of reassurance that will make you feel comforted, confident, and comprehending. A sense of equanimity should define these encounters. Reassurance is a large part of what physicians do and a substantial need for most people engaging our health-care system. To be able to deliver trusting reassurance requires confidence in one's analytic skills combined with an ability to be empathetic, to anticipate concerns (especially those that may be unspoken), to inform clearly, and to do so with an air of caring compassion. If you need reassurance or clarification around a specific concern, raise it explicitly—no significant need or concern should remain silent. A good physician will *listen* with an open heart and open mind. As Helen Keller once said, "Deafness is darker by far than blindness."

Hospitalist Physicians

A growing trend in the health-care delivery system is for a more discrete separation of acute hospital care from outpatient ambulatory care. Many physicians certified in internal medicine, for example, are working as "hospitalists" in this new model. They work only in the hospital setting, effectively coordinating the care of patients admitted by their primary care providers. So how might this affect your care?

There will probably always be a need for a primary care provider, someone who can "pull it all together." In a hospitalist model of care, if you require hospitalization, another physician team oversees your care in the hospital setting. Details of your care are communicated to your primary care provider at the time of your discharge from the hospital. Your primary care provider then resumes your outpatient care. This division of care has proven successful in recent years. It allows clinicians to focus on their offices and all of the care that occurs there. Hospitalist physicians can focus their skills on the acute care side, providing a more consistent presence in the hospital, coordinating care and services, and allowing more efficient use of time and resources. Some practices have physicians who work just in the hospital. Other practices may work with local hospitals that hire hospitalist physicians to provide this service. Regardless of the exact organization and delivery model, this appears to be a trend that is here to stay. Ultimately, as is true for all aspects of health-care delivery, its success depends on clear communication and continuity across the spectrum of care.

DO NOT MISS TAKE HOME POINTS

1. If you do not have a primary care provider, make it a priority to find one. Having the same physician-practice also caring for your spouse and family can have tremendous advantages.
2. Take a moment to consider the characteristics that are important to you in a physician-practice. This is one of the most important relationships in your life.

3. Try to get some recommendations from trusted friends, family, co-workers, or health-care personnel, such as experienced R.N.s, particularly in the emergency department or on the wards. These are often the best endorsements to have.

4. Physicians who have not been in practice as long are more likely to be taking new patients.

5. Write down appropriate questions before the encounter. Your goal should be to understand your primary care provider and his or her practice as much as it is the primary care provider's role to understand you.

6. If possible, make your first visit a complete physical exam to explore health maintenance, disease prevention (e.g., mammogram, colonoscopy, cholesterol, sugar, and other issues) and to gain a "feel" for the fit between you, your provider, and the practice.

7. If your first visit is more urgent and symptom-oriented, before you leave the office make a follow-up appointment for a complete physical .

8. If you have more questions than time allows, ask your provider how best to address your needs and concerns.

9. View your relationship with a physician-practice as a health partnership.

CHAPTER 2

THE PRE-HOSPITAL EMERGENCY SYSTEM

Those Critical First Moments

"When griping grief the heart doth wound, and doleful dumps the mind oppresses, then music, with her silver sound, with speedy help doth lend redress."

—William Shakespeare

THE OBJECTIVES of this chapter are:

- To understand how you and your family can benefit by greater awareness, understanding, and timely activation of your local pre-hospital system.
- To appreciate how you can contribute to the quality of pre-hospital care for your family, your workplace, and your community.

A Personal Story

My sister called one morning to let me know that my father was on his way to the hospital with symptoms of chest pain. She was living with my father at the time and quickly recognized the possibility of a heart problem. Because of her awareness and decisiveness my father was transported to our local hospital quickly. Within minutes she had called 911 and my father was taken to the nearest emergency department. There he was found to be having a large heart attack. A clot-dissolving drug, or tissue plasminogen activator (TPA) was administered. I lived almost three hours away and immediately headed for the hospital. In route, I called the emergency department for a brief update on my father's status. He was continuing to have pain despite his initial treatment; this concerned me greatly. He was subsequently airlifted to the University of Massachusetts Medical Center. I had attended medical school there, and this was an ironically painful way to be revisiting fond memories of my medical school experience. I rerouted my car and drove as quickly as possible to the Medical Center, where I arrived within minutes of the Life Flight transport. My sister soon met me there.

Upon arrival I learned that my father had had two cardiac arrests while in flight and had to be "shocked" for resuscitation. He was awake and alert when we met. I knew all to well how ominous the situation was and began to contemplate my father's mortality. At the same time I prayed for his survival with every ounce of hope in my being. All that could be done was being done. We talked. I held his hand, clinging to every precious moment. Despite all the heroic efforts possible, his blood pressure continued to drop and several hours after his arrival, he had another cardiac arrest. He could not be resuscitated. Before he died, while in the rapid spiral of near-death, he opened his eyes and said to my sister Nancy and me in a clear and strong tone, "I love you both."

I was struck by how clear and reassuring his tone was even though he was in shock. Shock is a serious medical condition characterized by a dangerously low blood pressure. Most people are not alert under these circumstances. This would be his last great earthly effort. These would be his last words. Moments later, he was dead.

It all happened so quickly. My father had endured a lot in his life and he was a survivor. He also firmly believed he would be reunited with my mother, who had died six years earlier. I have no doubt his faith has been affirmed. The pre-hospital system of care working at its very best added about twelve hours to my father's life. Those twelve hours allowed my sister and me to be with him, as we shared that transient last rally before his death. The three of us were able to be together one last time. How precious is life when you would have given anything for twelve additional hours?

The pre-hospital system refers to the network of first responders who are summoned to the scene in the event of an emergency. People's lives often depend on the quick reaction and competent care of emergency medical technicians (EMTs) and paramedics. Paramedics are EMTs with advanced training that allows them to perform more difficult pre-hospital medical procedures. Everything under the sun—from automobile accidents, heart attacks, drowning, childbirth—to burns and gunshot wounds all require immediate response and medical attention. EMTs and paramedics provide this vital attention as they care for and transport the sick or injured to the nearest medical facility. EMTs and paramedics may use special equipment such as backboards to immobilize patients before placing them on stretchers and securing them in the ambulance for transport to a medical facility. Usually, one EMT or paramedic drives while the other monitors the patient's vital signs and gives additional care as needed. Some EMTs work as part of the flight crews of helicopters that transport critically ill or injured patients to hospital trauma centers.

We are fortunate in this country to have a superb network of pre-hospital emergency personnel. Paramedics, EMTs, police, firefighters, and volunteers routinely carry out the task of bridging the "field," where the event is occurring, to the nearest emergency department (E.D.). These individuals are trained to assess, triage (prioritize the immediate needs of the patients), stabilize, treat, and transport to the nearest hospital in as little time as possible. In my experience, these professionals see their challenging tasks as a natural extension of their skills and responsibilities. They are energetic and focused, and they thrive under challenging and unpredictable circumstances. In many respects they are the unsung heroes of our health-care system. If you know such individuals or require their services, thank them for the good and important work they do.

The pre-hospital system can vary from community volunteers with EMT training to sophisticated systems including airlift for emergency transport. These systems can be contacted in most communities by dialing 911 on the telephone. For individuals who may be unable to access and dial 911 quickly, an emergency alert system such as a wearable call button can be obtained. Pressing this button immediately initiates a sequence of phone calls to family and emergency medical personnel.

It is the purpose of any pre-hospital system to provide timely evaluation, stabilization, treatment, and transport to the nearest emergency department. If you live alone, have mobility challenges such as difficulty walking, and are concerned about safe and easy access to a telephone, ask your physician about obtaining an emergency call button. Many insurers will cover this with adequate documentation of need. There are many manufacturers of emergency call devices. Your physician can help you find the vendor that best meets your needs.

People often find it difficult to decide when to call 911. I find that failure of the system falls into two common categories: The first is *failure to activate the system in a timely manner*. The second is *choosing to drive or have someone drive you to your local emergency department*.

Often these decisions are made to avoid the "fuss," cost, and attention that might be drawn to the scene by an ambulance siren resonating through the neighborhood. I have often heard people comment, "I didn't want to alarm everyone in the neighborhood and put people out for this." That might be reasonable for a relatively minor problem such as a musculoskeletal injury like a sprained knee, ankle, or back injury. However, many people avoid using the pre-hospital system for problems that require prompt and professional evaluation, treatment, and transport.

Two common examples are chest pain and possible symptoms of a stroke, such as weakness, numbness in arms or legs, and changes in speech. Timing is critical, as the degree of damage to the heart or to the brain can change quickly over short periods of time, profoundly impacting quality of life or life itself. Beneficial outcomes result from procedures carried out as quickly as possible. For example, for individuals having a heart attack, "clot-busting" medications or balloon angioplasty are most effective when done as soon as possible after onset of chest pain (although this can be up to twelve hours, within two hours yields the best results). For treatment of a stroke, the therapeutic "window of opportunity" is much smaller, up to three hours from the onset of symptoms, but best if under ninety minutes. It takes some time to perform an initial evaluation with questioning, examination, x-rays, cardiograms, and other tests before initiating treatment.

The point is that **timing is everything**. Recent statistics, for example demonstrate that only 5 to 10 percent of people who are eligible for clot-busting medication for a stroke actually receive it because they present beyond this narrow three-hour limit! We say in treating heart attacks, "time is muscle" (the heart is a very important muscle) and for strokes, certainly "time is brain." Often, time is life itself.

Rapid recognition of and response to a potentially serious problem is extremely important. Having trained professionals initiating evaluation and treatment from point of contact to the hospital is also crucial. Things change quickly, often requiring sophisticated intervention prior to arrival at the hospital. Driving yourself or having someone drive you to the hospital could place you and others in danger and possibly delay life-saving treatment.

Denial: The Reassuring Paradox

"By these things examine thyself. By whose rules am I act-ing; in whose name; in whose strength; in whose glory? What faith, humility, self-denial, and love of God and to man have there been in all my actions?"

—Jackie Mason

I find that people often delay evaluation and treatment or choose an al-ternative to their pre-hospital system for transportation due to the arch nemesis, denial. Denial can take a potentially serious set of circum-stances and reframe them in a falsely reassuring way. This brings me to another important health-care principal:

Denial is the enemy of the rational.

It is human nature to deny the possibility of a serious health problem when experiencing something unpleasant such as chest discomfort, lightheadedness, or a clumsy hand. "It's probably just some gas, indiges-tion, or a strained muscle." "It will probably feel better in the morning. I don't want to make a big deal out of it." "How could this be happen-ing to me?" "This is something that happens to other people, older peo-ple." Perhaps this sounds familiar. Accurate though our denial may ultimately be, its purpose is to reassure and to diminish fear and uncer-tainty. Denial does not readily engage rational and logical thinking be-cause that can quickly bring us to some frightening, undesirable realities. By its very nature it can be dangerously shortsighted. Denial is often rooted in sheer disbelief. Who wants to acknowledge the worst-case sce-nario or encounter a sudden, unexpected, and profound risk to life?

Reaching beyond denial can be very difficult. Help, however, is what you will find on the other side. Men are notorious deniers. Thank good-ness many have caring significant others who can prompt and guide the necessary evaluation and treatment. If I had a quarter for every guy I have met who said, "Doc, I wasn't all that concerned about it. My wife made me come to get it checked out," I would have enough saved for a nice vacation! I have met some men who are much more sensitized to the knocks and pings in their automobiles than to potentially dangerous signs and symptoms their bodies may be sending. A good question to ask when at risk for denial is *"How might my putting off checking this out affect me, my family, and my friends?"* Another way to think about this is *"What advice would I give someone I loved more than anything who was experiencing something similar?"* If a problem turns out to be nothing serious, that's terrific.

It is not always easy to recognize denial. The paradox is that those who are at greatest risk from denial are least likely to recognize it in themselves. When in doubt, get an opinion from someone you trust. Consider it a reality check. If you seek trusted advice, prepare yourself to follow through on it. At the very least, a little reassurance goes a long way.

Understand your pre-hospital emergency system. How do you access it? Where is the nearest hospital? Is there a list of people you would want contacted in the event of an emergency? Might you benefit from an emergency call button? Is there a family member or friend who regularly "checks in" if you live alone?

> *Loneliness and isolation should never be the reason*
> *a person fails to receive vital and timely care.*

For example, an eighty-four-year-old widow who is disengaged from the community and whose children are out of town may be at serious risk. An important problem may never get communicated to people who can help. If you know and care about someone who might be in that category (and believe me, there are many, many people who could fit this description), call and check in on them regularly. If you live out of town and are concerned about a loved one, have someone you know and trust check in on them. If you have a neighbor who is alone and infirm, keep a caring and watchful eye out for them. I have found that a stoic, independent, and determined mindset can effectively mask legitimate problems, never perceived through an occasional phone call from a distance. Seeing rather than simply hearing may more readily raise concerns. It is not my intention to make you sick with worry over a loved one living a distance from you. A picture, however, as seen through the eyes of a caring onlooker, is worth a thousand words. After all, we all need someone to look after us, don't we?

A few additional considerations: Are your physician's and family members' phone numbers listed clearly and visibly for others to see? Do you have a medic-alert bracelet, if necessary, to identify any important medical problems? Do you keep a list of medications in your wallet or pocketbook? Are your wishes for "heroic measures" such as cardiopulmonary resuscitation (CPR), defibrillation, or being put on a breathing machine clearly communicated? These can be put on a medic alert bracelet, added to your list of medications, and at a minimum should be documented in your medical record by your treating physician (see chapter 6, Advanced Care Planning). If EMTs or paramedics arrive on the scene and need to consider these interventions, they will be obligated to "do everything necessary" unless your wishes to do otherwise are spoken or plainly documented. Unfortunately, aggressive interventions are sometimes performed before it is learned that the individual never would have wanted them.

When Do I Activate the Pre-Hospital System?

It is not always easy to know when to engage pre-hospital emergency services. However, some problems or symptoms should raise immediate concern and consideration. Please realize that this is a short list of what may be many reasons to activate 911 or your local emergency medical system. Here are however, some of the more common and potentially serious problems or symptoms that should prompt rapid ambulance transport.

Chest discomfort

I say *discomfort* because people having heart-related symptoms often do not describe them as "pain." The feeling may be pressure, squeezing, or a strange or unusual sensation. You may notice something different or unusual in your jaw or left arm. Symptoms that should arouse suspicion may occur with activity and improve with rest, or change from a baseline pattern, for example occurring with lower levels of activity than usual or at rest. Additional red flags include shortness of breath, nausea, vomiting, sweating, lightheadedness, or pain traveling to the left or right arm or to the jaw. Many causes of chest discomfort have nothing to do with your heart. These include heartburn (or gastroesophageal reflux disease [GERD], also known as reflux) or a muscle strain of the chest wall. **Keep in mind that minor problems and more serious problems can sometimes be hard to distinguish on the basis of symptoms alone.**

If you have additional risks for heart disease, your suspicion of a possible heart problem should be heightened. Additional risks include:

- Prior history of heart problems
- Smoking
- High blood pressure
- Diabetes
- High cholesterol

- Family history (parent or sibling with heart problems at a young age, e.g. under age sixty)

Take a regular strength or baby aspirin until you can be more formally evaluated in your nearest emergency department.

Shortness of Breath

Difficulty breathing, particularly if not better in a matter of minutes, is a definite attention getter. There are few symptoms as frightening as air hunger. Again, many different medical problems can affect breathing. Some of these, such as a panic attack or a mild asthma attack, do not require immediate ambulance transport to your local emergency department. Warning signs of more serious trouble include:

- Shortness of breath that makes it difficult to speak a complete sentence without pausing
- Failure to improve after several minutes or after repeated use of your inhaler device, for example a "puffer" used with asthma or emphysema
- History of heart problems such as congestive heart failure (CHF)
- Increasing shortness of breath when lying flat; needing to prop yourself up on a few pillows
- Associated swelling in your feet, ankles, or legs in the days or weeks prior to the symptoms
- Progression over hours to days without relief
- Associated fever, cough, and increased phlegm production (signs and symptoms of pneumonia)
- History of lung disease, such as emphysema and smoking

Passing out or loss of consciousness for any reason

Loss of consciousness may be caused by non-serious reasons such as the sight of injuries or blood; however, passing out or losing consciousness can have serious causes that may need immediate attention, particularly if you have a history of heart problems. Passing out suddenly, without any warning symptoms such as lightheadedness or feeling faint, is of particular concern and deserves immediate attention.

Abdominal pain

Abdominal pain, particularly if severe and associated with nausea and vomiting and an inability to keep down fluids for more than twenty-four hours, or if you are pregnant, deserves immediate attention.

Symptoms of a possible stroke

Stroke symptoms may be **very subtle,** and many people having a stroke delay evaluation and treatment. Symptoms to watch for include:

- Diminished level of alertness
- Changes in speech
- Weakness in an arm or leg
- Changes in vision
- Sudden problems with balance or coordination
- Numbness or tingling in arms or legs
- Trouble swallowing
- Absolute worst headache of your life

Vomiting blood

Vomiting blood is often a symptom of a bleeding ulcer or bleeding gastritis (inflammation in the stomach). Vomited blood may look like coffee grounds. It does not always look red like blood from a fresh wound.

This is a sampling of the most common reasons to seek immediate care. If you have any doubts, call your physician's office. There should be a professional you can access quickly. You may get an automated message to dial 911 in the event of an emergency. If you reach a receptionist or answering service, say "I may be having an emergency and I need to talk to someone quickly." It is not always clear what constitutes an emergency. Always take the road of caution unless you are absolutely certain it is nothing serious. For symptoms such as those I have listed, do not hesitate. Remember, every minute counts.

The Chain of Survival

In my community and nationwide, there are efforts to enhance community awareness of what the American Heart Association and National Safety Council refer to as the "Chain of Survival." What follows is an outline of how this "chain" can save a life and how *you* can be an important contributor.

First Link—Early Access 911

a. An individual recognizes a serious or potentially serious health concern and activates 911.
b. Tape Dispatcher (EMD). Tape dispatchers obtain accurate information from callers and dispatch resources properly and efficiently. They allocate resources according to approved protocols. They give appropriate initial emergency medical instructions to callers.

Second Link—Early CPR

a. Early recognition of signs/symptoms
b. Recognition of unresponsiveness
c. Bystander intervention (call 911, safety, first aid, basic life support such as CPR)
d. Dispatcher directs instructions to the rescuers and EMS

This is a key link in the chain. In recent years, over 40 million Americans have been certified in basic life support (BLS). We can all contribute to the health of our communities by learning basic life support. It only takes a few hours to learn; it is safe and rarely causes significant injury to recipients. The goal of the American Heart Association is to reduce "call-to-CPR" time to a maximum of two to three minutes. CPR is easy to learn, interesting, and could save the life of someone precious. CPR has a greater chance of saving someone when started promptly, and can serve as a "bridge" until an Automatic External Defibrillator (AED) can be applied. All states have "Good Samaritan" laws that protect anyone trying to save the life of another. No one has ever been sued for attempting CPR during a cardiac arrest. Though you may feel uneasy doing mouth-to-mouth breathing or chest compressions, a person with no pulse and no ability to breathe will surely die without CPR. Though people often succumb despite CPR, early defibrillation with easy-to-use AED devices (see the third link) has the potential to save many lives! CPR can buy precious seconds until defibrillation is possible.

Third Link—Early Defibrillation

a. As noted, first responders are critical in the Chain of Survival. Aside from bystanders, first responders include police, fire and

EMTs or paramedics (EMTs with more advanced training in cardiac life support, airway management, and other more sophisticated interventions).

b. An AED is applied as soon as available to "shock" the patient with ventricular fibrillation. The device automatically detects this rhythm and instructs a shock in a clear step-by-step process. Best results are possible when an AED device is used within five minutes of the onset of ventricular fibrillation.

Learning to use an AED is easy and is often combined with basic life support training. *The most significant breakthrough in the world of pre-hospital care is the AED.* You are going to hear and see a lot about this device. AEDs are going to have a dramatic impact on the survival of people who experience cardiac arrest while in public places.

Here is a challenge and a plea:

If you want to do something great for yourself and for your community, learn CPR and become familiar with AEDs.

AEDs are automatic—the device determines whether a shock is necessary. Two adhesive pads are placed on the victim's chest and an "on" button is pushed on the device, attached to the pads. Simple, audible and visible instructions appear. This procedure can reverse a life-threatening and usually fatal heart rhythm disturbance called ventricular fibrillation. Timing is everything here. Early evidence suggests that most lay people can successfully apply an AED to an unconscious person and possibly save a life. Keep your eyes open for stories on AEDs. You will surely hear about them in your neighborhoods.

Although AEDs are portable (shoebox size or smaller) and easy to use, the challenge lies in balancing the costs (they are getting less expensive) with the enormous potential community benefit. AEDs should be readily available in public places, especially where large numbers of people come and go, such as airports, shopping malls, workplaces, schools, and sports arenas.

Figures 1 through 4 are provided courtesy of Philips Medical, Inc. They are not, of course, intended to be a substitute for an American Heart Association course in AED use. My intent here is to show you the basics. Familiarity could save a life.

I recently heard about a case in our community of a young woman

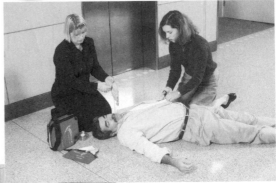

Figure 1. A typical
AED device.

Figure 2. Attending to an
unresponsive person and
finding an AED device.

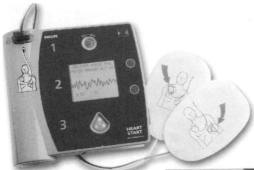

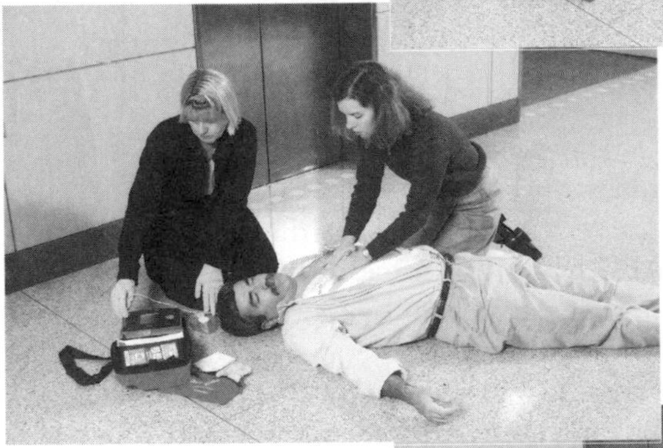

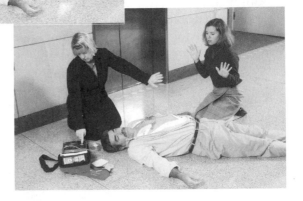

Figure 3. Placing the
defibrillator pads.

Figure 4. On command,
pressing the button
to defibrillate.

who was at a checkout counter of one of our local department stores. She collapsed and had a full cardiac arrest. An AED device was available. No one in the immediate vicinity of this young woman knew how to use the device! My daughter, who is twelve years old, could learn to use this in less than one hour. As every minute after a cardiac arrest is critical, people do less well if five to ten minutes pass without basic life support or AED intervention.

I know a young man, T.E., whose life was saved because his employer had an AED device where he worked and his co-workers were trained to use it. The "tipping point" between life and death can be so fine and so delicate. Cardiac arrests usually strike without warning. They need not lead down a certain, catastrophic, one-way street. Just ask T.E. and his family.

FOURTH LINK—PARAMEDIC/EMERGENCY DEPARTMENT

The last link involves having sophisticated training provided in the field by paramedics. As noted, paramedics are able to facilitate sophisticated interventions, including potential life-saving medications, prior to arrival at the Emergency Department, the final critical link in the resuscitation of potentially life-threatening emergencies.

The "Chain of Survival" will often mean the difference between life and death or survival with a more satisfactory quality of life. I have encountered many incredible stories of survival made possible by all that happened before arrival at the hospital.

DO NOT MISS TAKE HOME POINTS

1. Understand what you should and would do in the event of a medical emergency.
2. Recognize the common warning signs and symptoms that should prompt "911" activation.
3. Never drive yourself or have anyone drive you to the hospital if you are concerned about a potential medical emergency.
4. If you are concerned about a heart attack or stroke, *call 911 without delay.*
5. If you would benefit from having an emergency call button, get one.

6. Strongly consider learning CPR and AED use. A modest effort could make an enormous contribution to your family and to your community.

7. *Remember that denial is the enemy of the rational.*

CHAPTER 3

THE EMERGENCY DEPARTMENT

Organized Chaos

*"In the World Wide Web of Health Care, Emergency De-
partments are the Google®, the Yahoo®, the Gateway to the
System."*

—Mark Pettus

THE OBJECTIVES of this chapter are:

- To clarify the operations of an emergency department (E.D.).
- To go through a typical E.D. scenario from the viewpoint of a patient.
- To examine the potential "dispositions" or next steps after an emergency department evaluation.
- To examine alternatives to an evaluation in the emergency department that may be more suitable, depending on your individual circumstances.

Few areas of the health-care system are as busy, fast-paced, and interesting, for health-care providers and patients, as the emergency department. Emergency departments capture the incoming diversity of people, problems, and issues, all in need of evaluation, treatment, stabilization, triage, and disposition planning (planning the next steps). Many people are intrigued by the human drama of an emergency department (as depicted in the popular TV program *ER*). Though the drama of the television depiction is heightened, the accuracy on the set is not so far removed from real life. The ongoing activity, continuous movement, cacophony, and organized chaos are very much exemplified in the E.D. For sheer human drama, few places in the health-care system compare.

I have worked in our emergency department as an emergency staff physician. It was like being in a raft on white water rapids, dealing quickly with sick and needy people, unpredictable at every turn. It was both exhausting and exhilarating. As a physician, this was one of the most challenging roles I have ever been in. I have also spent a great deal of time in emergency departments admitting patients to our hospital for different types of medical problems. And like many of you, I have been a patient treated in an emergency department and have accompanied many loved ones as they were evaluated in emergency departments.

Almost all of us encounter an emergency department at some point in our lives. My primary goal in this chapter is to give you a "behind-the-scenes" look at a typical E.D. They can vary significantly in scope and service, depending on the setting. Small or large, the dynamics are comparable. Interactions are often emotional, tense, and transient. This is a place where people can share effectively in some of life's more noteworthy moments. Incredible bonds have the potential to develop in moments! Is it possible to enhance the quality of an E.D. visit? The answer is yes.

E.D. Operations

As I mentioned, E.D.s are very busy places. In fact, the volume of visits to emergency departments nationwide is increasing constantly. According to a study by the Center for Studying Health System Change, a policy research organization in Washington, D.C., in 2001, 108 million people went to emergency departments. This represents a 16 percent increase during the six-year period ending in 2001. Annual visits to the E.D. at my community hospital have gone from forty to sixty thousand in the last five years.

At times some E.D.s are so full, particularly in large inner city areas, that ambulances have to be diverted to other nearby facilities. Though this is an unusual event, the demand on most E.D.s is substantial. I think it is worth spending a short time on some of the reasons for this growing phenomenon. As overwhelming demand for emergency services outpaces staffing, you are more likely to experience long waits and possible delays.

So, why have E.D.s become busier places?

- As our society ages, more people have a growing number of chronic medical problems (we refer to them as "co-morbidities"); this creates a greater likelihood of needing medical evaluation and treatment.
- For people who do not have primary care physicians (e.g., internist, family practitioner, or pediatrician), the E.D. often becomes the default option for a "primary care" evaluation, even if not an emergency.
- People sometimes cannot be evaluated promptly by their own physicians (see the section on patient-centered access in chapter 1) because they can't get an appointment. Perhaps this sounds familiar. Most physicians are heavily booked, with minimal latitude and flexibility to get people into the office on short notice.
- Emergency Departments are always open—twenty-four hours a day, seven days a week.
- More medical problems are treated in the E.D. without admission to the hospital. Evaluations and treatments historically performed after admission are now initiated in the emergency department. This results in more involved evaluations, complex planning, treatment, and organization than ever before. As criteria for admission to the hospital have become more stringent, evaluations in the E.D. and planning for outpatient follow-up care has become more complex and time-consuming.
- The volume and complexity of medical problems evaluated and treated in the E.D. have increased as the prevalence of these problems has increased in our society; for example, diabetes, high cholesterol, heart disease, dementia, and other issues.
- In some instances, pre-authorization by primary care providers is no longer necessary, reducing the restrictions placed on going to the emergency department.
- Physicians, often concerned about potential litigation, feel safer recommending that a patient go to the E.D. for evaluation, despite what may be a low probability that the problem is an emergency.
- From a physician's perspective it is often easier and more convenient to have a patient evaluated in the E.D., where tests and interpretations can occur in a matter of hours, as opposed to possible delays with outpatient scheduling, testing, and interpretation.

- Most people desire the shortest measurable period of time between the onset of symptoms and a diagnosis and therapeutic resolution.

Emergency departments are equipped and staffed to deal with rapid evaluation, stabilization, diagnosis, and treatment of a wide range of medical problems. Some have more resources than others; for example, managing trauma. Patients with problems requiring a greater level of sophistication than is available are stabilized and subsequently transferred to another facility.

An E.D. is staffed with physicians trained to manage a wide range of medical problems; allied health professionals such as physician assistants or nurse practitioners; R.N.s; technical staff; and administrative assistants. Like most links in the health-care system chain, emergency department staff members must work effectively as individuals and as teams, collaborating, communicating, and rallying around specific tasks and responsibilities. In my experience, E.D. personnel (much like ICU/CCU, O.R., and recovery room staff) are attracted to the pace, activity, variety, and challenge. They think quickly on their feet. They thrive in a high volume, high complexity, unpredictable environment.

In the E.D. there are "stations," rooms or cubicles where individual patients and their families and friends are brought for evaluation. These settings can be very impersonal, in close quarters, near other patients, and secluded only by the thin veil of an aesthetically unappealing curtain, suspended by metal clips. When you don an inadequate hospital gown, you must be prepared (if possible) for an immediate abandonment of modesty.

Certain rooms and areas of the E.D. are equipped to evaluate and treat specific problems such as trauma or heart syndromes (e.g. a heart attack or angina). These areas contain sophisticated equipment for heart monitoring, blood pressure cuffs that automatically inflate and deflate, oxygen measurements, ventilators, and other equipment. Nurses and physicians work in concert to triage individuals to the most appropriate area in the department, based on the nature of the problems.

Intravenous lines (IVs), blood work, x-rays, and a wide assortment of medications are all applied as needed. Breathing treatments, given by mixing medication with moisturized oxygen for breathing problems such as asthma, may be given using nebulizers (also called NEBS or "updrafts").

An ambulance port allows individuals transported to the E.D. to be transferred directly into the department for evaluation and treatment. Phones will be ringing, beepers will be beeping, personnel will be scurrying about, conversations (some easily and unintentionally overheard) will be occurring everywhere. This is the landscape of the E.D. At times patients may feel forgotten or abandoned, particularly if staff has to respond quickly to a crisis—a trauma or a patient with dangerously low blood pressure or a critical breathing problem. It is an environment that can require patience, easier said than done if you do not feel well, are anxious, or hurting. E.D. personnel do all they can to be as prompt and attentive as volume and demand allow.

A Common Encounter

If you have never experienced an E.D., let me give you an example of a common scenario. While at work, Mrs. Smith develops a "funny" feeling in her chest. She has never experienced anything like this before. She has a history of high blood pressure and high cholesterol. Appropriately, her colleagues realize something is not right and call an ambulance (this is a critical step: see chapter 2 on pre-hospital care). Within minutes an ambulance arrives and EMTs place Mrs. Smith on a stretcher and apply oxygen through a small tube placed in the nostrils (a nasal cannula); they take her vital signs (blood pressure, pulse or heart rate, and blood oxygen (measured by placing a small clip on her finger).

Her pain is no longer present as they ask her a few routine questions about the intensity of her symptoms and about her medical history. She is placed on a portable heart monitor (sticky pads placed on the chest and extremities and connected with wires to the monitor). She is given a baby aspirin as a matter of routine.

En route to the hospital, the EMTs call in brief details and an update of Mrs. Smith's vital signs. A charge nurse and physician, receiving the call, ask further questions, give additional instructions, and triage Mrs. Smith to the "heart room." Soon thereafter, she arrives at the ambulance port of the E.D. Within ten minutes of arrival, Mrs. Smith will have her brief history repeated to the nurse, be placed on the E.D.'s heart monitor and oxygen (attached to the wall), have vital signs repeated, blood drawn for routine blood work, an EKG (or ECG—electrocardiogram) performed for the treating physician to see, and a "saline well" placed (an IV with a rubber tip from which more blood can be drawn, medicine given, or an IV started). As soon as possible, the treating physician will evaluate Mrs. Smith with a more detailed history and physical examination. She will be asked frequently about any recurrence of discomfort. Further testing, as needed, will be considered; for example, an x-ray of the chest. This is done with a portable machine at the bedside if the nature of the problem (usually chest pain or shortness of breath) requires keeping the individual stationary and under close observation.

Mrs. Smith's tests return reassuringly okay. However, because a heart problem cannot be entirely excluded, it is advised that she be observed in a special cardiac observation unit for twenty-four hours. She is subsequently transported to a floor in the hospital where she can be observed on a heart monitor, have blood work and ECGs repeated in twelve and twenty-four hours, and have a stress test, if she is stable, before she goes home. The emergency room physician contacts Mrs. Smith's primary care provider (or the covering physician after hours) to review the preliminary findings and the treatment plan. If the hospital is a teaching hospital, medical students or residents may be called to assist in the care (see chapter 19 on graduate medical education).

If you do not come into the E.D. directly by ambulance, you will register in the admission area and be seen by a triage nurse who will, as best he or she can, with the information given and the resources available, determine the order and urgency of your evaluation and treatment. This is no time to be stoic, shy, or in denial. If you are having any discomfort in your chest, neck, or arm (particularly your left arm); if you are short of breath; if you are feeling weak or numb on one side of your body; or if you feel like you may pass out, *speak up*. Only clear understanding and communication will allow medical staff to recognize an urgent problem. Even if it turns out to be nothing serious, or your mind is telling you "Don't worry . . . it can't be my heart," it is better to be safe. Minor problems and potentially serious problems can look the same in the early hours of their presentation!

After the Emergency Department Evaluation

The overwhelming majority of patients evaluated in the E.D. will be sent home with specific instructions for taking medications (prescribed or over the counter), limitations on activity, and following up, if necessary, with a primary care provider or consultant. Lab test results that are still pending at the time of your discharge from the department are usually communicated to you either directly by the E.D. staff or, after having been received, by your primary care provider. If you are prescribed medications at a time when finding an open pharmacy may not be possible, a small supply of medication is given to use until you can access a pharmacy.

All documentation from the E.D. encounter—nursing, physicians, allied health professionals, lab tests (blood work and x-rays) are forwarded to your primary care provider where the information is filed in your medical record. Again, this underscores the importance of having a primary care provider who can track all aspects of your care, which can easily become fragmented and lost in our convoluted system. The more fragmented your care becomes, the less likely it will be that any one individual will be able to provide guiding oversight and coordination. Communication regarding potentially important health issues is more likely to break down. This is not a good thing. It can lead to repetition of tests, harmful interactions between medications prescribed by different clinicians (see chapter 11 on taking medications), worse health outcomes, and much greater costs.

As you start to feel better, you will inevitably be tempted to discontinue the prescribed medication or depart from the recommended suggestions for activity modification. I know. Been there, done that, and on occasion I have paid the price. There are many problems for which you may be treated in the E.D. where stopping a medication (e.g., an antibiotic for an upper respiratory or sinus infection) could lead to a relapse or worsening of symptoms after initial improvement. Increasing your activity after a musculoskeletal injury (e.g., lower back strain, shoulder strain, or ankle sprain) will be a hard temptation to resist, as many of these injuries will begin to feel better in two or three days. This too could lead to a relapse of symptoms or aggravation of the initial injury that, in the end, could force you to delay your routine or miss more time from work than would have been the case had you adhered to the original plan.

If you are not sent home, the E.D. physician and staff will determine the best place in the hospital to admit you. It is possible there will be specialist consultants involved in your evaluation and in that disposition decision. For example, you may be admitted to a heart monitoring floor (called telemetry) or to the Intensive Care or Coronary Care Unit (ICU/CCU); behavioral health unit (e.g., for depression or suicidal thoughts), or to a surgery floor. Many floors in the hospital have categories of patients and problems that they deal with most frequently.

Less commonly, your discharge plan may involve a rehabilitation unit or skilled nursing unit if your problems are not acute enough (in the eyes of the health provider or your insurer) to require hospitalization, but are significant enough to create concern about your ability to return home safely, with enough support and functional capacity.

It is increasingly common for people to return home with supportive services such as visiting nursing care, physical and/or occupational therapy, a home health aide, a homemaker, or other assistance. It is important, under any circumstances, that you be a willing participant in any decision made with respect to your care (see chapter 9 on decision making) and that you understand the issues, the options, and the decisions.

Considering Alternatives to An Emergency Department Evaluation

First, I need to emphasize that E.D. staff are there to evaluate and treat *anyone* who feels the need and desire to be evaluated. I have observed however, many instances where the E.D. is chosen for convenience and availability. Some problems that are not "emergent" could be appropriately treated in another setting (primary care office, walk-in clinics, etc.). Some symptoms may become significantly better in a few days, no matter what you decide to do. Now, please do not get me wrong. It is not my intent to discourage any need for medical intervention. I do feel the need, however, to articulate a perspective that balances greater understanding regarding the desire to do all that is possible to feel well with the best available choices and resources. Waiting times in most E.D.s have increased considerably as the demand for resources has gone up more quickly than the supply. Waiting times, potential costs, and exposure to infectious diseases (there's no place like an E.D. waiting room for germ exposure) can be a real downside, particularly if the problem could be dealt with in an alternative fashion. E.D. staff must prioritize or "triage" the most serious of medical problems in an effort to avoid potentially serious delays in evaluation and treatment. The greater the volume of people needing to be seen, the greater potential there is for serious delay. Unintentional as this would be, of course, that is the nature of the beast.

That woman in the waiting room, for example, sitting quietly with vague discomfort in her left arm, may not be recognized as a potentially serious heart problem as triage staff scurry to get as much information as they can on the many people waiting to be seen. This woman sitting in the waiting area could be your sister, your mother, or your grandmother. Again, I do not mean to suggest that some medical problems are not worthy of attention. It is my intent and the purpose of this book to give you an "inside" perspective that can help you help yourself and those you love to use the system in as safe and effective a way as possible. It is my intent to assist you in reducing the inevitable frustration you may feel at a long wait, costly bill, and eventual common sense advice.

Here are some questions to consider before going to your local emergency department:

- Are my symptoms potentially serious?
- Will an evaluation likely change what I would otherwise do for myself?
- Is it worth waiting another twenty-four to forty-eight hours to see how I feel?
- Is there a possibility my primary provider's group or an alternative setting such as a walk-in clinic can evaluate me with less waiting time and perhaps lower costs?
- Is there anyone I know and trust with a medical background, such as an R.N., who can provide some guiding advice?

For example, the overwhelming majority of sore throats, cold symptoms, mild respiratory symptoms (e.g., cough or runny nose without shortness of breath), muscular injuries (e.g., lower back strain), will get better in a matter of days and do not require treatment beyond what you are capable of doing for yourself—rest, fluids, acetaminophen or ibuprofen, and decongestants or other over-the-counter (OTC) medication. Even that awful syndrome of nausea, vomiting, and diarrhea (in an otherwise healthy person) will usually turn the corner within a day or two. The challenge is to know what the usual course is of whatever you are experiencing, if possible. Departure from the typical should arouse suspicion.

For example, if you know that most sore throats and cold and cough symptoms are viral, do not respond to antibiotics, and turn the corner in one week with or without OTC symptom-oriented remedies, you are less likely to pursue an E.D. visit on the second day of your illness with symptoms of sore throat and sinus congestion. If your cough is now ten days old and getting worse, with fever and more sputum production, you are departing from the norm and should be evaluated for a bacterial infection. So how can you possibly know this? Educate yourself if possible. There are numerous sources of medical texts, Internet sources, and references for the lay public (see Chapter 15 on health-care literacy).

As I stated earlier, E.D.s are sometimes used as sources of primary care. Excellent though the care may be, this is not good utilization of our precious health-care resources. Patients who receive care only through the E.D. often see different providers; have no continuity, and have no opportunity for a relationship to develop with a provider. Many, many times I have heard people say they cannot get in to see their primary care provider quickly and they have no choice but to go to the E.D. That is a reality of our system that is sometimes unavoidable.

In my experience however, if you have a good, long-term relationship with a primary care provider, he or she will attempt to accommodate you (e.g., evaluate you within twenty-four hours as most basic medical problems can be safely treated the following day if a provider is not available on the same day). Your primary care provider can also help guide the decision to use the E.D., if in fact, this is a more appropriate place to be evaluated and treated, as it sometimes will be.

No one likes feeling poorly. We all want a quick turnaround. No one I have ever met could "afford to be sick." We are not a very patient culture. Our Jiffy-Lube, fast-food mindset, when it comes to health care, does not always serve us well. Healing can take time, and often will occur spontaneously, particularly with minor problems. The bottom line is *if you need to be seen, by all means, be seen.* And if the spirit moves you (and hopefully it will), express thanks for the constant commitment, support, service, and vital health-care roles that emergency department personnel play in our communities.

DO NOT MISS TAKE HOME POINTS

1. If you feel your problem is urgent, go to the nearest E.D. as soon as possible.
2. If you feel that your problem is a possible emergency, call 911.
3. For a problem that may not be urgent, consider alternatives to an E.D. visit such as a primary care office, walk-in clinic, or watchful waiting.
4. Make sure you understand your instructions prior to being discharged from the E.D.
5. Emergency departments are not designed to provide primary care.
6. The more resources available in the E.D. for the truly urgent and emergent, the better.

CHAPTER 4

COPING IN THE MIDST OF ILLNESS

"We could never learn to be brave and patient, if there were only joy in the world."

—Helen Keller

THE OBJECTIVES of this chapter are:

- To examine the many paths to hope and healing as you attempt to cope with the illness or loss of a loved one.
- To provide a source of strength by sharing the inspiring and courageous stories of people I have cared for who are experiencing challenging and difficult circumstances.
- To touch on the healing potential inherent in our positive emotions.

Illness and loss are the ultimate equalizers. They do not discriminate based upon age, gender, ethnicity, or socioeconomic class. It is true that many health problems, like diabetes, are strongly influenced by these factors. Illness can take many forms. It can strike without warning; it can be abrupt and unpredictable. It can be slow, progressive, certain, and at times unrelenting. It can be mild and it can be life threatening. It can be reversible or permanent. Illness, at some point in time, is unavoidable, and confronting illness is one of life's inevitabilities. Nothing

The most important questions that arise in our lives will not have clear answers.

can turn a life upside down more quickly than being ill, caring for someone who is sick, or losing a loved one.

Most medical problems are self-limited, that is, likely to improve over
time, usually with a full recovery. The human body has remarkable healing potential, with and without modern medical intervention. When we
deal with illness we become more aware of just how blessed we are to
have good health and to have those we love with us. We are reminded of
how thankful we should be just to feel well. Illness can serve as a sobering
reminder of how much we take our health for granted. It can leave our
glass looking half empty or it can open our eyes to the potential for positive life change, a glass half full.

The extent to which an illness challenges your ability to cope depends,
of course, on your circumstances. For example, appendicitis, with an anticipated full recovery in two to four weeks, is very different from a more
serious problem such as a heart attack or a stroke. The response to a
heart problem such as atrial fibrillation is different than a response to you
or a family member confronting a profound change in quality of life or
the possibility of death. From minor medical problems to the most life
threatening, there is inevitably a challenge in navigating life in a way that
was not anticipated before the illness or loss.

How we feel and react when dealing with illness reflects the physical,
mental, emotional, and spiritual dimensions of who we are. Our response to illness and loss is multidimensional. Rarely is it a simple matter. For example, an individual might experience physical symptoms
such as pain, nausea, or shortness of breath. These symptoms might
have emotional elements attached such as sadness, fear, anxiety, and
anger. These, in turn might affect mental capacity, making it difficult to
concentrate, recall detail, and reason. There might be spiritual symptoms of emptiness, isolation, and diminished meaning. Current research
suggests that changes in mood such as sadness or depression and pain
frequently occur together. Fibromyalgia is an example. People with fibromyalgia experience pain in several areas, including the upper back,
arms, and legs. Symptoms of depression and anxiety often co-exist.
While the cause of fibromyalgia is still uncertain, it is increasingly clear
that changes in central nervous system chemical messengers (called neurotransmitters) are likely to play a major role. These neurotransmitters,
can lead to pain *and* alterations in mood.

Having a serious illness or dealing with a loved one who is seriously ill
can serve as a painful reminder of the fine line in our lives that separates
harmony from chaos, serenity from turmoil, peace from angst, faith from
doubt, certainty from uncertainty, and light from darkness.

I have experienced serious illness and death in those I have loved in my family and those I have cared for in my professional life. I have seen sudden, shocking, and unfair circumstances thrust upon the unprepared, and I have seen the most remarkable of recoveries! I have weathered and seen many others weather the darkest of storms. I have experienced the power and strength of the human spirit and the suffering inherent in illness or loss. I have seen faith, determination, and purpose overcome seemingly insurmountable obstacles. I have seen light emerge from the darkest of places. I have observed the spark of life refusing to be extinguished. I have seen a readiness to let go.

Many patients and families I have known have graciously opened the doors to their lives. In choosing to enter and in sharing the journey, I have observed many powerful resources for coping. I have seen, in this interesting laboratory of life, the "faith factor" at its very best. I have seen the power of the human connection at work. Nurturing relationships become a rainbow of comfort and hope in the midst of dark skies. It is in this personal space that I have experienced our inherent capacity for healing and coping, regardless of the circumstances or the ultimate outcome. It is what I have consistently found in this tender space that serves as the basis for these words of encouragement as you or a loved one struggle to cope with illness.

I sympathize deeply if you are confronting a challenging time in your life; such challenges seem unfair and yet inevitable. It is very hard to move forward in the project of healing without first attempting to reconfigure perceptions of fairness and unfairness. We can identify factors that increase the risk of certain events occurring in our lives; for example, high blood pressure, diabetes, high blood fats, and smoking as risk factors for heart disease and stroke. And though ignoring these risks and living an unhealthy lifestyle may leave many thinking a bad outcome is fair retribution, there are some individuals who simply appear to be luckier than others. Good genes? Perhaps. Lucky? I think so.

On Fairness, Indifference, and Luck

Though most of the information in this chapter is positive, I need to start with some darker sentiments on dealing with illness or loss. Faithful and hopeful though I tend to be in my personal and professional mindset, what I am about to say may seem cynical. It applies more often to serious crises that arrive uninvited in our lives. I offer the following observations—perhaps you will see that you are not alone in your feelings.

1. Take one day at a time.
2. Forget about fairness, deserving, and undeserving. It just does not work that way even though it seems it should. Very bad things happen to very good people.
3. In the midst of illness and crisis, the rest of the world will eventually move forward with an unintentional indifference to your circumstances. The wounds of others may heal faster than yours.
4. If there is an eternal, universal energy of life that transcends this existence (and absence of proof is not proof of absence), we have a lot to be hopeful about.
5. If there is an eternal, universal life force that transcends this existence (and I'm a believer), it is not an energy that micromanages our lives.
6. We micromanage our own lives.
7. The human being is a masterful creation.
8. Pray, at a minimum, for good luck.

Consider this true story. It speaks painfully to the fine line that really does define the distance between life and loss. It shatters the notion of fairness and boasts of random indifference. It also speaks to love's enduring strength and the resilience of the human spirit. I was working in our emergency department one evening when the pre-hospital emergency dispatcher rang out an imminent arrival. The EMTs were transporting a sixty-year-old man who had experienced a cardiac arrest just moments before at a local bowling alley. It was a Thursday, just another cold, snowy, Berkshire winter evening.

The individual being transported had eaten supper with his family, including his wife of twenty-eight years and his three school-aged children. It would be the last time they would see him alive. All was routine as he proceeded to do what he had done every winter Thursday evening for the last several years. He went to join his buddies at the local bowling alley. Perhaps tonight there would be a personal high score or a team best. Perhaps there would be a great comeback in the last frame, against all odds. Perhaps the "boys" of the Thursday night bowling league would bowl like they had never bowled before.

The ambulance siren became progressively louder. The ambulance port automatic doors slid open and a stretcher rolled forward with two EMTs focused and desperately engaged, attempting to save this man's life. I was the emergency department physician in charge on this particular evening. The patient had no pulse or heartbeat. He was not breathing, and he was being supported with a synthetic plastic football-sized bag, being squeezed to deliver oxygen to his lungs. A tube was in the opening of the lungs to allow delivery of oxygen and release of carbon dioxide. Here was a fellow who had been bowling as usual just fifteen minutes earlier. He had not had a pulse since. He was wearing his bowling shirt with his name embroidered above the left chest pocket. He was still wearing his bowling shoes. This is probably what he wore every week on Thursday night at this time. His life could not be saved. Death would have the last word. He would not return home to see his family and children. He would not return to bowl with his buddies. He would not show up for work on Friday morning. He probably never knew what hit him. And just like that . . . it was over. Death did not care that there was much more to do and say in his life. Death was indifferent to his being a devoted, loving father and husband. It did not matter in these circumstances that he was kind, giving, and a contributor to his community.

The activity in the emergency department continued, indifferent to the painful, sudden, and shocking circumstances before me. People continued to arrive, sick and in need of assistance. The ambulance dispatcher continued to ring out. The activity around me was painfully indifferent to what I was feeling in my heart. One of our staff nurses notified me of the arrival of the man's family. I vividly remember walking toward our "quiet room," a small island in the middle of a sea of organized chaos, where a private and personal conversation could take place. There I would meet his wife and three children. The look on my face communicated clearly, without words, the worst of all possible messages. I had dropped a bomb into the lives of this beautiful family. We embraced each other. All I could do was to look into the eyes of his kids, see the eyes of my children, and briefly be in the moment. My message was sad and true, empathetic and empty. In an instant, his wife's life would never be the same. Her strength and courage were a vision of control, giving her children a lifeline to cling to. Her spirit, though shattered, remained buoyant, allowing her children to grasp and remain afloat despite the weight of their shared grief. Nothing fair about this, is there?

How do we respond to the universal outcry of "Why me? Why us? Why now? What did I/we do to deserve this? How can such awful circumstances fall upon the good and loving?" Our expectation that good things happen to good people and bad things happen to bad people in no way describes many difficult experiences in our lives. The experience of having a heart attack, being diagnosed with cancer, losing mobility from Parkinson's, or losing mental capacity from Alzheimer's, is not related to what is fair or unfair. There is no solace in the expectation of fairness when it comes to the unexpected loss of a loved one.

Some events in our lives are not governed by principles of reciprocity. I say some because I do strongly believe that kindness, love, compassion, forgiveness, and reconciliation do come back to us in exponential ways. Ancient worldviews have stood the test of time as testimony to the power and truth of this positively reinforcing cycle of energy. Disease and death seem devoid of such governance. Sure, we can influence some outcomes by the choices we make in life. The choices we make have a huge impact on our lives. Fairness, however, may be indifferent to these choices as our lives unfold.

Anger, abandonment, and resentment are sometimes byproducts of our attempts to reconcile what should be to what is. If you find your faith shaken, it is understandable. A universal and dynamic energy, if you are inclined to believe in one, is not a force that controls outcomes good or bad. It simply exists. It has taken me a while to come to grips with this in my own life. As I witnessed my parents struggling with many health problems, I could not help but think that life was showing them way too little respect. This was woefully unfair. I found my faith in fairness challenged and shaken. These were good, caring people, suffering and shortchanged. I searched with pain and exhaustion for sources of reason, responsibility, and reconciliation.

What has become increasingly clear to me is that faith, hope, and reconciliation are not always found in answers and justification but instead in the awareness that something more profound is at play in our lives. While life's circumstances may leave us broken and lost, we are drawn forward by love and by purpose. We are lifted by love, friendship, and relationships. We become more mindful of what those we have lost would want most from us. Perhaps they would whisper in our ear . . . "Move on, I'll be waiting." It is in an awareness of the present that we indeed are alive. Perhaps, and I must say I am really counting on this, the end is not the end at all. Is it possible that life as we know it is just a prelude? Is it possible we are sprinting with purpose, fear, and insecurity to the starting blocks instead of the finish line?

Before I shift my perspective in a more positive direction, I want to touch briefly on the experience of indifference. It is true that what is most meaningful to us usually does not affect most of the world around us. Of course, those who love and care about you will be affected deeply by your circumstances. Your personal wounds, however, will take longer to heal as the rest of the world moves on with life. You may find your circumstances "suspended in time," a whirlwind of fog, settling only slowly. You may find yourself more isolated due to your circumstances because friends and family are uncertain how best to behave. You may find yourself, at a time when you need to be held and understood most, struggling with attempts to reach out. Some around you, in an effort to deal with their own feelings and issues, will tiptoe around, avoid, or mask what is most necessary to say and share. Health-care professionals may enter and pass through your life, caring and professional, but unaware of their inability to connect with you or your family. At a time when you need most to have others support you, you may find yourself needing to support others. You may have to help others be more comfortable in their feelings about you and your circumstances. You may need to find more time for yourself and your thoughts, helping others to be mindful of the delicate balance between support and space. No matter how still and surreal our lives become, the rest of the world goes on around us. This may be an added source of frustration as you attempt to cope with your circumstances. It is also an opportunity to help others understand you and to create the most positive energy possible as the process of healing moves forward.

On Love

"One word frees us of all the weight and pain of life: That word is love."

—Sophocles

My son Alex is almost twelve years old and has Down syndrome. When he was five, he began to have problems with recurrent nausea and vomiting. He would improve for a short time only to have his symptoms return. He had a series of tests that after a few very long months led to the diagnosis of a severe narrowing of his small intestine. This was something he was born with. Until his symptoms appeared, there was no way to know of its existence. Serious though this could have been, my wife and I were relieved that an answer had been found. Within two days he had surgery and the problem was repaired. I will never forget how he appeared after surgery. He was so small, dwarfed by the technology surrounding and attached to him. He had an IV in his arm, that was taped to a Styrofoam board to prevent him from bending it; a tube through his nostril into his stomach; oxygen into his nostrils; a small tube providing anesthesia into his spinal canal, and a tube placed through his penis into his bladder. My wife and I felt heartbroken, afraid, out of control, weary, and even a little angry that our sweet child had to go through all of this. This certainly was not fair! He looked overwhelmed, scared, uncomfortable, and confused. Because of some delays in his language development it was impossible to help him clearly understand what was happening and what was to happen. Love was our language. Love was our primary source of communication. Love was clearly transcending this harsh reality. Alex was awash in it. He felt it. He understood it. I could see it in his eyes and he could see it in ours. We could feel it in our shared human touch. It sustained my wife and me. Our shared love was perpetually in the moment.

While his care was excellent, the turmoil, anxiety, and time-altering nature of our singular experience were immersed in the busy routine of just another day on the pediatric inpatient service. For those working with and around us this was all a matter of routine. For us, it was once in a lifetime! I am always reminded that routine health-care exchanges for me as a physician are anything but routine for those I am caring for.

The pain we feel when we see someone we care deeply about confronting illness mirrors the depth of our love for that individual. We are givers and we are recipients. Our pain is shared pain. Our suffering is shared suffering. Love deepens our reality and serves to remind us of our purpose. It sustains us in the deepest and darkest of times. Love transcends our senses. Love is a divine presence, an adhesive when our lives begin to unravel. The love I have seen expressed and shared in family after family, regardless of the circumstances, regardless of the people involved, is incredibly powerful and universal. Love's expression is timeless and, when unrestrained, opens the door to healing. While this may not immediately undo your burden in the midst of a tumultuous time, it will eventually take hold and ease your pain. It will calm. In love there is hope. What is there to live for if not for love? There is simply no force in our existence greater than that of love. I realize this is hardly a novel insight. No force, no disease process, and no misfortune, no matter how great, no matter how painful, can overwhelm love.

It has been several years now since my parents died. Progressive illness, in its indifference, had the last word at much too young an age for both my parents. Not a day goes by that I do not think about them. Some deep wounds continue slowly to heal. My love for them has transcended their physical passing, and I still feel very connected to their spiritual essence. Their deaths were not, in any way, the end of a growing relationship. My two beautiful children, Anna and Alex, are now thirteen and eleven years of age respectively. As I share in their journey, I am frequently filled with overwhelming emotions of pride and love, as any parent would be. This is what parenting is all about. I consider the notion that many times as a child, I must have filled my parents' hearts with the exact same feelings. These emotions after all are universal. The notion of being responsible for creating such joy brings a smile to my face and fills my heart. Only as a parent could I connect this feeling with what my parents must have felt when I was younger. Love is the connection. It allows my relationship with my parents to continue to grow, alive and meaningful, years after their death. This connection has been like an old friend, bridging the past with the present.

If you or a loved one are ill, whether the illness is serious or not, find the words to express your love. Never underestimate the potential for greater mutual understanding. I have on many occasions encountered broken, distant, and dysfunctional families. I do not mean to sound judgmental. This is just the way it is. I have seen many families struggle with wounds, some deeply rooted. Conflict, when dealing with illness and loss, has the potential to deepen these divides. Anger, silence, distance, and disrespect can be unrelenting burdens. These are negative emotions that perpetually consume, never allowing the pieces to become whole. If there are negative emotions that consume your life, particularly in response to illness or loss, you must look for ways to transform them.

If you feel you need help with this, and most of us do, talk to friends, family, a nurse, pastoral care person, or your physician. Remember that the doors most begging to be opened are the doors we often tiptoe by. Health-care professionals may not recognize the vital need "to go there," waiting instead for an invitation to enter and failing to recognize the subtle, soft, and nonverbal messages to pause and be in the moment. The best invitations to enter may take the form of a tear, a laugh, a look, or even silence.

I have seen remarkable healing when family members or families and health-care professionals choose to enter this "space." I have also seen painful wounds deepen unfairly and unnecessarily as a consequence of allowing deep hurt to stand in the way of forgiveness. Love is the ultimate therapy. Illness or loss can create a tremendous void in one's life. Love unleashes a flood of positive emotions that opens doors to greater understanding, meaning, reconciliation, and better health outcomes. Love is the foundation upon which joy and hope reside. There is no substitute for the loving support of friends and family when coping with illness or dealing with loss. There is an inherent human need to share our grief, to share our pain, and to share our journey. There is no substitute for loving friends and family being present, in the moment, lifting our spirits.

Another challenge to effective coping is the strong desire not to disrupt the lives of others. People can be very stoic, often reluctant to ask for help or uncomfortable expressing feelings of fear, need, and despair. "I don't want to burden others. They have enough going on in their lives."

It is not uncommon for me to hear parents say this about their children. There is a paradox I have often observed in times of illness, loss and the challenge to cope:

Those who need most to be held are, at times, least likely to reach out. Those who need most to reach out are, at times, least likely to hold.

Sadly, many people are isolated and lonely when coping with illness. If someone you know and care about, friend or family, appears to be in need, do not wait for an invitation. Reach out. Be present. Be in the moment. Embrace. It's not about saying all the right things. Love speaks for itself.

On Gratitude

"Gratitude unlocks the fullness of life.
It turns what we have into enough and more.
It turns denial into acceptance, chaos to order, and confusion
*   to clarity.*
It can turn a meal into a fast, a house into a home and a
*   stranger into a friend.*
Gratitude makes sense of our past, brings peace for today
*   and creates a vision for tomorrow."*

—Melodie Beattie

It is naïve to suggest that feeling grateful should come naturally when experiencing illness or loss. Gratitude is not the first sentiment that usually comes to heart. I have observed and experienced, however, opportunities for gratitude taking hold and transforming what can be very difficult circumstances. Gratitude can be an important path to healing. Gratitude is really about transformation and it can enter one's life in subtle ways.

The distinction between healing and curing is worthy of reemphasis in the context of reflecting on gratitude. It is possible that the illness you or a loved one are confronting cannot be cured. You may have diabetes, heart disease, a stroke, or cancer, problems for which cures remains elusive. When someone is cured they are returned to the state they were in before the problem came up in the first place. Returning to normal is not possible for many of the illnesses that we see and experience in life and modern medicine today.

To heal implies something very different. The word *heal* is derived from the Old English word *hal*—to make whole, to mend. Healing, in my view, implies a greater awareness and realization of peace and wholeness. I see it as a reconciliatory sense of contentment. Healing is acceptance. Healing is awareness. It is an awareness that the essence of who we are as people, our spirit, if you will, has the remarkable potential to transcend what may appear to be physically and emotionally broken, quite whole and intact. Ancient wisdom reminds us why they call it ancient wisdom. It is remarkable and true. Ancient worldviews such as the monotheistic faiths of Judaism, Islam, and Christianity, as well as Buddhism and Hinduism, share an appreciation for the interconnectedness of all life. These worldviews see the project of healing as naturally intersecting with one's spirituality. It is in this domain that we feel our connectedness with each other. It is in this domain that our lives are viewed as divine gifts to be nurtured, respected, and valued. Although manifested differently around the world, most cultures have developed linguistic and cultural methods for expressing gratitude.

I recently met an individual who exemplified the healing nature of gratitude. Mr. Jones was a patient on our inpatient rehabilitation unit. He lived outside our immediate area and did not have a local primary care provider. As he had several medical problems in his history, our rehabilitation team asked for my help with his management. He was there to focus on regaining his strength and functional independence. My first step in this process was to thoroughly review the medical records and all other available medical information. These are stories about the individual, though they read more like a medical biography. Mr. Jones was in his late fifties. He had had diabetes for over thirty years and had experienced most of the devastating complications that can accompany this disease. His vision was limited. He had a history of heart disease. His kidney function had failed, requiring dialysis for survival a few years prior. He now had a kidney transplant from his daughter, allowing him independence from dialysis. One year ago his left leg had been amputated because of circulation problems, pain, and infection. Just before I saw him, he had had his right leg amputated below the knee. Now this is a pretty devastating history.

It is my habit, after reviewing a record, to form an image of the human being I am about to encounter. This is an image that considers the physical, mental, emotional, and spiritual. My instincts have been pretty accurate in matching my image of the individual with the reality. My image of Mr. Jones was that of a man who would be in bed, appearing much older than his stated age. I thought he would be weary and despondent from the setbacks he had encountered through the years. My image was that of a man who would likely be less than enthusiastic about having yet another physician enter his life, asking the same tired old questions, forcing yet another examination of all that was unfair and unjust. When I entered the room, Mr. Jones was sitting up in his wheelchair, alert, upbeat, and very glad to see me. "I heard you were coming and I know you're here to look into my medical problems," he said "Ask and do whatever you must."

He spoke joyfully of the love he felt from and for his wife and family and of the purpose they gave to his life. He spoke of the challenges he had overcome after his first amputation that would prepare him well for his current situation. He had confidence in his ability to manage with a prosthesis, an artificial leg. He spoke of the miraculous experience of having the kidney of his daughter inside him and how thankful he was for this precious gift and his independence from dialysis. He spoke of his friends, his life and his purpose with an indifference (indifference can be positive) to his current circumstances. It was as if the complications of his diabetes were beside the point. His recent amputation was more of a detour than an obstacle. Mr. Jones's glass of life was indeed half full. He embodied gratitude. He exemplified the distinction between healed and cured. I believe that Mr. Jones did much more for me than I did for him. This has been true of many people I have cared for. Mr. Jones was able to transcend the limits of unfairness. He was able to transform the egregious indifference of events in his life to an indifference to the circumstances themselves. As a physician, I am intrigued by what makes possible a perspective such as this. I saw these same characteristics in my parents.

There has been growing interest in the connection between positive emotions like gratitude and love and meaningful health outcomes. There is a clear connection between these dimensions of how we see our lives and our circumstances, and how we heal. There is a clear connection between our senses of appreciation and how well we cope, respond, and ultimately fare. Robert Emmons and Michael McCullough have found in their research that people who are able to cultivate a sense of gratitude in their lives, particularly under trying circumstances, have a greater sense of well-being, fewer physical symptoms, increased alertness and energy, improved immune function, and brighter perceptions of emotional and physical health and well-being. As you confront the challenge of coping in a very difficult time, consider, in a quiet, contemplative way, the sources of light in your life for which you are truly grateful.

Is it possible to allow more light to enter? If you are able, write down a few of the things that have happened today for which you are truly grateful. You may find that that for which we are most grateful is often that which we most take for granted. As a psalmist once said:

> *"This is the day which the Lord hath made: we will rejoice and be glad in it."*
>
> —Psalm 118:24

On Forgiveness

"There is no revenge so complete as forgiveness."

—Josh Billings

People can be very hard on themselves and others. Our perceptions can easily become fixed, deeply rooted, and resistant to change. The lens through which we view our lives is filtered by our experiences, backgrounds, and feelings. We see the world as we are, not necessarily as it is. We tend to be much more generous in our assessment of self than we are in our assessment of others. Perhaps this sounds familiar?

When the stability of our lives is shaken by illness, we are forced to confront a confusing and often contradictory set of internal messages. Our love may be mixed with anger; our caring may be mixed with a sense of resentment; our grief may be immersed in guilt. Our need to reach out may be hindered by shame. We will all experience the tendency to look back and contemplate the many "what ifs" in our lives. As the Danish philosopher Kierkegaard once said, "We understand our lives by looking back. We live our lives by looking forward."

It is very hard not to dwell on what a loved one or we could have done better or differently. Forgiveness is a powerful liberator. Forgiveness opens the door to a reality less burdened, less mired down in negativity and the debilitating emotions that can be all-consuming. There is interesting research examining the role of forgiveness in health. It has been shown that people who are unforgiving are more likely to struggle with symptoms of anxiety, psychosomatic problems, and heart disease. Research has also demonstrated that people who are unable to forgive themselves or others are more prone to experience symptoms of depression and social isolation. This is particularly troubling as illness itself can force people into an isolated and lonely existence. Data also show that acts of forgiveness can result in better health outcomes, better coping with stress, and less anxiety and depression. Hmmm.

Forgiveness enhances interpersonal functioning and social support. This is essential in promoting healing, wellness, and positive health outcomes. People sometimes punish themselves with guilt or the perception that illness is an act of punishment. If our actions are responsible for all the events in our lives, I must have done something to deserve this. Somehow I must be responsible for this. This perspective can prove an enormous obstacle to healing, reaching out to others, or seeking timely medical treatment. The resentment and isolation inherent in an inability to forgive self and others diminishes self-esteem and self-worth. This demoralizing and debilitating mindset interferes with adequate self-care and can increase the risk of health problems.

Forgiveness is not about giving in. Forgiveness is about letting go. Forgiveness is the suture that closes the wound by liberating healing energy. We are all imperfect. It is in this awareness that the grace of love takes hold, love for ourselves and love for others. It is in this difficult moment of choice that forgiveness presents itself. I do not mean to suggest that forgiveness should come easily or will immediately erase all anger and pain like a wet sponge erasing chalk on a chalkboard. If you are confronting a serious illness or loss, consider to what extent your feelings—physical, emotional, mental, and spiritual—are burdened by emotions that have at their root a need to forgive or seek forgiveness. You may be surprised. Healing is a complex process made easier and more effective by unloading as much negativity as possible, and fostering a positive spirit. Though the impact of this process may take some time, you may notice an immediate difference. Remember the difference between healing and curing!

Forgiveness opens the door to hope. Hope leads to a path of transformation and new beginnings. Forgiveness enables the process of coping to be shared. Forgiveness liberates the healing love of others to fully enter our lives and take hold.

On Hope

"The past is a source of knowledge, and the future is a source of hope. Love of the past implies faith in the future."

—Stephen Ambrose

Experiencing illness can feel like entering a dark and frightening tunnel. The light in your life may be diminished or even extinguished. The path is uncertain. Each step is met with fear. The potential to feel hopeful in the midst of fear, uncertainty, and physical, emotional, and spiritual distress is not easily realized. Hope, in the lives of those I have cared for, is a source of light, illuminating a darkened space. The metaphor of light and darkness seems fitting here. People without hope or with diminished hope describe their worlds as dark. They sometimes describe sadness and feeling lost and adrift.

Hopelessness may reflect the overwhelming nature of your circumstances. It may be a symptom of depression, a treatable health problem. Depression is usually expressed as a combination of symptoms characterized by hopelessness, loss of pleasure, and sadness. Reflect on your circumstances. Undoubtedly they are having a major biologic impact affecting the way you feel. For example, anxiety is usually felt as deep fear, impending doom, trouble sleeping, air hunger, palpitations, and restlessness. Treating depression and anxiety with counseling and medication may very effectively improve the way you feel. These problems can be unforgiving and are manifestations of chemical imbalance and coping patterns that are common and consuming. Depression and/or anxiety may have been present before your current circumstances. It is estimated that as many as 5 percent of all adults, at any one time, are suffering from symptoms of depression. This is a staggering statistic! While most individuals with depression respond nicely to therapy, many are unrecognized and consequently not treated.

I have seen many sources of hope emerge under very trying circumstances. These sources can be illuminating by their very nature, having the effect of lifting the increasingly heavy burden of your circumstances, in a way that brightens, comforts, and soothes. I have touched on many of them. Love and gratitude, for example, can significantly alter the lens through which we view our circumstances. Spiritual or faith-based worldviews, though at times a potential source of conflict, can serve as a context within which to re-examine our perspectives. In the words of Dr. James Griffith, "Spirituality can powerfully protect against such demoralization. It helps someone not to feel alone, with the presence of one's spiritual community, God, saints, or ancestors. It furnishes rituals, prayer, and practices for attuning mind and body to a reality not bound by present circumstances. It sustains purpose and mobilizes hope."

The Cartesian mind-body separation is no longer supported by our contemporary understanding of brain biochemistry and psychoneuroimmunology, a fancy term for how our thoughts and emotions are linked with brain and bodily function. It is clear that our emotions, regardless of their ultimate source, have a biologic expression that can profoundly alter how we feel and ultimately how we do.

Hope is embodied in our innate need for purpose, value, and meaning. In the words of Abraham Twershi, a physician, ordained rabbi, and associate professor of psychiatry, University of Pittsburgh School of Medicine, "Finding a goal and purpose to one's existence can encourage a person to strive more energetically for recovery and enable one to better cope with suffering." A greater sensitivity and understanding of the needs of individuals who are ill or confronting illness in a loved one can add purpose in the midst of suffering. It is in this purpose that the light of hope emerges. The freedom to contemplate issues of meaning and purpose should always be based on the will of individuals and their families. Depending on the nature of the illness, these concerns may not be relevant; for example, during a minor medical problem with anticipation of a full recovery.

Thomas Aquinas spoke of hope as a special desire, characterized by a special type of object. The object of hope had to be clearly good, apparent in the future, difficult to attain, yet possible to attain. I have yet to encounter a clinical scenario that was "hopeless" when looked at in this way. For example, I have discussed decisions with many individuals around discontinuing dialysis therapy. This is an incredible decision to make. It is a decision that you think would always be an agonizing one as it inevitably leads to death, usually in a matter of weeks. While it can indeed be an agonizing decision for all involved, I have been moved by the grace with which some people pass through this process. We all desire not to die, *and* our eventual mortality is certain. In the darkest of moments and places I have experienced the emergence of hope. People have shared with me their contentment in how their lives have played out. They express a sense of completeness in their lives and the hope that this will forever sustain those they love. I have seen people speak of death with a sense of preparedness. I have seen hope expressed in the dying through the purpose and meaning that their lives have attained. I have seen and experienced in my father, on the threshold of his death, the hope expressed of reuniting with the spirits of those he loved who had gone before him. He was certain of this. I have seen and felt expressions of hope in the potential for the human spirit to rally under the most trying of circumstances. People have often expressed hope in the context of joy they have in their relationships, their pets, their passion for art, music, and literature, the places they have been and the places they hope to see some day.

Love is the ultimate source of hope. While sources of hope in your life may not readily diminish the pain of your current circumstances, they will allow you to survive another day and to survive what can be an indifferent reality as life goes on around you. I truly believe that in life and in death, regardless of one's circumstances along the way, we eventually arrive at the place we always wanted to be.

On Humor

"Humor is the great thing, the saving thing. The minute it crops up, all our irritations and resentments slip away and a sunny spirit takes their place."

—Mark Twain

I cannot imagine where I would be without a sense of humor. It's a great feeling to have humor in your heart. My kids think I am a complete nut. There is absolutely nothing like a good belly laugh—the kind of irrepressible laughter that brings tears to your eyes. Humor is definitely therapeutic. Who doesn't feel better after a good laugh? People do sometimes see, in the midst of a painful time, a biting absurdity in their reality or in the responses of people around them. "Here's the kidney stone, Dr. Pettus, the one you asked me to look for," said a patient. "While doing the Hell Dance, this popped out of my penis. I hope you're happy. Now you can add this to your rock collection!" Now I thought this was a pretty witty and clever way of expressing an awful experience with therapeutic humor and sarcasm.

Many of the people I have cared for are older. Like many physicians, I tend to reflexively speak louder to what is often a hard-of-hearing patient. One day, as I was making rounds in our critical care unit, I came upon a man, who was lying, very ill, with his eyes closed. I positioned myself close to his ear and asked him how he was doing. His eyes opened wide as he looked at me, startled, and said, "I may be dying, but I'm not deaf!" He was quite right. Inappropriate though it may have seemed, I had to laugh and it brought a smile to his face. Levity can be a real icebreaker when dealing with health-care professionals and vice versa. Humor is an excellent antidote to stress and tension.

A patient I once cared for had had an amputation of his leg. He was waiting for a prosthesis that can sometimes take several weeks. One Friday evening on rounds, I asked him what his plans were for the weekend. He looked at me and smiled, "I'm thinking of taking my wife dancing, but I'm not sure what will happen if I shake a leg." We shared a great laugh, one that connected us. I have always admired people who could transcend the pain of their circumstances with a smile or expression of humor. Humor is an elevator for the mood. If your mood is on the ground floor, humor can take you to the penthouse. It is also very contagious. Humor can be an excellent means of coping and channeling fear, anxiety, and pressure. When it comes to coping with illness, surround yourself with loving, compassionate, sensitive, and caring people, particularly those with a good sense of humor. It is okay to laugh. It is okay to smile. A smile is the shortest distance between two people.

A nurse in our ICU orchestrated one of the funniest encounters I have ever had as a physician. This R.N., as you will soon see, had a great sense of humor. My pager went off one weekend afternoon and I immediately recognized the telephone extension as coming from our ICU. The page required prompt attention, given the severity of illness I encountered there as a kidney specialist. When I returned the page this particular nurse answered sounding very worried.

"Mark," he said, direct and focused. "The patient you saw earlier this morning looks worse. He is making less urine and something is very wrong with the urine he's producing," (something a kidney specialist would be interested in) he said, genuinely concerned. "It has gold streaks in it. I don't like it. I've never seen anything quite like it."

He cleverly skirted specific questions. This was an experienced R.N. and I did not like the way he sounded. "I'll be right up, Bob," I replied.

On arrival at the ICU I went to the patient's bedside where Bob was nervously pacing. I bent to look into the catheter bag that was draining urine. Bob intercepted me before I could actually see the urine catheter bag.

"Here's a sterile container for a sample," he said. "You may want to see if something is growing in it." As I bent to look closely, I did a double take. I could not believe my eyes! I looked again. There were three goldfish swimming around, mouths bobbing up against the side of the urine bag.

"Damn," I said looking into Bob's smiling face, bordering on unrestrained laughter, "I forgot to bring my net." It was a moment of shared laughter I will never forget. It was also just what we both needed. The patient, who had given permission for this prank, seemed grateful for the opportunity to share a lighthearted moment. He went on to a full recovery.

On Pets

"Animals are such agreeable friends—they ask no questions, they pass no criticisms."

—George Eliot

When it comes to loving, nonjudgmental, and steadfast companionship, pets rule! I must say I have a bias as a longtime dog lover. I have cared for many patients whose pets were the most important living souls in their lives. I have heard the same sentiments expressed over and over again. "My pet knows when something isn't right with me. My pet is so comforting to me. My pet welcomes me like he hasn't seen me in years. I feel so good when I'm holding my pet, etc." Some hospitals and clinics are beginning to use pets in a therapeutic capacity. Pet therapy, as it is referred to, attempts to facilitate healing by bringing specially trained dogs, for example, into hospital settings.

I always enjoy seeing these animals walking in our hospital hallways. I notice an immediate lift in my spirit when around our therapeutic pets, as I'm sure many of our patients do. I am convinced that pets connect with us on an "energy level" that cannot be seen, though definitely felt. Some dogs, for example, can sense seizures before they occur in their owners. They definitely seem to appreciate changes in mood. I am certain that my mother's dog did much more for her mood than her psychiatrist or Zoloft ever did. I was very thankful for her psychiatrist and her Zoloft, but for people with and without human companionship, pets are a great source of support. They are a buffer to isolation and loneliness. They never hold a grudge. They do not attach conditions and contingencies to the emotions they express. Perhaps they are trying to tell us something.

Other Sources of Comfort When Coping with Illness

I have found many other sources of comfort and strength in my personal and professional life. Mindfulness practices of yoga and meditation are ancient practices that effectively serve as sources of peace and healing. They are proven to have profoundly positive effects on those individuals who respect and practice them. Mindfulness meditation involves deep breathing and heightened attention to physical and emotional sensations, with the goal of easing stress and pain. There is a growing body of medical evidence supporting the benefits of meditation in many types of chronic disease, including cancer.

Jon Kabat-Zinn directs the stress reduction clinic at the University of Massachusetts Medical Center. He introduced this program in 1979, and now more than 240 programs exist in the United States. His technique is somewhat different than traditional forms of meditation. Most traditional forms of meditation focus on the release of all external thoughts while entering into a passive state of relaxation. In mindfulness meditation, focusing on the process of breathing is also key. In addition, however, the individual attends to all thoughts, feelings, images, and sensations as they arise. The goal here is to become more acutely aware of the details in one's awareness, including sensations of pain and stress. The goal is to develop another context to accept what one is feeling. Discomfort is managed more effectively as one "relaxes into it" instead of struggling to avoid or diminish it. According to Dr. Kabat-Zinn, patients learn to pay closer attention to the present moment. In doing this they can separate the physical experience of pain from emotions such as anger, resentment, and fear.

The most common method for practicing mindfulness meditation is the "body scan." In this technique a person sits or lies comfortably, directing his or her awareness of the sensations of breathing throughout the entire body, from head to toe. Any discomfort noted during the deep breathing body scan is "let go."

If the soul had an appetite, music would surely be one of the entrees most often requested. Writing can also be profoundly therapeutic. Experiencing nature and the outdoors can be marvelously soothing. Nothing lifts my spirits like a walk in the woods or watching nature's glorious dance at our bird feeder. When one takes a moment to examine the potential for human creativity and expression in music, art, dance, and literature, a comforting light of hope emerges. When one examines the boundless beauty, intricacy, and balance of nature within which we coexist, a feeling of peace and connectedness takes hold. We are reminded that we are never alone in this earthly existence. We are reminded that our journeys are woven and our being, under any circumstances, is rich with meaning and purpose.

Caring for the Caregiver

Caring for caregivers is an area of growing relevance and importance in our aging society. Serving a loved one as a caregiver is an enormous responsibility. As our society ages, many of us will confront circumstances where a spouse, parent, or grandparent develops health problems requiring care. There is no greater labor of love than providing care. These efforts can present many demanding challenges, often resulting in neglect of the caregiver's own health and wellness.

My sister Nancy and I were caregivers for my parents in the last few years of their lives. I have cared for many individuals whose family members or spouses pushed the limits of human endurance, resilience, patience, and strength in their caregiver roles. While you may be confronting a situation as a caregiver that you "would have no other way," the responsibility can create physical and emotional challenges that have the potential to significantly impact your health. In an ironic way, feelings of guilt, shame, and resentment can emerge and transcend deep acts of love.

Let me give you an example. As my sister cared for my mother, an incredible effort that allowed my mother to be in her home, nurtured and sustained, she frequently found herself physically exhausted. She worked full time in a demanding job and had, in addition, unrelenting responsibility for my mother. On the other hand, the option of placing my mother in a nursing home was unacceptable. Assistance was necessary for bathing, meal preparation, medication dispensing, blood sugar monitoring, transportation, and other activities. As with a parent caring for a young child, there would be inevitable moments of impatience, anger, frustration, sadness, and overwhelming fatigue. These were clear and understandable reactions not to my mother, but to the circumstances. Under such perpetual stress and fatigue, feelings, thoughts, and words sometimes emerge that obscure the satisfaction, joy, and contentment of caring for a loved one.

This is an important message: *Do not confuse feelings that reflect a reaction to circumstances beyond your control with feelings for the loved one you are caring for.* For example, there is a huge difference between anger directed toward circumstances that have diminished one's independence and safety and feelings of anger directed toward the individual you are caring for. Acts of love, under perpetually demanding circumstances, do not always feel positive. As many caregivers also work, are married, and have children, potential consequences affect vital relationships in our lives. Your spouse or children may need more of your time and energy. Your boss, unaware of your circumstances at home, may seem indifferent as he or she makes casual comments about your performance. You may be forced to put on hold activities that bring you joy such as exercise, reading, or travel. As you react with frustration, impatience, sadness, or anger, you come out the other side feeling guilt or shame.

Dr. Aaron Lazare, a psychiatrist and Chancellor of The University of Massachusetts Medical School, has spent years studying such self-conscious emotions. These emotions and others, like humiliation and embarrassment, are at the core of people's existence. As Dr. Lazare would suggest, shame is the feeling that you are less than you want to be or ought to be. The expectation of loving satisfaction, total control, and harmony in one's life—marriage, work, parental, and care giving roles—is usually impossible to meet, as the caregiver navigates an ocean of rough waters. We feel diminished as the needs of others exceed our supply of patience, energy, and understanding. Shame, in this context, implies judgment of one's self. It is failure in the eyes of the beholder. Guilt, on the other hand, is an emotion that comes from a person regarding his or her actions as wrong; for example, raising one's voice or using profanity. As Dr. Lazare would say, "In shame people are concerned with their diminished self-esteem, whereas in guilt people are more concerned with their effects on others." The challenge is to respond to these telling emotions in positive ways, for example, exploring options for respite, apologies, or social and emotional support.

My sister's heroic expression of love for my mother sustained my mother's life in a way that simply would not have been possible otherwise. Caregivers are on a mission to restore and sustain comfort, dignity, independence, and purpose. You and your family member are partners, fighting the obstacles, rejoicing the triumphs, and mourning the setbacks. You are partners in a journey both sustaining and consuming. You fight the good fight. My sister could not have allowed it to be any other way. That's what is to be a caregiver. It is to openly share a deep part of oneself with another. It is both sustaining and consuming. In the end, the caregiver must survive. Is that not how an individual being cared for would want it? The caregiver must maintain an awareness of the delicate balance of caring and needing care.

It is not hard to understand how our health and wellness can become compromised under such circumstances. It has also been my experience that many auxiliary health-care providers may not be as aware, empathetic, and supportive of the primary caregiver as they could be. The predominant focus is on the person being cared for, not the caregiver.

It is also very difficult for caregivers to reach out to others for fear they will be sharing a burden that is too much to ask. While it may be better to give than to receive, the joy of giving for one individual is made possible by the willingness of another to receive. While relinquishing care for oneself may be an inevitable consequence of being a caregiver, it can undermine, over the long haul, your ability to feel well, stay focused, and provide effective support. I realize there are no easy answers or solutions here. Here are some thoughts to consider as your labor of love attempts to navigate the path of caregiver.

- The healthier you are, the more effective you will be as caregiver.
- Are you as good a caregiver to yourself as you are your loved one?
- Consider whether you are eligible for or can afford some help in the home, such as a housekeeper, health aid, or a personal care attendant.
- Are you reaching out to other friends and family as much as possible? Remember that the joy of giving is made possible by a willingness to receive. Do not let stubborn pride interfere with the potential for others to give.
- Talk to your physician about options for respite care that may allow a brief reprieve from your circumstances. Small degrees of respite have large effects on attitude and energy!
- Explore the option of day-habilitation or social centers. These can be supportive environments for your loved one and reduce the potential for isolation.
- Reach out for emotional and spiritual support. You may find it beneficial to talk with a counselor or clergy member.
- If you are experiencing symptoms of anxiety, such as insomnia and irritability, or depression, such as sadness, despair, and loss of joy, you may need more specific treatment. These are common and unrecognized symptoms that may respond wonderfully to therapy and medication.
- If possible, share your feelings with the person you are caring for. Potentially debilitating emotions of guilt and shame can be transformed through acknowledged love, understanding, forgiveness, and apology.
- When the going gets tough, be partners in the journey.

DO NOT MISS TAKE HOME POINTS

1. Dealing with illness and loss is inevitable.
2. Tap into the loving resources of family and friendship in your life.
3. If possible, keep a journal of your feelings, experiences, and the sources of gratitude in your life.
4. Leave nothing that needs to be said unspoken.

5. Forgiveness has the potential to heal and comfort.
6. Find the courage to reach out.
7. Find the courage to ask to be embraced.
8. Positive emotions have the potential to illuminate our lives.
9. If you are a caregiver, pace yourself. No shared journey is more challenging, noble, and meaningful.

CHAPTER 5

THE ICU/CCU
EXPERIENCE
Surviving the Storm

"Have courage for the great sorrows of life and patience for the small ones; and when you have laboriously accomplished your daily task, go to sleep in peace. God is awake."

—Victor Hugo

THE OBJECTIVES of this chapter are:

- To provide an overview of the basic medical technology commonly encountered in an ICU/CCU setting.
- To provide an overview of the many health-care professionals involved in the care of critically ill individuals.
- To provide insights and suggestions that will allow you to better understand and cope with a challenging ICU/CCU experience.

While in the automotive department of a local retail store I came across a fellow who approached me with a smile on his face and his arm extended for a handshake. "Do you remember me, Dr. Pettus?" he asked. "You took care of me almost eight years ago. I work here now." He raised his shirtsleeve and showed me his arm. "We put this here because you thought I might need dialysis for a long time." He pointed to a scar where he had surgery for what is called a fistula, used for people requiring hemodialysis. I saw that he was wearing hearing aids and within moments I remembered who he was.

Late one night my beeper went off, paging me to our emergency department. A young man in his thirties had been found lying unresponsive on the floor by a friend. An ambulance was called and he was brought to our local hospital. Because he was not breathing well on his own when the EMTs arrived a tube was placed in his lungs and he was later placed on a ventilator. He required many IVs for fluids and medications. He was also placed on a heart monitor. When his blood work came back, it was apparent he had significant kidney damage and many other "metabolic" abnormalities. Given his critical condition, he was admitted to the intensive care unit for further evaluation and management.

After a few hours it became apparent that he had tried to commit suicide by drinking antifreeze. This is a very potent poison that can be life threatening in even very small quantities—three or four ounces. His parents were, of course, in shock and distraught by the notion that his despair had left him no choice but to attempt to take his life. Depression was a problem that other family members had confronted. I assumed the care of this individual and soon after his arrival to the hospital arranged for him to have dialysis. This was the only way to effectively remove the antifreeze from his system. Every minute was critical, as I was not sure how much time had passed before he was found. I placed a special intravenous in his neck for dialysis. At the time of my initial evaluation, I had deep reservations and uncertainty about what the eventual outcome would be. He remained in our ICU for three weeks, requiring regular dialysis, breathing with assistance from a ventilator, receiving numerous intravenous medications, and receiving nutrition from a tube we placed through his nose into his stomach. He developed pneumonia as an additional complication. After several days he began to wake up.

I would learn that before his suicide attempt, he was having relationship and financial problems that became overwhelming. As an auto mechanic he had regular access to antifreeze. After about two weeks he was able to come off the ventilator and breathe on his own. His kidneys began to recover at about four weeks and he was able to be taken off dialysis. He also began to eat, and the tube we had placed in his stomach for nutrition was removed. After almost one month from his presentation, he was discharged from the hospital with his only physical problem being diminished hearing. This was an unfortunate and irreversible effect from the antifreeze toxicity.

There were numerous discussions with our staff and his family about his medical progress and many remaining physical and emotional issues. His parents were forced to confront many concerns relative to their son's mental health. They were forced to examine wounds, unresolved, from years past. The patient, never intending to wake up, had much to contemplate as he confronted a second chance at life. He had fully intended to take his life. His life was spared. Our psychiatry staff was actively involved in the care of this individual and his family. There were countless other people involved in his care, including pre-hospital personnel, emergency department staff, ICU and dialysis staff, consultants in various medical specialties, and many other health-care personnel. It was the collective efforts of many that saved this young man's life. It was great to see him years later, alive and well. He was clearly thriving and grateful to be around.

There are few health-care experiences more frightening and overwhelming than being in the coronary care or intensive care unit or having a loved one there. The very nature of any illness or injury severe enough to warrant an admission to the ICU is cause for tremendous concern, eliciting inordinate fear and overwhelming uncertainty. A modern ICU epitomizes the sophistication of medicine in its technological, pharmacological, and intellectual complexity. The human and technological resources invested in the care of individuals in the ICU/CCU are unlike any place else in the health-care system. For sheer human drama, there are few environments quite like it.

Reasons to Be in an ICU/CCU

People are admitted to or transferred into an ICU/CCU because the seriousness and complexity of their medical problems require the most sophisticated support and individualized attention available. The decision to have an individual in the ICU/CCU implies that comparable care cannot be found in other hospital areas. Examples of this sophisticated clinical support include:

- The need to be on a breathing machine.
- The need for medications to raise a dangerously low blood pressure.
- The need to monitor the heart closely because of a heart attack or the potential for a serious heart rhythm disturbance such as ventricular fibrillation (V.Fib).
- The need for a clot-busting drug as treatment of a heart attack or stroke.
- The need for special care after a major operation, such as repair of an abdominal aortic aneurysm, or a problem with severe bleeding, such as a bleeding ulcer.

Who Are the People Working in an ICU?

The ICU/CCU has a confusing array of people coming and going, often making it difficult to know who is who. More health-care personnel are involved with the care of a patient in the ICU/CCU than anywhere else in the health-care system. The nurses are very experienced and usually responsible for only one or two patients, given the complexity of the problems they are managing. Nurses are an enormous source of caring support and information as they monitor their patients constantly during their shifts. ICU/CCU nurses are incredibly skilled and dedicated, and require a certain "bravado" to thrive in crisis settings. This is true in other clinical arenas like the emergency department, operative and postoperative units, and in dialysis units. Nurses here are focused and sharp as observers and providers of care and communication. Nurses arriving for a new shift receive an extensive "sign-out" of the events that occurred during the preceding shift, such as changes in medication, vital signs, lab results, procedures, testing, consultant reports, and information discussed during rounds.

Many physicians, including residents in training and medical students (see chapter 19 on medical education), also come and go for various reasons. There should be a primary doctor coordinating the care. This will be either a primary care physician who had a prior relationship with the patient or an ICU specialist, known as an "Intensivist." They coordinate the work of the many other health-care professionals who may be involved. Other involved physicians are usually specialists called in to assist with a particular area of concern. They bring specific expertise, adding important insights in the evaluation and management of the critically ill. Specialists commonly seen in an ICU/CCU setting include:

- **Cardiologists** are experts in the evaluation, diagnosis, and treatment of heart problems, including heart attacks, angina (heart pain at risk for a heart attack), congestive heart failure (difficulty breathing from fluid in the lungs), and serious heart rhythm disturbances. Some cardiologists receive special training for interventions such as cardiac catheterization (placing a wire into a coronary artery) and balloon angioplasty with stenting. Angioplasty opens up a narrowed or blocked area and a stent is inserted to help prevent the area from closing down again.
- **Nephrologists** are experts in the evaluation, diagnosis, and management of kidney problems, usually kidney failure that occurs from a serious underlying medical problem. The kidneys are necessary to

filter the blood of impurities that are continuously being produced by the body's metabolism. Kidneys also allow elimination of excess water and salt from our bodies. Deteriorating kidney function can impact virtually every other organ system in the body. If kidney function deteriorates to less that 10 to 15 percent of normal, dialysis is considered. Dialysis involves cleaning the blood and removing water by using an artificial kidney-dialysis machine. Hemodialysis does the work that the kidneys are unable to do. It is life sustaining, as a person could die without adequate kidney function for a prolonged time, usually days to weeks. Requiring dialysis does not necessarily mean that one's kidney function is not going to improve. It can take days to sometimes several weeks for kidney function to turn around.

- **Infectious Disease or "ID" Specialists** are experts in infectious diseases assist in the evaluation, diagnosis, and treatment of serious infections. These infections may occur anywhere in the body; for example pneumonia in the lungs or an abscess in the abdomen. ID consultants are expert at helping with diagnosis and antibiotic treatment of infections. They will advise how best to establish what is causing an infection and which antibiotic or antibiotics are necessary to clear the infection.

- **Pulmonologists** are experts in the evaluation and management of lung problems. They are often called upon to assist with individuals on ventilators who are unable to breathe on their own or who have complicated pneumonias. They assist with the evaluation and management of a wide range of problems in the lungs that affect the ability to deliver oxygen to the body and to remove carbon dioxide that the body produces. For difficult diagnoses, pulmonologists often perform a procedure known as bronchoscopy. While the patient is under sedation, a small fiber optic tube is placed in the lungs for direct visualization, sampling for different types of infection, and biopsy for diagnosing infection, tumors, or other conditions.

Many lung specialists also have special training as *intensivists*. This involves highly sophisticated training with certification in critical care medicine. Intensivists apply their skills in all aspects of critical illness, from ventilator management, blood pressure monitoring and support, to nutrition and other areas. *If you have a loved one in the ICU, it is prudent to inquire if an intensivist is necessary and available to coordinate care.* Many larger, tertiary care centers that deal with all types of complex medical problems staff their ICUs with intensivists who coordinate, with other medical staff, the care of all critically ill patients. I think of intensivists as the "quarterbacks" of the ICU team.

- **Gastroenterologists** are experts in stomach, intestinal, and liver problems. In an ICU they are usually called to assist with diagnosis and treatment of severe bleeding, such as bleeding ulcers or other sources of bleeding from the intestinal tract. Much as a pulmonologist uses bronchoscopy to visualize what is happening in the lungs, gastroenterologists use a similar type of fiberoptic scope to look into the esophagus, stomach, and first part of the small intestine. This is called EGD or (brace yourself) esophagogastroduodenoscopy. They can often identify and treat sources of serious bleeding. If bleeding is occurring from the rectum, a colonoscopy is used.
- **Neurologists** are specialists in diseases that affect the brain or nervous system, such as stroke, muscle weakness from other causes, or severe seizure disorders. Neurologists are central to the coordination of stroke care, especially if a clot-dissolving drug like TPA (tissue plasminogen activator) is used. When a neurologist is involved in critical care it is usually because of a serious stroke, bleeding into the brain, or an immune problem causing quickly progressing and profound muscle weakness.

The specialists described are examples of common medical subspecialties (as distinct from surgical subspecialties) necessary to manage the critically ill. They also have training and certification in internal medicine (adult medicine) that allows them to add both focused and broad perspective in the care of the critically ill. The point of emphasis is that many minds are at work here. And though you may not see a particular specialist as you visit a loved one in the ICU/CCU setting, much is happening behind the scenes.

There are also surgeons with varying degrees of specialty training (as in internal medicine) applying their skills to any problem that may require an operation or care after an operation.

- **General surgeons** treat a wide range of surgical problems such as appendectomies, removing gall bladders (cholecystectomy), and removing parts of the colon for cancer or diverticulitis (inflammation with infection of the colon).
- **Neurosurgeons** most commonly evaluate and treat ICU problems involving trauma to the head requiring evacuation of blood, or treatment for strokes that have serious bleeding complications, cre-

ating too much pressure in the brain. They are also asked to evaluate surgical removal of tumors, repair of brain aneurysms, and other surgeries.

- **Cardiothoracic Surgeons** evaluate and operate, when benefits outweigh the risks, on problems involving the heart or lungs, such as removal of a tumor, repairing damage from trauma, or removing a collection of blood or infection fluid. They perform bypass operations for people with severe coronary artery disease from blocked or near-blocked arteries in the heart that will not respond sufficiently to medications or balloon angioplasty; they replace heart valves damaged by infection, heart attacks, or mechanical changes.

- **Vascular surgeons** operate on arterial blood vessels such as aneurysms in the abdomen or blocked arteries in the legs or neck. Their skills are essential in stopping life-threatening bleeding from aneurysms in the abdomen or restoring circulation to a "clogged artery."

- **Orthopedic surgeons,** affectionately referred to as "orthopods" by their colleagues, are experts in the repair and stabilization of broken bones. In the ICU setting, this is usually in the context of trauma such as an unstable broken leg, arm, or pelvis. Timely surgical repair of serious injuries to the skeletal system is essential to ensure structural (bone shape and architecture) and functional (ability to use) integrity.

- **Trauma surgeons** I think of as the surgical equivalents of intensivists for the individual who has sustained multiple traumatic injuries, perhaps in a serious motor vehicle accident. Trauma surgeons are experts in transforming the chaos of complex injuries from head to toes to systematic clarity, ensuring that no area of possible injury is overlooked in the rapid process of evaluation and management. They have special training in all aspects of care as it relates to the victim who has sustained multiple injuries. They, too, are the quarterbacks on the team of many surgeons involved in the care of the critically ill trauma victim.

Behind the scenes are many expert clinicians who are integral to the care of the critically ill. One example is the **radiologist**. Radiologists not only interpret the many x-ray images necessary in the diagnosis and management of the critically ill, they also perform many procedures that lessen the need for potential surgery, such as draining an infected abscess or unblocking a clogged artery in the leg with a balloon (known as angioplasty). **Pathologists** interpret enormous volumes of blood work, evaluate biopsies, prepare blood for transfusions, and perform other tasks.

Many other health professionals are present in the ICU/CCU: R.N.s; nursing specialists in IV therapy (starting and caring for intravenous), dialysis, and nutrition; respiratory therapists (assisting with ventilator care and breathing treatments); radiology technicians (taking x-rays); and others. It is almost impossible to fathom the resources involved in the care of the ICU/CCU patient! I have observed some truly unbelievable recoveries in this setting. They are a tribute to the unrelenting efforts of the many incredible professionals involved. The whole is truly greater than the sum of its parts. It is also a testimony to the remarkable inherent potential for healing of our bodies.

What Is All this Technology?

It can be rather intimidating to observe all the technology "invading" the space of an individual in the ICU/CCU. Each has a specific purpose. Technology you are likely to encounter includes:

- **Breathing Machines (Ventilators).** These machines actually breathe for or assist individuals unable to breathe on their own. They are attached to a tube placed into the trachea (the large airway just below our vocal cords). This is called an endotracheal or "ET" tube. Because it goes beyond the vocal cords, individuals requiring one are unable to speak. If an ET tube is in place for more than about ten days, a tracheotomy will be considered. This is a surgical procedure where a tube is placed through the skin, below the "Adam's apple," into the trachea. The reason for this is that an ET tube placed through the mouth or nose into the trachea can permanently damage the airway if left in for a prolonged period. A tracheotomy can allow more prolonged assistance and management while on a ventilator. It may be used for several weeks, months, or years, if necessary.
- **Heart monitor.** Most people are familiar with this portable television-like device. It is attached to sticky pads on the chest, allowing a continuous heart rhythm to be observed at the bedside. There are also monitors around the nurses' station and in the patient's room. Also displayed on the heart monitor are continuous readings of oxygen levels, referred to as a "FOX" or finger oximetry. This is a small clamp-like device placed on a fingertip that continuously reads oxygen levels in the blood. Monitors also provide continuous

readings of heart rate and blood pressure. Nurses observe these monitors carefully for important changes in vital signs. Alarms on the monitors will signal potentially serious changes in the heart rhythm, pulse rate, blood pressure, or oxygen level.

- **Intravenous (IVs).** There will probably be several IV tubes connecting various medications to an individual's veins. These IVs are often in one or both arms. IVs in the neck area are usually used if a person's veins on the arm are too small or insufficient to provide appropriate access. These are located on the sides of the neck or under the collarbone, called IJ (internal jugular) and subclavean, respectively. They are often used for providing nutritional support called total parenteral nutrition (TPN). TPN appears as yellow bags of fluid, able to provide the equivalent of three meals per day. These neck IVs are also used for dialysis. They allow connection to a machine that clears the blood of impurities if the kidneys are not working adequately. Another type of special IV is referred to as the P.I.C.C. This is a long IV that is placed into the arm, usually at the inner fold of the elbow, where blood is usually drawn. It is "threaded" into the veins in the neck area under the skin. P.I.C.C. lines are an excellent alternative to IVs placed in the neck for people who may need IV access for several days to weeks. They are also helpful in individuals whose veins will otherwise "wear out" from repeated blood sticks or infusion IV fluids and medication.

Most people in the ICU/CCU have several IV bags hanging at one time, going through a pump that precisely controls the amount that is infusing into the individual. Common ingredients in these sterile plastic containers include:

- ❖ Sugar/salt/water for people unable to drink fluids and to treat or prevent dehydration
- ❖ Antibiotics to treat infection
- ❖ "Pressors," medications to raise blood pressure when dangerously low
- ❖ "Anti-arrhythmics," medications to treat or prevent potentially dangerous disturbances in heart rhythm
- ❖ Heparin, a blood thinner given to prevent blood clots (also given as a shot under the skin)
- ❖ Nutrition TPN, usually a yellow or white solution
- ❖ Sedatives, often used to help calm and soothe individuals
- ❖ Insulin to treat people with very high blood sugar levels

- Foley catheter is a tube placed in the bladder to drain it of urine. This is often necessary in the ICU/CCU when a patient is unable to urinate.
- Venous boots are plastic, air inflated "boots" that repeatedly inflate and deflate on the patient's legs. This is to keep the blood circulating in order to diminish the risk of blood clots or phlebitis.

Challenges Encountered in the ICU/CCU— Suggestions for More Effective Navigation

INFORMATION IS INCOMPLETE AND HARD TO UNDERSTAND.

Suggestions:

1. Identify key people responsible for care, for example, the primary nurse, physician in charge, and consultants involved.
2. Write down names, phone numbers (including pager numbers), questions, and key information as you receive it. It can be very hard to recall or comprehend a lot of information when under stress and when a lot is happening quickly. This is extremely important!
3. Identify a family representative to facilitate sharing of information or to serve as the family spokesperson. This will help health-care providers focus their communication on a specific individual. Communicating with many family members, though at times necessary, can be fragmented and harder to interpret in a clear and consistent way.
4. Consider a larger family meeting (see chapter 7 on the family meeting), inviting key physician providers, a nurse who knows your family member well, and family members who are "closest" to the situation. Other people, including clergy and social service personnel, may be appropriate as well.
5. Find out when the best times to call or "connect" with a nurse or physician might be. Write down questions in advance, when possible, to maximize use of everyone's precious time. A good general question to ask after you have addressed all of the issues you can think of is: *"Can you think of anything that would be important for me/us to know about that we did not think to ask?"*

Invest in an understanding relationship with key health-care providers to facilitate effective and meaningful therapeutic partnerships. "Closeness" between you and the ICU/CCU staff will definitely make the experience more effective. This is true in every aspect of the health-care encounter and the main point of *The Savvy Patient*.

FRUSTRATION WITH LIMITED VISITING HOURS

Visiting hours in all hospital settings, particularly in the ICU/CCU, have historically been limited, to allow as much rest as possible for patients and often because of the many bedside procedures and interventions required for patients in the ICU/CCU. These procedures require strict maintenance of a "sterile field," as in an operating room. The ICU/CCU staff must limit people coming and going as necessary to decrease the risk of infectious exposure to the individual patient. Rigid though the visiting hours may seem, they are well intentioned. However, thinking is beginning to shift significantly with respect to these standards. The therapeutic importance of family and friends at the bedside is enormous. Communication between providers of care and family is made easier by such a presence. Many hospitals are now piloting such changes with great success. Hospitals are beginning to explore more flexible policies on visitation. The balance here is in recognizing the benefits of having family present with the need to ensure the best care possible. I think it is fair to say that for many hospitals there are better options to achieve both than the current policies.

If more time seems necessary, negotiate this with your loved one's primary R.N. (the R.N. most involved with you or your loved one's care) or with the ICU/CCU nursing director. In my experience, latitude around these policies is often possible depending upon the individual circumstances.

Suggestions:

1. Take advantage of unsettling moments in the waiting areas to bond with family, friends, or family members of other patients. These can be isolated, difficult, and very challenging circumstances. The presence of another individual who can relate to your circumstances, sharing this difficult experience, can be comforting and mutually supportive.
2. While waiting, write down questions to ask.

3. Consider a walk to a courtyard, surrounding gardens, or hospital chapel for momentary peace, reflection, and comfort.

Make sure the nurses and physicians know how they can reach you, for example by page or cellular telephone, if you are leaving the waiting area.

Exhaustion

Having a loved one in the ICU/CCU is exhausting physically, emotionally, and spiritually. Although easier said than done, try to pace yourself. At times these circumstances can become prolonged and unrelenting. Attempt to balance sleep with wakefulness. Try to eat a balanced diet. If you have several family members, try visiting in shifts. You will need your health to rally effectively in the long run. It's okay to reach out for help with meal preparation, shopping, and daily activities often neglected. I find that most people struggle to ask for help. I also find that most people are very willing to help those in need.

When a loved one is critically ill you will naturally extend yourself beyond imaginable limits because of your love and care. Exhaustion sets in quickly. These experiences resemble a marathon more than they do a sprint. Perhaps there are family and friends ready and able to extend themselves fully because of the love they have for you. Confronting critical illness or any acute or protracted illness can be unforgiving by nature. The ride can be, and usually is, characterized by many ups and downs. Just when the sailing begins to smooth out, stormy weather reappears. Your circumstances will feel unfair. There may be more questions than answers. Keep the faith. Find strength in love. Most importantly, take care of yourself.

Confronting Unexpected Changes in Clinical Status

While we always hope that sustained improvements and satisfactory recovery will occur after initial stabilization, the nature of the medical problems that cause critical illness can be rapidly changing and unpredictable. Under normal circumstances, the heart, brain, liver, lungs, and kidneys are precisely fine-tuned and are able to quickly adapt in a way that maintains harmony and homeostasis, that is, balance and precision. Critical illness, regardless of the underlying cause takes a boat sitting on calm waters and throws it into the unbalanced center of a severe storm. Unfortunately, it is not uncommon for initial improvement in a patient's clinical status to be followed by a setback, because of the disruption of this homeostasis. For example, a person admitted to the ICU and placed on a breathing machine because of a severe pneumonia may begin to improve considerably by the second or third day, as antibiotics, IV fluid, and improved oxygen delivery begin to turn things around. The individual may be more awake, temperature down, WBC (white blood count—a marker of the body fighting infection), down, and reliance on the ventilator decreasing. On day four a serious heart problem such as a heart attack or rhythm disturbance occurs. The heart may have been stable prior to the burden of "physiologic stress" that the pneumonia caused. This burden may become too much for an otherwise vulnerable heart. This vulnerability may or may not have been apparent prior to the pneumonia developing.

I have treated many critically ill patients. As I mentioned previously, the potential for the human body to endure and heal can be most remarkable. As many people in the ICU/CCU setting have other chronic medical problems, an "insult" in one part of the body can have a ripple or domino effect elsewhere. As treating clinicians we are always on guard for this potential vulnerability to be unmasked by a critical event. Though many complications or setbacks can be dealt with, there is a point beyond which the momentum may be too great to turn around. This is of course the worst-case scenario.

Prepare for what may feel like a roller coaster ride. Ideally, the course will be smooth, steady, and sustained. Hopefully any further complications can be effectively dealt with. If, after a week or two, there is not much progress, regroup with your family and providers to examine where you are, what your options for further treatment are, and what the likely outcomes are.

While we always do and pray for the best, we are sometimes forced to revisit what can be a hard-to-predict reality. The landscape can shift quickly and fault lines, hitherto unrecognized, declare themselves.

DO NOT MISS TAKE HOME POINTS

1. Pace yourself, as having a loved one critically ill can be all-consuming.
2. Try to rest and care for yourself as best as you can. Hard though it may be, allow yourself to be supported by others who love and care about you. One has to feel comfortable receiving in order to give.
3. Keep a notebook to write down important contact providers, medical information, and questions.

4. Appoint someone in your family as the spokesperson to communicate with the health-care team.

5. Get to know the primary nurse responsible for your loved one's care. This is one of the key relationships in the encounter!

6. Request a family meeting with key clinical providers to address complicated medical decisions that need to be made.

7. Determine whether advance directives have been appropriately addressed. (See chapter 6.)

8. Consider whether you would benefit from other support personnel—social services, clergy, and behavioral health specialists such as clinical psychologists or psychiatrists whose purpose is to help support you and your family's emotional needs.

CHAPTER 6

ADVANCE CARE PLANNING
Understanding Advance Directives and Acting as a Proxy/Agent

"A man cannot be comfortable without his own approval."

—Mark Twain

THE OBJECTIVES of this chapter are:

- Understanding the purpose and importance of the health-care proxy as a legal advance directive.
- Understanding the situations under which the health-care proxy form is used.
- Understanding the types of decisions a proxy or agent would have to consider if a loved one were unable to speak for himself or herself.
- Appreciating the importance of sharing your thoughts about what quality of life means to you and what you would want or not want done depending on your values, preferences, and wishes.
- Providing suggestions and insights that will assist with this process for you and your family.

At some point in our lives we will inevitably confront the difficult decision of what treatment we want, for ourselves and perhaps for our loved ones, when facing potentially life-threatening problems. Advance care planning is the process of initiating awareness, thought, and discussion about preferences for care with respect to such circumstances.

The ethical principles of autonomy, informed consent, and self-determination are basic to any health-care decision process. *Autonomy* ensures the right of free will. In other words, no one can impose an intervention, such as a diagnostic test or treatment that goes against your wishes. *Informed consent* means that any medical decision should be based on as much knowledge as possible of the situation. Being informed implies that you have been given an explanation of the issues and have carefully considered the risks and benefits of diagnostic testing and/or treatment under consideration. It also means, of course, that you agree with the decision being made. *Self-determination* is the principle that allows you and your loved ones the right to accept or refuse treatment, based on your values, preferences, and wishes.

There are different methods for making clear one's wishes concerning advance directives about treatment. It is important to spend some time in the absence of an emergency situation, carefully and thoughtfully reflecting on these issues. These decisions encompass many dimensions of our lives, reflecting our understanding, values, preferences, and life experiences. They speak to the depths of our physical, emotional, and spiritual being. Formulating advance directives are the ultimate acts of self-advocacy. It is important to share your thoughts with trusted people in your life who could express your wishes with a deep and personal understanding. These are individuals you would trust to speak for you if you become unable to speak for yourself.

I have had many discussions with patients and families about advance directive planning and decision making. Clarity with respect to advance directives can markedly enhance critical decisions that might otherwise leave family members conflicted and painfully uncertain about the best course to take. Loved ones often experience overwhelming guilt and grief as they attempt to navigate these decisions under duress. As traumatic as the circumstances necessitating the implementation of advance directives will be, families who feel prepared experience a greater sense of control, certainty, and understanding. To be caught by surprise or to confront conflict regarding wishes of a family member, who cannot competently express his or her desires, is a difficult burden to bear.

There are different mechanisms for written documentation in advance care planning. Based on a recent study published in the journal *Gerontologist* in 2002, all states have durable power of attorney for health-care statutes. This is commonly referred to as a *health-care proxy*. This is a document that identifies an agent (or proxy) and an alternative agent who would be appointed to speak on your behalf *only* if you were unable to competently speak for yourself. An example of a Massachusetts Health-

Care Proxy Form is provided at the end of this chapter. By "competent" I mean able to understand clearly and weigh your options. Competency also implies that you clearly understand the consequences of the decision or decisions you are making. The assigned proxy or agent is most often a spouse, sibling, or child. This individual would make medical decisions on your behalf. In instances where immediate family is not an option, a more remote relative, close friend, or attorney can fill this important role.

It is important to consider what an acceptable quality of life means to you and what conditions would constitute an unacceptable quality of life. For example, is there a point beyond which your life would not be worth living, for example, being unable to care for yourself, requiring ongoing dialysis treatments, losing your capacity to think and engage others? Most of us prefer not to think about such questions, particularly when all is well in our lives. Is the current quality of your life such that you would never want treatment if your heart or breathing were to stop? It is naïve to think these are easy situations to contemplate hypothetically. It is also naïve to believe that our thinking might not shift dramatically when actually confronting such circumstances. This said, in my experience, most people truly do have clear thoughts regarding the "what-ifs" and are usually consistent in applying these wishes when necessary. Let me give you a real-life example.

I was caring for an eighty-two-year-old man who had advanced Alzheimer's disease; he was unable to competently understand and make an informed decision as his kidneys deteriorated. He was confronting dialysis treatments that ultimately would enable him to continue living. Without them he would die in a matter of weeks. He had recently had a stroke and was no longer able to ambulate, work in his garden (a lifelong passion, according to his wife), or care for himself independently. He could no longer drive. His wife of fifty-six years was his proxy and had discussed these issues with her husband when he was healthier and much more lucid. Despite the pain of having to make such an enormous decision, she understood her husband's wishes. "My husband would never want his life prolonged in this way, Dr. Pettus," she said with a resigned and poignant awareness of the man before us. She decided dialysis would not be appropriate for him.

It is important to note that Health-Care Proxy forms do not stipulate specific "dos" or "don'ts" for medical treatment. They simply appoint an individual to articulate your wishes *only* if you are unable. All states but three—New York, Massachusetts, and Michigan—have living will statutes. These three states, however, have recognized living wills in case law. Living wills provide more specific instructions for future care under various circumstances. State laws vary on the terms around which the conditions of the living will are applied, for example, terminal illness (less than six months to live) or a state of unconsciousness, that is, a coma. As of this writing, thirteen states have statutory forms that combine both types of directives in one document. Some patients who have not filled out a health-care proxy or living will do have clear documentation in a physician's record of conversations regarding advance directives. This is usually an acceptable basis for making decisions.

At a minimum, all individuals should fill out a durable power of attorney for health-care status (Health-Care Proxy Form). Decisions that most people need to understand and consider under these circumstances include:

- Treatment options if the heart stops beating. These options would include, for example, CPR, electrical cardioversion or "shock," as is done for ventricular defibrillation.
- Treatment for patients unable to breathe on their own. This option would include having a tube (endotracheal or ET tube) placed through the nose or mouth into the lungs and connected to a mechanical ventilator that would provide oxygen and breathe for the individual. This decision could also involve removing from a ventilator a person who has no meaningful chance of recovery.
- Kidney dialysis: This a treatment to clean the blood of waste products and excess fluid when an individual's own kidneys can no longer do so sufficiently to sustain life. Decisions here could include whether to start dialysis or possibly whether to discontinue it.
- Nutrition: This can be given intravenously (IV) or more commonly through a tube placed in through the abdominal wall. This is called a PEG or percutaneous (through the skin) endoscopic (placed using a fiber optic scope that looks into the stomach) gastrostomy (an approximately one-inch-long incision that goes through the stomach and abdominal surface). A PEG allows provision of nutrients and fluids directly into the stomach if a person is unable to eat and drink normally.

Studies have shown that treatment decisions with respect to end-of-life care are often not adequately addressed by physicians or expressed by patients. Many individuals have not completed an advance care document even though they are clear that they would never want "their suffering prolonged." For example, in a study of physicians published in *The Journal of the American Medical Association*, 53 percent of doctors did not know when their patients wanted to avoid cardiopulmonary resuscitation. In addition, 59 percent of patients who did not want aggressive measures reported getting care inconsistent with their wishes. On a similar theme, in a report published in *The Journal of the American Geriatrics Society*, 35 percent of patients who wanted care focusing on comfort reported getting care contrary to their wishes.

The federal Patient Self-Determination Act of 1990 requires hospitals, health maintenance organizations, nursing homes, and hospices to inform patients of their rights to accept or refuse treatment at the time of admission; to ask if a patient has an advance directive; and to provide documents to be completed and entered into the medical record.

The Difference Between "DNR" and "Do Nothing"

Many people who would not want CPR or to be put on a ventilator in the event of a cardiopulmonary arrest (cessation of heartbeat and breathing) may have concerns that other aspects of their care will not be fully addressed. DNR (Do Not Resuscitate) status does not mean there would be no other treatment. Other necessary treatment might include pain medication, oxygen, antibiotics, intravenous fluid, and blood transfusions. It is important to discuss available treatment options and to determine with your provider which would be appropriate.

Under any circumstances, your comfort or the comfort of your loved one should not be compromised. This is essential, as available data clearly points to the fact that people who are confronting terminal illness or a potentially life-threatening event desire more than anything to have their wishes respected and their comfort and dignity ensured. Some advice regarding advance care planning:

1. Do not wait until you are critically ill to contemplate your wishes. Communicate them to your family. Consider whom you would trust to speak on your behalf.
2. Health-care proxies are not just for older people. My wife and I filled out our proxy forms. They are in our medical records at our primary care provider's office. We also have copies in our personal files. My proxy is my wife and my alternate is my sister. You should be able to obtain a form at your physician's office or at your local hospital. Lawyers can be involved in executing advance directives, but are not required.

3. Try to allow time to discuss your wishes with your physician and your family. Do not hesitate to introduce the topic, as others may not feel comfortable raising it on their own.

4. If you and your family are struggling with what decisions to make for a loved one who is critically ill, it is essential that you let your loved one's physician provider know of your need to sit and review the clinical status in detail. I have often found a *family meeting* (see chapter 7, The Family Meeting) to be the most effective process for communicating these issues and concerns in a way that builds understanding, clarity, and consensus. Questions I have often been asked that sometime shed clearer light on a complicated matter include:

   a) **Do you think my loved one will improve to the same level as prior to this illness?**
   If not, is it possible to say what he or she will be capable of doing or unable to do? The response to this is never a certainty, although depending on the clinical circumstances, a physician may know that complete recovery is very unlikely, or still very possible.

   b) **What has your experience been in treating other people like this under similar circumstances?**
   While individual circumstances may vary from average outcomes, experienced physicians readily recognize patterns and may feel comfortable sharing information that can shed more light on your circumstances.

   c) **What would you do if you were in my position?**
   This can be a difficult question for physicians, and some may not feel comfortable answering it. I do think it is a reasonable question to ask. Many family members have expressed to me their comfort and deep appreciation for sharing on such a level.

You should never feel locked into a decision. You can change your health-care agent or alternative by notifying your physician. If you are a proxy, you may feel the need to change a decision based on your comfort level and clinical circumstances.

The need to make critical decisions can sometimes occur quickly and unexpectedly. Loved ones are left stunned, shocked, and at times, unable to reconcile such enormously important decisions. A decision to "hold back" on more aggressive intervention may leave you feeling as if you are surrendering or abandoning your loved one. Grief takes on the added burden of guilt. Physicians involved with your loved one's care may be uncertain about the prognosis or immediate outlook. It is *very important* to know that a decision to place someone on a ventilator or to electrically shock their heart does not preclude a subsequent decision to refrain or withdraw heroic measures. For example, you and your loved one's physician may share uncertainty about the outlook. Often the outlook becomes clearer in a short time (days to weeks). Doing "everything" until uncertainty becomes more certain may be the best option. Decisions can be made to withdraw ventilator support, not to do CPR or shock the heart again, or to withdraw dialysis if the kidneys are not improving in an expected and acceptable period of time.

I offer one last thought on this topic. I have seen many families (and physicians too) anguish over these decisions. We are at times distraught or guilt-ridden by an outcome such as a decision to withhold support, possibly hastening death. We may painfully regret a decision to do everything, leading to a prolongation of suffering and unacceptable quality of life. Modern health care offers more interventional options than ever. More responsibility is placed on families to make complex, difficult decisions under maximum stress (see chapter 9 for more details on medical decision making). You may be caught between a rock and a hard place. It is very important to share the burden of the decision-making process. It is important to distinguish giving up from letting go. It is essential to protect your family relationships, as conflict sometimes emerges and unfairly fractures families under these trying circumstances. All providers (physicians, R.N.s, social workers, clergy, and others) need to both treat *and* advocate effectively for compassionate decision making.

In my opinion, a "right" or "wrong" decision is determined not so much by the outcome as by the process by which the decision is made. This process requires frequent and timely provision of necessary information. It requires clear understanding. It requires speaking from the heart. It requires a trusting sense of one's deepest instincts and feelings.

If you find yourself torn before or after the fact, ask yourself:

- If my loved one could whisper in my ear, what would he or she be telling me?
- What does my heart and soul say to me? (Trust your gut instincts.)

- Do I need to discuss this more and perhaps with others, such as pastoral/spiritual care providers?
- Have I asked all the questions I need to ask?
- Have my questions been addressed to the best extent possible?
- Are there any other family or friends who need to be included in the decision-making process?
- Is there anyone I know and trust who has been in a similar situation and could relate to my circumstances?
- What was the trend, if any, in my loved one's quality of life before this current situation presented itself?

It can be much harder to let go when someone you love had a fine quality of life before a catastrophic event as compared to a quality of life that may have been declining significantly and irreversibly. Proper attention to advance care planning will hopefully create a greater sense of peace and control as you navigate these difficult waters. As in any critical medical decision, it is paradoxical that a decision grounded in deep love can cause torment, guilt, and uncertainty. It is so hard to separate the angst of the decision from the angst of the circumstances necessitating the decision. In the end you are forced to cope with both. And in the end, those we love and on whose behalf we are deciding would be thankful. Of this I am certain.

Example of a Health-Care Proxy Form

Health-Care Proxy

1

I, _____

hereby appoint

_____

(name, home address and telephone number)

_____

_____

as my health-care agent to make any and all health-care decisions for me, except to the extent that I state otherwise. This proxy shall take effect only when and if I become unable to make my own health-care decisions.

2
Optional: Alternate Agent
If the person I appoint is unable, unwilling or unavailable to act as my health-care agent, I hereby appoint

_____

(name, home address and telephone number)

_____

_____

as my health-care agent to make any and all health-care decisions for me, except to the extent that I state otherwise.

3
Unless I revoke it or state an expiration date or circumstances under which it will expire, this proxy shall remain in effect indefinitely. (_Optional: If you want this proxy to expire, state the date or conditions here._) This proxy shall expire (_specify date or conditions_):

_____

_____

4
Optional: I direct my health-care agent to make health-care decisions according to my wishes and limitations, as he or she knows or as stated below. (_If you want to limit your agent's authority to make health-care decisions for you or to give specific instructions, you may state your wishes or limitations here._) I direct my health-care agent to make health-care decisions in accordance with the following limitations and/or instructions (_attach additional pages as necessary_):

_____

_____

In order for your agent to make health-care decisions for you about artificial nutrition and hydration (_nourishment and water provided by feeding tube and intravenous line_), your agent must reasonably know your wishes. You can either tell your agent what your wishes are or include them in this section. See instructions for sample language that you could use if you choose to include your wishes on this form, including your wishes about artificial nutrition and hydration.

5
Your Identification (*please print*)

Your Name _____

Your Signature _____ Date _____

Your Address Address _____

_____

6
Optional: Organ and/or Tissue Donation
I hereby make an anatomical gift, to be effective upon my death, of: (check any that apply)

☐ Any needed organs and/or tissues

☐ The following organs and/or tissues _____

_____

Limitations _____

If you do not state your wishes or instructions about organ and/or tissue donation on this form, it will not be taken to mean that you do not wish to make a donation or prevent a person, who is otherwise authorized by law, to consent to a donation on your behalf.

Your Signature _____ Date _____

7
Statement by Witnesses (*Witnesses must be 18 years of age or older and cannot be the health-care agent or alternate.*)

I declare that the person who signed this document is personally known to me and appears to be of sound mind and acting of his or her own free will. He or she signed (or asked another to sign for him or her) this document in my presence.

Date _____

Name of Witness 1

(print) _____

Signature _____

Address _____

_____

Date _____

Name of Witness 2

(print) _____

Signature _____

Address _____

_____

DO NOT MISS TAKE HOME POINTS

- Signing the form gives the person you choose (your agent) the authority to make health-care decisions for you if you are unable to make them yourself.
- Your proxy (agent) should have a clear understanding of your wishes, values, and preferences as they relate to your health and quality of life. It is essential that you discuss these issues, explore any change of heart that may occur, and have the consent of your proxy before signing the form.
- As long as you are able, you will always have the right to make health-care decisions for yourself.
- You do not need a lawyer to fill out a health-care proxy form.
- You may choose as proxy any adult eighteen years or older, including a family member or close friend.
- If you name your spouse as your proxy and later become divorced, you may need to update your wishes or any changes and date them on your form.
- You have the right to change your proxy at any time.
- Appointing a health-care proxy is voluntary, but strongly recommended.
- You will need two witnesses, not including your chosen proxy.
- It is not recommended that you choose your doctor as your proxy as he or she will be in the difficult position of both serving as your agent and providing your medical care.
- It is a good idea to give a copy of your completed health-care proxy form to your agent, your doctor, your attorney, and other family members.
- Make your feelings and wishes clear to family and to your doctor regarding cardiopulmonary resuscitation.
- Consider wearing a medical bracelet with this information, as mistaken resuscitation sometimes happens because of communication failure.

CHAPTER 7

THE FAMILY MEETING

Where Do We Go From Here?

"The truth is more important than the facts."

—Frank Lloyd Wright

THE OBJECTIVES of this chapter are:

- To review common circumstances where a family meeting may be of some value to you.
- To review the essential elements of the family meeting.
- To review the necessary steps to ensure an effective family meeting.

Few processes are as useful and effective as the family meeting to clarify and reconcile difficult health-care decisions. While family meetings usually occur in the hospital, or acute care setting, they can also occur in the clinic or physician's private office.

Family meetings are preplanned, organized gatherings that may include several participants:

- Patient and family members
- Primary care provider and often, if available, key consultants involved in the care
- Nurses, for example the primary nurse or clinical nurse leader (charge nurse)
- Social worker
- Case manager, an individual, sometimes a social worker or R.N., who is skilled in exploring options for future care; identifying the

needs of an individual by having discussions with involved health-care providers; examining available resources for continued care; and assisting in exploring the care planning options based on medical needs, available resources, and patient and family preferences.

- Clergy member or pastoral care provider. As mentioned previously, this can be an essential contribution to the discussion of health, as one's spiritual perspective can profoundly influence understanding, coping, and decision making.

Deciding who should attend a family meeting depends on your specific needs and circumstances. There should be agreement between the medical provider and the patient and immediate family as to who should be present. This is important, as your treating physician can arrange for key people to be present and informed of the current issues. I have found family meetings to be a very effective way to address more challenging and difficult medical decisions. The primary purpose of the family meeting is to learn as much as possible about the facts and to discover the "truths," as they relate to your individual circumstances. Examples of situations where a family meeting might prove beneficial are:

- Critical illness when the complexity of the problems, the prognosis, and the diagnosis and treatment options are overwhelming and unclear
- Contemplating discharge from the hospital to home after a significant medical problem or complex hospital course
- Contemplating the transfer of care from one facility to another, for example from a community hospital to a larger tertiary care facility for more specialized care
- Addressing differences of opinion and understanding, usually between family members and patients or between providers of care and families, regarding major issues such as advanced life support, the decision to start dialysis, to be placed on a breathing machine (ventilator), or to have CPR (cardiopulmonary resuscitation) or a "shock" to start the heart, or to have major surgery
- Decisions regarding nursing home placement
- Addressing anger or conflict regarding quality of care received or poor communication (see chapter 16 on managing conflict)
- Decisions regarding palliative care or hospice care, when confronting a terminal illness, usually with a diagnosis for survival of less than six months

Family meetings can be vital in establishing clarity around:

- An understanding of health-care issues for the patient and closest of kin
- Improved understanding by the health-care providers of the wishes, values, and preferences for care by patients and their families
- Improved communication regarding complex and challenging health-care issues
- Reconciliation of physical, emotional, and spiritual wounds realized in the moment of serious illness
- Improved mutual understanding between health-care providers, patients, and families
- Facilitating a more meaningful therapeutic bond between providers, patients, and families by spending an "undivided moment" to share thoughts, concerns, and interests
- Allowing physicians involved in the care of your loved one to build consensus around shared goals, facilitating communication and clarity

An Example of a Family Meeting

Mrs. Brown is an eighty-eight-year-old woman who was admitted to our hospital after falling and breaking her arm and elbow. Prior to this, she had been a vigorous, independent woman who was widowed and was able to care for herself with the assistance of two loving nieces. She had no children and her nieces were her closest relatives.

I was asked to see Mrs. Brown because her primary care provider practiced in a town distant from our hospital. Mrs. Brown was admitted to our orthopedic team and was going to be taken to the operating room later in the day to repair her broken arm. It is routine to address any other medical problems to ensure safety and stability prior to surgery. Mrs. Brown had a history of high blood pressure and osteoporosis ("thinning" of the bones) and was prescribed medication by her local primary care provider for these medical problems. They would require continued management during her stay with us. My role was to oversee that.

When I, a total stranger, entered Mrs. Brown's room, I encountered a graceful, sweet woman, sharp as a knife, who forced a smile through the pain of her broken bones. She shared the frustration of her fall and mentioned that her falls were occurring with greater frequency at home. I soon discovered that she had lost more than twenty pounds over the last few months, had a diminished appetite and had been increasingly weak. She was finding it more difficult to manage, despite the loving care and attention provided by her nieces. There was a look of poignant understanding in her eyes, of total awareness and preparedness that only the wisdom of eighty-eight years could produce. This was a familiar look, one patients have shared countless times with me.

Though she was admitted with a severely broken arm after a fall (this is not at all uncommon, though most broken bones I see are at the hip), her larger sphere of issues were much more significant. I believe we were both, in a silent uncertain way, asking ourselves the same questions.

Would she be able to return home, perhaps ever, under these circumstances?

Why was she losing so much weight and finding herself increasingly weaker?

Could she have another health problem that would overshadow her broken arm?

Is she on the verge of descending "the slippery slide," a metaphor for rapidly failing health status?

What are her expectations for recovery and functional independence?

What are her thoughts and preferences regarding advanced life support, if necessary?

How will I be able to address her physical, emotional, and spiritual needs?

Does surgery on the arm make sense if we are confronting an uncertain and possibly limited prognosis?

How "connected" are the nieces to her life and what role would they want to play in the difficult decisions I knew we were confronting?

As you can see, a seemingly straightforward and common healthcare scenario can bring up many critically important questions. Because of her weight loss and diminished appetite, an ultrasound (see chapter 18 on tests for more details about ultrasound) of her abdomen had been ordered. A large mass, most certainly a tumor, was found in her pancreas. This was an ominous finding indeed. I suggested a family meeting and within hours her nieces, her orthopedic surgeon, a medical resident in training, and I met to address these issues. We met at Mrs. Brown's bedside.

I told her that she had a large tumor in her abdomen. We reviewed the available treatment options, none of which were likely to prolong her life and all of which would likely carry significant risks to her comfort and quality of life.

"I have lived a long and wonderful life, Dr. Pettus," she said with conviction and resolve. "My nieces are more important to me than any-one. I would not want surgery or chemotherapy for a tumor." Her nieces asked several questions and lovingly supported her decisions.

"Mrs. Brown, what do you think about returning home?" I asked, careful to first hear her views, realizing that returning home might not be possible.

"My nieces cannot be with me twenty-four hours a day. It is too much to ask. I know there are some facilities (she meant nursing homes) in my hometown."

Her nieces realized that her care would exceed their capacity and seemed prepared to accept a local nursing home. With the participa-tion of our orthopedic provider, we mutually agreed that surgery on her arm would pose an unacceptable risk, relative to the benefits given the "big picture." Surgery was deferred accordingly. I examined her faith background. She had been a member of a faith community for years, and her nieces were going to notify her pastor of the circum-stances. Her faith community would provide spiritual support as she contemplated skilled nursing placement. She did not desire resuscita-tive measures in the event her heart stopped. Hospice was contacted and would arrange to provide palliative care at the facility to which she was transferred.

By arranging to consult all key participants in Mrs. Brown's life and with her centered awareness and understanding, we were able to openly discuss and agree upon some major issues now confronting her, her fam-ily, her orthopedic providers, and me. *Significant potential for under-standing and healing can occur in the context of a family meeting.* The difference between curing and healing is enormous and cannot be over-stated. I will elaborate on this distinction in chapter 8, Spirituality, Reli-gion, and Health. I certainly could not cure Mrs. Brown by restoring a normal arm or an abdomen without a large tumor.

This true scenario illustrates how a family meeting allowed us all to "connect" with open and honest sharing of information and feelings. This allowed an important understanding of the options, preferences, and wishes of Mrs. Brown and her nieces to emerge. It enabled develop-ment of a peaceful and harmonious consensus. Difficult and painful though these issues were, clear and compassionate communication al-lowed peace and understanding to emerge from pain and uncertainty. The ability of patients and families to reconcile or begin to reconcile such profound multidimensional issues, through such a process, is often underestimated and underappreciated by medical providers, patients, and families.

If a family meeting can help, what can I do to make this happen?
I have initiated most of the family meetings I have been involved in. After all, patients and families may not realize the potential benefits of a family meeting and may not be aware of its potential as an option. *One does not know what one does not know.* Families may feel uncomfortable asking busy doctors to organize and convene such a meeting. If you feel a family meeting might help you or your loved ones to better navigate a "stormy sea" of medical issues, consider the following points.

DO NOT MISS TAKE HOME POINTS

1. Ask your primary care provider to arrange a time to meet with your family. If this is uncomfortable for you, ask your primary nurse, social worker, or case manager involved in your care to discuss this with your treating physician.
2. Consider whom you would want to attend the meeting (e.g. select family members, pastoral care providers, nursing personnel, important consultants).
3. All critical discussions regarding patient care should be *centered on the patient*. The patient should be included, if possible.
4. Arrange a time that is convenient for all, especially the physician. It is important to be as flexible as possible in order to bring people together. It may be easier, for example, for your physician to meet in the evening after office hours, or earlier in the morning, before the busy day begins.
5. Write down your questions in advance. Consider your objectives and try to have them met during the meeting. Prepare specific questions by discussing them with family members beforehand. For example:

   - What are the main medical problems we are confronting?
   - Is there any way of knowing how long he/she will need to be on a ventilator?
   - What has your experience been in treating people with problems like this?
   - How long might it take before we have a clearer sense of what is likely to happen?
   - If _____ were to happen, what options would we need to consider for further evaluation and treatment?

- If _____ were to happen, we would want or not want _____.
- If I have a question about my loved one's kidneys or lungs, whom should I call? Often a different physician specialist will be involved and will be able to more accurately address your concerns as they relate to their area of expertise.
- Who will be on call for your group over the weekend? Who will be covering for you while you're away? How would I reach them?

6. Assign a person to represent the family. This will simplify communication and diminish confusion. The communication between your treating physicians, health-care team, and your family will be more efficient and accurate. Information will be channeled through key parties whom others can look to as sources of information.

7. Take notes. Write down anything that is important or may be forgotten. These can be overwhelming circumstances. It will not be possible to retain, remember, and understand all of the information you are receiving. It will also be challenging to recall "who said what."

8. If something is not clear, ask for a more detailed explanation. Mutual understanding is a key objective of the family meeting. I have never encountered a physician who was unwilling to meet with a family to discuss important issues. While this may require an investment of time, in my experience, the time invested is often much less than the time it would take to effectively address these issues by alternative means such as repeated phone calls; sharing similar information with several family members; the time it takes to defuse anger with respect to issues that could have been communicated more clearly; and time regarding management decisions that could have been avoided by a better understanding of values, wishes, and preferences. The family meeting is about communication and understanding. All parties involved will benefit greatly.

CHAPTER 8

SPIRITUALITY, RELIGION, AND HEALTH

Is This a Match Made in Heaven?

"Nothing in life is more wonderful than faith . . . mysterious, indefinable, known only by its effects."

—William Osler, M.D.

THE OBJECTIVES of this chapter are:

- To explore the medical evidence linking faith-based, religious, and spiritual practice with health outcomes.
- To explore the disparity between the extent that spirituality is central in the lives of many Americans and the infrequency with which spiritual issues are explored in the context of health care.

A young physician was vacationing in the Caribbean with his family. Early one morning while his family was still asleep, he ventured out for a peaceful walk on the beach. The beautiful teal Caribbean waters stretched as far as the eye could see. The sun was rising above the horizon. A gentle breeze danced in and around the slender, graceful palms. The peace and beauty were almost overwhelming as the young physician sat alone on the white sand. While he gazed out over the ocean, he was drawn to a soft, barely audible sound in the distance . . . "Ask and I shall answer," it whispered. At first he thought this was a deception of nature, a sound created by the ocean breeze dancing with the palms. Again, and this time with more intensity, the voice returned . . . "Ask and I shall answer."

"Who is this?" the young doctor asked, looking out over the water in disbelief. No answer. "Is it you . . . God?"

After a moment, the voice from beyond responded, "Yes, it is me . . . it is God."

The young physician was stunned, replying, "God, this is miraculous! I cannot believe you are talking to me."

God replied, "Ask any question, and I will answer it."

Without giving it much thought, the physician asked, "God, my family and I love coming here, to this place in the Caribbean. However, I am so afraid of flying. I wonder if you could build a bridge connecting the island to the mainland?" A long pause ensued.

"I must say," responded God, "I have not given this opportunity to too many mortals. I am a little disappointed in the quality of your question. Sure, I can build that bridge. It will be a very big project. It will take a lot of steel, concrete, and sophisticated engineering. Those Caribbean depths and currents are pretty tricky. But I can do it. I am God, after all."

The young physician, feeling guilty about the self-serving nature of his request, responded, "God, I am sorry about that selfish request. Would it be possible to have one more chance? Would it be possible to ask another question?"

God graciously replied, "Sure, I understand. What is your question?"

"Well," replied the physician, "I've been a doctor for quite a few years. I'm concerned about our health-care system. Many people are without insurance. Many cannot afford necessary medications. People are not always treated equally. Many people feel our system has become too confusing and impersonal. Can you give me some ideas that will help me fix our health-care system?"

There was a long silence and then a response, "Do you want that bridge to be four lanes or six lanes?"

You may be wondering what a topic like this is doing in a book about improving the effectiveness of your health-care experience. I will start to answer that question with an admitted bias: I was raised in a Congregational Protestant setting and my parents' religious faith played an important role in their lives. Our shared faith was particularly important as my parents confronted many health problems. While my faith has played an important role in my personal life, it has been greatly nurtured and affirmed by my experiences as a physician. Often I have looked to God for guidance in all I do as a parent, spouse, friend, and physician. I must emphasize that it is not my intent here to push religion. Issues of religion and spirituality are personal. This is a place that should not be entered without a significant degree of sensitivity and open-mindedness.

I have had a longstanding interest in the potential health benefits of spiritual and religious practice, and I lecture a great deal on this subject. Much is now being researched and published in this interesting area.

When I was a medical student and resident there was no formal instruction, discussion, or curriculum addressing spirituality. It was a topic nowhere near the radar screen. Any discussion of religion or spirituality in the context of a health-care encounter was best left to the individual and the clergy. In fact, the only time prayer came up when I was in medical school was prior to taking exams. I quickly realized these were not the kinds of prayer God had much interest in listening to, nor did they affect my test scores.

It can take a long time for a culture to shift, particularly one as deeply rooted and time honored as the tradition of medicine. As a medical resident, I became more fully immersed in the complicated tapestry of the human condition. I began to confront, with greater regularity, the universality of suffering, illness, and tragedy. I experienced the power of love, hope, and the tremendous resilience of the human soul. I saw firsthand the spirit's marvelous potential for lifting and healing. I began to enter the lives of total strangers routinely. What we shared was our common humanity. As the Dalai Lama once said, "The practice of compassion allows us to see how much alike we really are." I began to appreciate patient care on a deeper level, as an opportunity to share a journey—interesting, uncertain, frightening, but always meaningful. Becoming more skilled at diagnosis and treatment was surely an important aspect of that experience, as it continues to be for me today. However, something, much more remarkable and consistent transcended these medical encounters.

After I completed my training I was pretty well prepared to recognize physical wounds. I am damn good at recognizing broken kidneys. Spiritual wounds, on the other hand, are much more subtle and profound in their effects. There is no x-ray or blood test that can "pick up" a broken spirit. It is nothing like a broken bone or laceration on the skin. The nature of spiritual wounds sometimes makes them difficult to recognize and talk about. I have found that they rarely jump out and say, "Here I am, I need to be fixed." So how does a spiritual wound manifest itself? It usually takes the form of:

- Loss of meaning
- Loss of purpose
- Loss of hope
- Shame

- Guilt
- Isolation and loneliness
- Abandonment

Awareness, understanding, and supporting the spiritual dimension of one's life is essential to the healing process.

Illness is the great equalizer. I have treated custodians, Nobel laureates, and orchestra conductors. I have entered the lives of the young, the old, and the ethnically diverse. The stories I have experienced in these diverse lives offered remarkable opportunity. These allowed me to see the universality of our experience as human beings with greater clarity. Though the names, faces, and backgrounds were often very different, the expressions of love, fear, hope, and faith were not at all unique. Entering into a moment of pain, fear, uncertainty, joy, gratitude, sadness, and grief began to look familiar, even though the lives of those I was caring for were remarkably varied, and on the surface seemed quite dissimilar.

I have been brought to many places where intangible "connections" prevail. By connection I mean an interpersonal bond that is shared by individuals experiencing the moment, in the same way, place, and time. These are connections felt and not seen. These are connections that are not readily explained or defined by the science I have spent years learning and refining. For many medical encounters, I could just as easily have left the science at the door. The following story is an example.

A close friend is currently confronting a terminal cancer at the age of thirty-seven. He was diagnosed with a different cancer at the age of twenty and told he would not likely survive more than six months. He was cured of that and now confronts a separate, unrelated malignancy. He is a deeply spiritual man, having committed his life to such activities as mindfulness meditation, prayer, and macrobiotic nutrition. He has studied with the Dalai Lama, and fully extended all dimensions of his life in the project of helping others to heal. Recently a group of twenty people gathered in a local chapel with him to reflect and to share in the mobilization and transfer of healing love and energy. We sat in a circle. My friend, in too much pain to sit for prolonged periods of time, was surrounded by comfortable pillows, allowing him to shift positions as needed. He looked tired and worn. This incredibly vibrant and compassionate soul was struggling to transcend a body fatigued and in pain. As we shared our deepest feelings, meditated, prayed, and reflected, the bond between us was strong. I could not remember ever feeling so connected to others and to my dear friend.

Near the end of our meditation, my friend played three recorded songs, each with a positive and strong message. The last of the three songs was

"I Will Survive" by Donna Summer. Weak and uncomfortable, my friend stood in the center of our circle and together we sang and danced. One at a time we entered the circle to dance, connected physically and spiritually, lifted, as our friend gently danced in perfect rhythm. His arms and legs were moving as they had not in many months. A look of contentment emerged on his worn face. A beaming smile transcended his discomfort. Healing was so clearly at work here. I felt it. We all felt it. It was indescribable.

Another story I will never forget is that of E. B. He was a veteran of World War II and experienced significant physical and emotional trauma from battle. He would relive these memories for the rest of his life. E. B. was a sweet, gentle man who beamed when talking about his wife and daughter. He had several chronic medical conditions, one involving his kidneys, for which I followed him closely for many years. His was a name I would see on my day's schedule and feel very good about, as he was a friend in addition to being a patient. He had shared many stories about the war, his family, sports, and other aspects of his life. He gratefully placed his life in my hands (and those of my partners) with an openly expressed trust. After many years of reasonable health, and having overcome many trials and tribulations, E. B. and I confronted his mortality. Near the end of his life he developed serious heart complications, breathing problems requiring that he be on a ventilator, and dangerously low blood pressure, requiring medications to support it. His kidneys were failing and I could see that his weary fight was reaching an end.

As you might gather, I do believe in some form of afterlife. I do believe there is an energy, divine and immense, that emerges from our tired bodies, whole and complete. I love Elizabeth Kubler-Ross's metaphor of the butterfly emerging from the aged and weathered cocoon.

There are instincts physicians and nurses develop with experience. They guide our thinking and actions. I sensed the imminence of E. B.'s death. I was doing all possible within his wishes to sustain him. He became unconscious, as he lay motionless in our CCU. I reached his daughter, whom I had heard so much about and had never met. She traveled a few hours to get to the hospital, accompanied by her husband. She was aware of her father's critical condition. She gracefully prepared to say "goodbye" to him. Together we stood at his bedside. She asked if he was comfortable and as I looked at E. B., an aura of peace and equanimity prevailed. As his heart rate slowed further, his daughter took one of her father's hands to hold. She reached for my hand as I held his other hand. Together we stood connected, father, daughter, and physician. We held hands and looked on in silence as his heart rhythm on the monitor said its final goodbye. This leg in his journey had come to an end. As we stood there I could feel E. B.'s presence. It was as if he stood with us, looking down at the tired physical frame that had housed his spirit for many years. There was an incredible sense of peace and spiritual sharing between us that day. Weeks later I received a letter from E. B.'s daughter. She shared exactly the same feelings I had experienced.

I have experienced this many times in the people I have treated during the process of death and dying. There is a dimension that transcends our physical boundaries. From my perspective, experiences around death and dying inherently invite opportunities to "see" the human spirit. I have observed many people's ability to sense death, often with an aura of peace and expectation. In modern medicine we view death as an event. Death is not an event. Death is a process. Though the process of dying may have discomfort associated with it, the readiness of the spirit to transcend this, I believe, occurs far in advance of death itself (medically defined by absence of a pulse or heartbeat and spontaneous respirations).

We need to demystify the process of dying with an emphasis on comfort and shared compassion. People confronting their mortality often have much to share about this inevitable aspect of our existence. Painful and difficult though these circumstances are, they offer incredible opportunities for witnessing the strength, resilience, hope, and faith inherent in the human spirit.

We are a death-phobic society. So ineffective has modern medicine's approach to palliative care and the death process been that the hospice movement was created. Physicians refer individuals and families to hospice when treatment options are limited and the prognosis felt to be less than six months. Hospice care can be provided in homes, hospitals, and nursing home facilities, depending on the circumstances and the resources available in the community. Care is provided by skilled teams. Hospice support is not about death. It is about nurturing all aspects of the individual—physical, emotional, and spiritual—while alive. Hospice embraces every moment of life with total respect and integrity. Hospice care applies a patient- and family-centered approach allowing individual values, wishes, and preferences to be fully respected in a "self-determined" manner. Hospice also provides bereavement support for caregivers. As a society we need to have more dialogue regarding these important issues. Such discussions, uncomfortable though they may feel, provide greater insight into what our shared humanity is all about.

Certainly my experiences as a physician have raised many difficult questions about meaning. I have been sobered by the unpredictable fine line between life and death, hope and despair, and healing and curing. It is in this domain, in all its wonder, mystery, and universality that the worlds of faith, spirituality, and science have converged. What a remarkable and interesting place!

The overwhelming majority of people I have treated nurture and express a religious or spiritual dimension that is critical in their lives. It may strongly influence the way they care for themselves and the way they cope. It may provide a context within which they understand and interpret their health, wellness, or illness. These issues are of personal importance to providers of care as well. Physicians are people too. A growing body of evidence suggests that belief in God is common in the lives of most Americans. There is a growing body of medical evidence that religious or spiritual practices may confer beneficial health outcomes. Many studies suggest that as many as two out of three people, in certain circumstances, would want their physicians to inquire about their faith beliefs and even consider praying with them! Have you prayed with your physician lately?

I need to make the distinction between religion and spirituality, as they can be very different. I view religion as an organized set of teachings, doctrines, rituals, and practices that facilitate closeness to God. Most of the people I have treated observe one of the monotheistic faith traditions—Christianity, Judaism, or Islam. Many studies in the medical literature examine the potential health benefits of religious faith, in part because these practices can be "measured," with arguable accuracy, by worship attendance, use of devotionals, prayer, and other practices. Spirituality, on the other hand, is much harder for science to wrap its arms around. I think of spirituality as that which adds depth and meaning to our lives. Another way to think of spirituality is as a quest for understanding, meaning, and purpose that nurtures a deeper connection to values that may or may not lead to the development of religious rituals and community. Spiritual practices are attuned to a deeper or higher consciousness, inherently connected to a divine life force or energy. Our spirituality defines the "soul" of who we are as human beings. Our biology is the fine orchestra conducted by this divine energy.

Spirituality is a more individual experience, though it can be manifested through community or religious participation. It does not, however, necessarily have anything to do with God. Meditation and relaxation techniques can be deeply spiritual experiences and have nothing to do with organized religion. Pets, music, art, and literature, for example, can elicit in us a deeper spiritual awareness. My mother Agnes had a wonderful pet dog, a Shitzu named Zachary. Zachary did as much for her mood, spirit, and faith as her Prozac ever did! The combination of the two, I believe, was more powerful than either alone.

So what does any of this have to do with health-care encounters? Studies suggest that 90 to 95 percent of Americans believe in God. Many people, about 60 to 75 percent, feel that faith plays an important role in their health and wellness. Our societal response to the events of September 11, 2001 speaks to the inherent need to understand and to put pain and suffering into some context. I believe that as a society we were moved to a depth of sadness, grief, and uncertainty that made more visible our shared experience in life and our innate "connectedness" to each other. Pre-existing boundaries of color and socioeconomic class were diminished. As I looked into the eyes of others, I could sense something connecting us, unspoken and undeniably real. Often I have seen this same spiritual dimension emerge in the context of confronting serious illness.

Other medical studies demonstrate the important role that prayer, perhaps the most common form of meditation practiced worldwide, plays in how people respond to illness and how they cope when ill. The more significant the medical problems, the more likely people are to pray and desire to be prayed for.

For many Americans, expressions of faith through prayer or worship are the first and most significant response to an illness. As many as two out of three people say they would want their physician to address this aspect of their life during illness. Addressing religious/spiritual issues can range from simply inquiring about the role faith plays in your life, arranging for pastoral care visitation, to actually having a physician pray with you. Rarely, less than 10 percent of the time, do issues of religious faith or spirituality come up in the context of a health-care encounter. What this clearly suggests is a pervasive disconnect between the role that faith plays in the lives of most people, in sickness and in health, and the extent to which these issues are addressed by treating clinicians.

I have on occasion, prayed with a patient or family, at their request. I am not suggesting that this is appropriate for all types of health-care encounters. After a talk I gave in our community

Faith is the foundation upon which the therapeutic relationship between a physician and patient rests. I have never had a patient encounter where I did not want the individual and the family to believe in me. Nor, to my knowledge, has any patient I have cared for ever desired anything but my total faith in our ability to share a therapeutic bond.

on this topic, a woman who was listening intently approached me. She said she had thought many times about asking her primary care provider to pray with her and felt uncomfortable bringing it up. "Why do you feel uncomfortable asking your doctor to pray with you?" I asked.

"Oh, he's very busy and I'm not sure how he will respond." This is the typical response I hear when talking to people about discussing religious or spiritual issues with their physicians.

"What's the worst that can happen?" I usually ask. "You might be surprised by the response to your invitation." It is interesting that this can be such an awkward and delicate door to open. Breaking the ice is often just what a physician needs to feel more comfortable sharing in this way. He or she may in fact find faith and prayer to be of great importance in their lives but may be uneasy talking about it. I later learned that this woman, before a necessary hip replacement operation, asked her primary care provider to pray with her while she was in his office. He graciously obliged, and I know with certainty that their relationship was taken to a deeper level. This could easily have been a missed opportunity for sharing.

Some very provocative evidence indicates that faith practices can facilitate healing from illness. Remember the critical distinction between curing and healing. Evidence strongly suggests that faith-based and spiritual practices may reduce complications after surgery; help with recovery from depression; play an enormous comforting role in end-of-life care; improve the immune response; improve symptoms of anxiety; reduce the risk of teen pregnancy, drug use, criminal behavior, and suicide; and perhaps even prolong life expectancy!

Children are remarkably spiritual beings. Even very young children have clear ideas about divine realities, faith, and prayer. Religious traditions may play an important role in the moral and social development of parents and their children. These beliefs and contexts are important to understand, as they often influence ideas of sickness, suffering, coping, and healing. The pediatric/adolescent literature in medicine is recognizing the importance of this intersection between coping and spirituality. Many common issues such as nighttime fear, behavioral health problems, domestic abuse, hospitalization, disability (intellectual, cognitive, physical, and developmental), substance abuse, terminal illness, and cultural challenges can be better understood and more effectively addressed by a greater appreciation of this connection.

For example, prayer in individuals with AIDS has been shown to reduce physician visits and hospitalizations and to improve mood. Interleukin 6, an immune protein that is involved in the inflammatory process and can be associated with disease activity, is reduced considerably in individuals who attend worship once per week. Spiritual support is fundamental to the provision of palliative and end-of-life care. Studies have consistently shown that religious/spiritual beliefs and practices are positively correlated with life satisfaction, happiness, and diminished anxiety and pain, even though length of survival is not changed. This is another example of the important difference between healing and curing.

There is some evidence that if you pray for someone physically distant from you (intercessory prayer), both the "prayer" and the "prayee" experience a heightened sense of wellness. Studies from Duke University have shown that health outcomes in individuals with depression were strongly and positively predicted by the extent to which their religious faith was a central motivating force in their lives. The Cochrane Database of Systematic Reviews is an objective, vigorous, and critical appraisal of the medical literature as it relates to various medical topics. On the issue of prayer it suggests, "The evidence that exists is compelling enough to justify further study . . . any effect may be beyond present scientific understanding."

A clear correlation exists between religious and spiritual practices and health outcomes. I need to add that the aforementioned health benefits from the "faith factor" depend more on the individual intensity of one's spiritual commitment than on the particularity of one's faith tradition. Of course these more recent insights would have come as no surprise to Jesus in the Christian tradition, Moses Maimonides from the Jewish tradition, or Avicenna from the Muslim tradition, to name a few noteworthy spiritual/healing authorities of the last three thousand years. Hindu, Buddhist, and shaman traditions all see healing as intersecting with one's spiritual identity and journey. As Ben Franklin once said, "God heals and the doctor takes the fees."

To balance this perspective, many of these studies have come under scrutiny for their methodologies, lack of scientific rigor, quality, and interpretation. I agree with these observations, and yet the studies are compelling. These findings have been consistent with what I have observed as a physician, and what I have observed in the lives of my parents, who confronted many spiritually challenging medical problems. These observations are also consistent with what hundreds of patients and families have shared with me. As I have seen many times, when peoples' health and the world around them are crumbling, faith is the adhesive that keeps things intact. Prayer is the most common source of comfort I have found and observed in this context.

These studies certainly do not confirm the presence of God or a divine force. A person of faith, as I am, does not require proof to believe. Absence of proof is not proof of absence. Faith is something you feel from within, more than something you can easily measure from without. Even if you are an atheist or skeptic, there is very good evidence that the social support offered by communities of faith, the lifestyles of many spiritual and religious practices, and the "buffer" from isolation and loneliness inherent in spiritual and religious practice are health promoting. There is clear evidence for this and it is intuitive. Being part of nurturing communities of people is more likely to promote healthier outcomes than loneliness and isolation.

A "non-self" construct for examining life and all its complexities, particularly when you are ill, allows a transcendence of pain and suffering by offering a context of hope and meaning. There is excellent medical evidence to support the power of mind-body integration. Herb Benson, director of the Mind-Body Institute at Harvard, long ago recognized the biologic potential of the relaxation response. Harvard's continuing medical education course on spirituality and medicine is among the most popular of their outstanding offerings. Prayer and meditation can decrease levels of "stress" hormones and lower blood pressure and respiratory rate. Positive emotions embodied in world faith traditions, such as love, hope, forgiveness, and kindness stimulate parts of the brain that can have profoundly positive effects on our immune system, and many other mediators of inflammation, emotional, and physiologic stress.

Stephanie Brown, a researcher at the Institute for Social Research at the University of Michigan, and her colleagues have found that by helping others, people help themselves, improving their mental health, their physical well-being, and possibly their longevity. The ancient wisdom that giving is better than receiving just may have been a prescription for good health, in addition to its altruistic virtues, which can more than stand on their own. As Carolyn Schwartz, a social scientist states, "when you open your heart to other people to listen and care about them, it changes the way you look at the world and you're happier." Much will be learned in the near future with respect to the biologic and physiologic effects of love, kindness, and altruism. Undoubtedly there will be effects on stress hormones, brain messenger proteins, and the immune system. This is one of the most fascinating areas of research today.

Even if one were to reduce current evidence to the placebo effect, there is no greater, more enduring, and more consistent clinical observation than that which connects the power of belief with beneficial health outcomes. I view the placebo effect as the most powerful scientific observation ever. The placebo effect speaks to the marvelous and mysterious interconnectedness between our mind, our emotions, our thoughts, our spirits, our biology, and our health. A professional, reputable scientific study that is looking at the benefit of a particular treatment must include a placebo comparison. It has long been recognized that as many as one of three people who receive a placebo, or treatment without any active ingredient, such as a sugar pill, will experience a benefit similar to the experimental treatment. For any experimental treatment to be beneficial, it has to prove to be better than a placebo. This is a truly remarkable phenomenon, fascinating and not well understood. It is clear that a focused and uncritical belief or faith in the potential benefit of a treatment, even if the treatment is lacking an "active ingredient," can unleash a cascade of biologic effects that produce, in some instances, a profound change in feeling.

To believe, to truly believe unconditionally, unleashes a cascade of biologic effects that are still not well understood. These effects have the remarkable potential for health promotion and disease treatment.

More than a mind-body phenomenon, these observations affirm the beautifully integrated tapestry of all that it is to be human, physical, emotional, mental, and spiritual. They are indeed one—not separated at all. People who are attuned to this in their lives have healthier perspectives and, clearly, a greater sense of wellness. Physicians and other health-care providers who are attuned to this seamless integration are, in my opinion, more effective in their therapeutic alliances with patients.

I know there are some people who feel strongly that any physician who opens this door and examines the other side is challenging the limits of ethical appropriateness and expertise. In fairness, I could not agree more that issues of religious expression, faith, and spirituality are deeply personal and are not appropriate to address in all health-care encounters. The importance of these issues in someone I am treating for a sinus infection is not the same as in someone with whom I am discussing initiation of dialysis. I also agree and feel strongly that a physician's personal views on these matters should never be forced on an unwitting, vulnerable, or disinterested individual. This is a sacred domain and should be carefully and delicately navigated. The power imbalance between a patient in need of care and a healer, trusted with answers and insights, must never be exploited in service to the physician's beliefs. I do, however, feel strongly that these are critical issues, and under certain circumstances are "ripe" for inquiry and sharing. At a minimum, clinicians should inquire about the role faith or spirituality plays in the lives of those they are treating. If the answer is "none," leave it at that. Particularly when confronting a serious medical problem, it is critical to consider what gives meaning to people. This may have nothing to do with religion. In my experience, particularly in dealing with acute and critical illness, life-sustaining interventions like dialysis, advance directives, organ donation, and the death process, matters that awaken thoughts of meaning and purpose are almost *always* relevant and vital to individuals.

As a kidney specialist I have frequently dealt with extremely challenging bio-psycho-social-spiritual matters. I cannot begin to fathom my role as an effective physician healer without some consideration of meaning and spirituality in addressing these matters. When teaching medical students (third and fourth year medical students from the University of Massachusetts Medical School train in our hospital) and residents (we have approximately thirty residents training and becoming primary care internists), we review actual cases and apply the acronym F.I.C.A. (developed by Christina Puchalski, GWish Foundation, *The George Washington Institute for Spirituality and Health* (www.gwish.org) to facilitate the taking of a spiritual history. This tool offers physicians and nurses a template to initiate the dialogue regarding these important issues. Perhaps as a health-care consumer, you can contemplate these issues yourself and feel more comfortable discussing them with your providers of care. F.I.C.A. asks the following questions*:

F—Faith and Belief
"Do you consider yourself spiritual or religious?" or "Do you have spiritual beliefs that help you cope with stress?" If the patient responds "No," the physician might ask, "What gives your life meaning?" Sometimes patients respond with answers such as *family, career*, or *nature*.

I—Importance
"What importance does your faith or belief have in our life? Have your beliefs influenced how you take care of yourself in this illness? What role do your beliefs play in regaining your health?"

C—Community
"Are you part of a spiritual or religious community? Is this of support to you and how? Is there a group of people you really love

---

*Copyrighted. Obtained with permission from Christina M. Puchalski, M.D.

or who are important to you?" Communities such as churches, temples, and mosques, or a group of like-minded friends, can serve as strong support systems for some patients.

A—Address in Care
"How would you like me, your health-care provider, to address these issues in your healthcare?"

Again, the conversation may end after the "F." Many people may wish to have a pastor or rabbi from their faith community contacted. They may want to pray with a hospital chaplain or receive communion. They may want to pray with a nurse or physician. We may plan a family meeting to address some of these issues. (See chapter 7, The Family Meeting).

Here's an example of how profoundly important these issues can be. Some time ago, I cared for E. C., a woman in her sixties. She had problems with depression and was receiving therapy from a counselor. In addition, she was taking antidepressants. She had kidney failure and required dialysis to stay alive. She had been on dialysis for years and was slowly failing to the extent that the combination of her emotional and physical problems forced her to move from her apartment of many years to a local nursing home. She was clearly suffering, and I found myself deeply saddened by her painful demise. She had no family in the area. Despite our best efforts the quality of her life continued to decline.

During a hospitalization for an infection, she became quite tearful and said to me, "Dr. Pettus, I simply can't go on any more. For a long, long time I've thought of stopping dialysis. It's a decision that torments me."

"That's a horrible place to be, E. C.," I replied. "Tell me more about how you are feeling? How do you see your life right now?"

E. C. went on to say tearfully, "I have been suffering. I'm not afraid to die and I have felt ready for some time."

"Why do you feel tormented?" I asked.

She replied, "What would God think of me, choosing to end my life this way?" E. C. felt that the decision to discontinue dialysis would make God angry, and her relationship with God was much too important to allow that to happen. When I explored this with her in more detail, I learned that she was a member of a local faith community. Many members of this congregation were, in fact, her closest friends. Her church was her family. She had a close relationship with her pastor, who knew her well, though it was difficult for her to share these feelings with him. My partner and I contacted her pastor, who spent time with her in the hospital reconciling her faith and conflicting views with respect to stopping dialysis.

She had a psychiatric evaluation and clearly was competent in her understanding and wishes. I met with her and her pastor and some members of her church, who visited her regularly upon hearing she was in the hospital. She decided to stop dialysis. She was visibly at greater peace knowing that God loved her unconditionally no matter what she decided. She had reconciled the greatest source of torment in her life at that time. Her spiritual wounds were given the opportunity to heal as her weary physical body gave way. She died soon thereafter with those she knew and loved at her bedside, softly singing the hymns that had so often lifted her spirits.

For E. C., her faith was both a source of support and of conflict. This is not uncommon; faith practices can have a negative side as well as a positive. If we had failed to recognize the opportunity to understand this, we never would have been able to address what was the most important concern in her life.

So what are the obstacles that create this disparity between the importance that faith practices play in the lives of most people and the extent to which they are addressed in the health-care encounter?

For physicians:

- Minimal attention paid to this during formal training in medical school and in residency
- Inadequate skills in addressing matters of spirituality
- Lack of awareness of the resources available to provide support such as pastoral care
- Lack of interest or insight in this area
- Discomfort discussing such "sensitive" issues
- Feeling that it is an inappropriate area to "visit" under any circumstances, that it is best left to spiritual healers
- Lack of awareness of the importance spiritual, faith, and religious practices and perspectives play in the lives of patients and families

I frequently speak in public about the spirituality-health connection. When I ask people why they do not raise these issues with their physicians and why matters of faith are not explored more openly, the responses usually fall into one of these categories.

For Patients/Families:

- Perception that physicians are too busy to delve into these matters
- Uncertainty and sensitivity to how a physician may respond

- Uncertainty about how important this is to the physician
- Awkwardness and discomfort raising these issues because they usually do not come up in health-care encounters
- Feeling that these issues are inappropriate to discuss
- Not an important issue to them personally

Interestingly, while many physicians may find areas of faith and spirituality important, they are less likely to address them unless a patient brings up the subject. While most patients find areas of faith and spirituality to be very important, they are less likely to mention them unless their physician brings them up in conversation.

It seems that physicians and their patients are silently engaged in a delicate and shared tiptoe on the periphery, so close to a more meaningful spiritual dance in the middle of the dance floor.

It is interesting what our culture is willing to comfortably embrace. I do feel that greater awareness and sensitivity to matters of religion and spirituality are permeating the medical culture. Almost two out of three medical schools now have a formal curriculum that helps medical students develop skills to be more aware and effective in these areas. I recently received a grant to develop a spirituality-medicine curriculum in our residency program. I feel that it has been very successful.

Here is an example of our learning objectives and a sampling of the feedback from our medical residents with respect to the one-year curriculum:

Basis for Developing a
Spirituality-Medicine Curriculum

- As humans treating humans we are brought "closer" by a sharper awareness and understanding of the role that spirituality plays in our own lives and in the lives of those we treat.
- We develop a broader perspective on health and healing.
- We explore the available resources for helping patients and their families better understand and cope with illness.
- We respond to the growing social imperative for more holistic approaches to health maintenance, disease prevention, and treatment.

A Survey of Our Medical Residents:

1. Spirituality plays an important role in the lives of people I treat.

Not important	0%
Somewhat important	30%
Important	45%
Very Important	25%

2. Patients' views regarding spirituality can influence the way they view their illness/wellness.

Not important	0%
Somewhat important	10%
Important	40%
Very Important	50%

3. Spirituality plans an important role in my life.

Not important	10%
Somewhat important	15%
Important	20%
Very Important	55%

4. I feel comfortable addressing spirituality with my patients.

Not at all	5%
Somewhat	20%
Depends on circumstances	20%
Always, if circumstances are appropriate	55%

There is clearly growing interest in this area. Just as we are still improving the efficacy of our dialogue in areas of death and sexuality, it will take a while before spiritual issues become a more consistent and comfortable area of discussion in modern health care. As for the personal nature of spirituality, we are who we are. Anyone who has ever had a colonoscopy, given birth, undressed from stem to stern for a complete physical, had a prostate exam, or had a catheter placed in his bladder, in my experience, is not likely to view a few basic questions about faith as invasive or too personal.

What advice can I give you?

- If you are at all curious about practices that place greater emphasis on more mindful awareness, greater balance, and the mind-body connection, consider meditation and/or yoga. One does not have to look far these days to find a good class, book, or video. Classes offer the benefit of structure, guidance, and social support.
- If you are a member of a faith community, or curious about a particular faith community, visit a local church, mosque, or synagogue. Examine, with greater awareness, how you feel before and after. Find a pastoral care leader who speaks in a way that is appealing and feels right to you.
- If prayer feels right, pray more often.
- If these matters are important to you, find the courage to ask your health-care provider how he or she feels about them and how they can help you connect with resources that may be available in the hospital or in the community, if appropriate. If you do not raise your spiritual voice, you may not be called upon and it may not be heard. I think most physicians, even if somewhat uncomfortable or caught off guard, will understand the importance of this. It is also possible that something very special may transpire. Perhaps you can even teach your physician the F.I.C.A. acronym.
- If you or a loved one are in the hospital, and are a member of a faith community, call or have someone call your pastor. If you are not a member of a specific faith community, hospitals usually have pastoral care staff on call to assist with your spiritual needs if you wish.
- If you are confronting an illness in the hospital or at home, surround yourself with whatever it takes to lift your spirits and promote your health. This may be having important people in your life nearby; pets; photographs; music; sources of humor; or human touch. The spirit has many doors. Open as many as you can.
- Forgiveness is a powerful, challenging, and remarkable opportunity to facilitate healing and to lift the spirit. In my experience, many deep spiritual wounds have at their core relational or internal conflicts that are deep-seated and seemingly impossible to let go of. Forgiveness, difficult though it can be, is liberating.
- If you or family members are confronting an advanced chronic illness or a "terminal" illness (one that could progress to death in a matter of months), consider a hospice referral. Evidence suggests that physicians refer to hospice late in the course of illness, often resulting in a shorter time for services. There are many reasons for

late referral. Sometimes physicians feel an individual has longer to live than he or she actually does. This can be very hard to predict. There may be difficulty having an open conversation about death, dying, and terminal illness. A discussion of a terminal prognosis is often seen as an undermining of hope. This is a difficult balance. Hope emerges in the sharing of the journey. Hope is in the assurance that you will never be abandoned. Hope is in the peace and comfort of knowing that those who love and care about you are connected. Hope is in the promise of physical, emotional, and spiritual comfort. If you are wondering about the appropriateness of hospice services and the subject has not been brought up, discuss it with your primary care provider or your oncologist.

- In matters of faith, leave nothing unsaid. There are simply no obstacles that love cannot overcome.

As C. S. Lewis said in *Reflection on the Psalms:* "Praise almost seems to be inner health made audible."

DO NOT MISS TAKE HOME POINTS

1. If spiritual or religious practices are important to you, inquire about available resources to assist in meeting your needs.
2. How do your spiritual/religious views influence your understanding and response to illness, e.g. coping and decision-making, as they relate to you or your loved one's circumstances?
3. If you are a member of a faith community, do not hesitate to reach out for support, prayer, and comfort.
4. If you desire, has your faith community's pastoral care person or a hospital chaplain been notified of your circumstances? Given the Health Insurance Portability and Accountability Act (HIPPA), federal regulations that were adopted to ensure patient privacy and confidentiality, anticipate that you or a family member will need to give permission for others to be notified of your health status.
5. Find out where the chapel is in your hospital. This can be a peaceful and comforting place to pray and reflect.
6. If matters of faith, religion, or spirituality are important and relevant to your health, mention this to your physician.

CHAPTER 9

MAKING DIFFICULT MEDICAL DECISIONS
Knowing What Questions to Ask

"Defining moments force us to find a balance between our hearts in all their idealism, our minds in all their knowledge, and our lives in their messy reality."

—Joseph L. Badaracco, Jr.

THE OBJECTIVES of this chapter are:

- To review the process of medical decision making.
- To highlight the necessary elements of an effective decision-making process.
- To provide sample questions that will increase the likelihood that you will have the best information available in making a medical decision.

Inevitably, we will all confront the need to make some very difficult decisions regarding our health and wellness. These decisions may be about our own lives or about the lives of people we love dearly. As you well know, medicine has become much more complex. For us as physicians and for you or your loved ones as patients, there are often many options to contemplate regarding diagnostic tests and treatments. More responsibility is placed on individuals and families to make these challenging decisions. There may be several possible paths to get from "A to B." The options that must be considered are often complicated and difficult to understand. At times, there will be significant uncertainty as to the consequences of a chosen path. The stakes are often enormous and the time available to make these decisions sometimes very short.

How can you be sure which path is the best for you or your loved one? I have had many discussions with patients and their families regarding medical decisions with profound implications for quality of life and life itself. I have learned a lot from these experiences, both as a physician and from personal decisions made regarding my parents' health and livelihood. I have found that difficult medical decisions fall into a few basic categories.

HOW BEST TO TREAT?

Some decisions relate to a type of therapy for a particular problem, for example, surgery, radiation therapy and/or chemotherapy, dialysis, use of a particular medication or medications, or comfort care (while comfort is always a priority under any circumstance, it may sometimes be chosen as the only treatment, as with a terminal illness).

HOW BEST TO DIAGNOSE?

Diagnostic decisions examine the options available for trying to find out what is causing the underlying problem or problems. Common examples include blood tests, a biopsy (taking a sample of tissue for analysis), cardiac catheterization, some type of x-ray or imaging study, and surgery.

WHAT IS THE BEST DISPOSITION OR NEXT STEPS?

This usually refers to the options available for providing the safest environment for day-to-day living. These options can include being at home with extra support, such as family, a homemaker, health aide, physical and occupational therapists, and personal care attendants. They may require being in a more supervised and supported setting such as assisted living or a nursing home. Another example of a decision in this category would be the transfer of care to another facility. They may also include decision options as the patient prepares to be discharged from the hospital—for example, going directly home with or without support; going to a rehabilitation unit for a few weeks to get stronger before going home; going to a skilled nursing unit as a longer bridge to home (perhaps several weeks to a few months) or going to a skilled nursing facility, or nursing home, forever. These can be very difficult decisions.

Would I want life-sustaining or "heroic" measures, if necessary?

Please refer to chapter 6 on advance directives for a review of this important topic. These critical decisions address what you would want if your breathing or heart were to stop or become dangerously unable to keep you alive.

Should we withdraw life-sustaining interventions?

I have been involved with many of these decisions. There are none more difficult, given the circumstances during which they are made and given their consequences. However, sometimes such decisions are necessary. They usually involve removing an individual from a breathing machine (ventilator) or from dialysis when there is little or no hope for an acceptable recovery.

There are of course, many other types of decisions that can surface. Most of the really difficult ones, however, will fall into these categories.

Any medical decision should be thought of as a negotiation process between your physician and you. It is a process that should be defined by timely, open, and clear sharing of information that is sufficiently understood by everyone involved.

Of course, everyone involved desires the best outcome possible. There are varying degrees of certainty as to how good an outcome might be. For example, a surgeon can be pretty certain that most of the time, removing an inflamed gallbladder will provide excellent results, resolution of symptoms and, except for the expected time for recovery, a low likelihood of serious complications. The decision to have the surgery is based on this understanding and is usually associated with a good outcome.

> *It is the quality of this process that ultimately determines how good the decision is.*

A person with a history of heart disease and an enlarging aneurysm in need of surgery may, after a careful and complete discussion, decide to proceed with surgery, only to have a bad outcome; for example, suffering a stroke, kidney failure, or death. I would not consider this a bad decision if the risks and benefits had been considered carefully, and if there were a good understanding, consistent with the informed wishes, values, and preferences of the individual. I would not consider this a bad decision if all available options were reviewed and the eventual one chosen was felt to be the best available under the circumstances. Sometimes a bad decision may have a good outcome; for example, failing to see an orthopedic surgeon for a minor fracture or broken bone that ends up healing satisfactorily. Alternatively, a good decision may have a bad outcome; for example, the decision to have a bypass operation that leads to a serious complication like kidney failure, requiring dialysis. So what constitutes a good decision-making process? Here are some elements critical to building the foundation upon which any important decision is made.

Communication

It is very important that the information you are receiving is as clear as possible. It is equally important that your concerns, questions, and preferences are communicated clearly to those responsible for you or your loved one's care. The flow of information should be open, honest, and as specific as possible. Clear communication cannot be taken for granted. Evidence would suggest that patients and families frequently do not grasp what is being communicated to them. It is important to recognize and remedy any potential barriers to effective communication. Examples of such barriers include:

- Excessive use by health-care providers of medical jargon
- Insufficient skill mix to address challenging conversations effectively
- Lack of awareness by you or your physician with respect to the *gap* between perceived and actual understanding
- Excessive waiting time
- Differences of opinion between you and your physician
- Noise, lack of privacy, too many or too few key participants present
- Pain or emotional discomfort that interferes with focused sharing of information and an ability to grasp the facts
- Ethnic/cultural, for example, language or differences in cultural understanding and expression

Relationships

A trusting relationship is at the heart of the decision-making process. You may not have known your physician well enough or long enough to establish a close relationship. I have found however, that most people have good instincts about the quality of a conversation with a physician, even a total stranger. A trusting relationship can be nurtured and developed quickly when the quality of the exchange is good and meaningful.

You must make clear how you view the roles and responsibilities you and your family wish to have in the process. Some people need more control than others. Some families prefer to have the treating physician simply do what he or she feels is best. Some people prefer or need to have family speaking and acting on their behalf. These are very important differences in roles and expectations that need to be made as clear as possible, because they provide an important framework for the medical decision-making process.

Content

As with communication, some people need/want to know as much as possible. Other people may desire to know very little when it comes to making decisions. There is often a great deal of information to be shared and discussed in the context of the decision-making process. Do you feel comfortable you have all the information necessary? Do you have specific concerns that the content shared has not addressed? Do you feel comfortable that the risks, benefits, and available options have been covered? This is critical to examine.

UNDERSTANDING

It is common for physicians to assume a patient's or family's understanding is complete when in fact it may be very deficient. You may feel that the physician's understanding of your interests, concerns, and fears is clear when in fact there may be considerable gaps. Recapitulating or paraphrasing what you hear is an effective way to affirm this clarity. It not only demonstrates your understanding, it also allows the physician to identify an issue that is misunderstood. For example:

> PATIENT/FAMILY: Dr. Pettus, what I hear you saying is that my father needs dialysis because his kidneys are working at less than 10 percent of normal and he could die without this treatment. His kidneys are "gone" and there is not much anyone can do to turn them around! (The family's understanding is that this is likely to be a permanent problem.)
> DR. PETTUS: It is true that his kidneys are not working very well at all and this can be life threatening. Dialysis can help do the work his kidneys are unable to do. It is possible, if his infection gets better and his heart stronger, that his kidneys may recover to the ex-

tent that he can get by without dialysis. His kidneys are "gone" right now, but not necessarily forever. We will have to carefully see what the next few weeks bring. The long-term prognosis may be more clear at that time."

Separating fact from fiction, certainty from uncertainty, and misunderstanding from understanding is so important in this process.

Expectations

It is important to clarify expectations to the extent the situation allows. It is also important to appreciate that there will always be an element of uncertainty. Often, I have found that anger, bitterness, guilt, and deep distress emerge from large disparities between expectation and reality. These gaps are sometimes unavoidable as unexpected outcomes and unforeseen complications are inherent in any medical illness. Many times, however, these gaps occur because of a lack of clarity regarding expectations and possible outcomes. For example, a physician may, because of uneasiness, lack of important data, or inherent optimism, overestimate a prognosis or fail to consider and communicate a potential complication. The likelihood of an individual needing "transitional" care, for example, a two-week rehabilitation stay after a total hip replacement, may be understood by the providing physician, but not clearly communicated to the patient. The patient expecting to be home within a few days confronts the necessity of spending more

An effective decision-making process should attempt to minimize the expectation-reality gap.

time in the hospital before going home. This is not a serious concern, though it provides an example of well-intentioned people failing to make expectations clear.

As with any negotiation process, communication is a two-way street. It is important for patients and families to make their expectations and concerns candid and clear as well. Let me give you some examples of how this can and does play out on a daily basis. An individual's expectation of how well he or she will do at home is far greater than the realistic likelihood of how well he or she will do. Or the person may be very concerned about how safely he or she can navigate at home, but be reluctant to share those concerns and expectations. This might occur because a person does not want to burden family or friends, delay discharge from the hospital to home, accrue added expenses by staying in the hospital, or confront placement in a nursing home.

Another example: Perhaps a person is about to be discharged from the hospital after being treated for pneumonia. The expectation of the health-care providers is that things are much better, the prognosis good, and the plan to continue medications at home is indeed the best plan. The "unspoken" concerns and expectation of the individual are: "Who will pick up and pay for my prescriptions? Who will prepare my meals until I am stronger? Will I be able to climb the stairs to my bedroom? Will this nausea I'm feeling interfere with my ability to keep fluids down? How will I get to my primary care provider's office or to the laboratory to get my blood work done after I am discharged?"

Though there are resources available to help identify and deal with these very important issues, the extent to which a shared awareness of these issues exists and needs to be addressed may not be well understood.

As you move forward, commit to staying as clear and well informed as possible. If you or your family is confronting a difficult medical decision, here are some questions to consider asking the physicians and nurses involved in the care.

- Dr. _____, to the best of your knowledge, what is going on at this time?
- Are there other consultants involved? If so, what are their impressions?
- Would it help for me to discuss this with anyone else?
- What are the most common risks?
- How often do they occur?
- I know you cannot predict the future with certainty. If a hundred people like me or my loved one were to have this done, how many might have one or more of the complications you mentioned?
- What are the likely benefits of moving forward with this??
- If a hundred people in my or my loved one's position were to have this, how many, as an approximate average, would have this likely benefit?

Often in medicine we use statistics like 90 percent, not realizing that many people might not understand that "percent" in this case means ninety out of one hundred. Or we use more ambiguous expressions of risk/benefit like "unlikely," "rare," "uncommon," or "commonly." Precise answers may not be possible. However, to the extent that they are, it can only be helpful to put things in better perspective. Commit to narrowing the expectation-reality gap.

- Have we considered every reasonable option available?
- Can you recommend resources where I can review more information about this?
- To the extent that you feel comfortable and able, what are your expectations, in the near future and in the weeks and months ahead?
- To what extent are you and/or others uncertain about the best way to go? This is both a very difficult *and* a fair question, in my view.
- What can I/we do to better prepare for this important decision?
- Is there any further advice you could give me to assist in making this decision—for example, talking to someone who has confronted something similar; friends/family who can provide loving support; pastoral care professionals to provide spiritual support?
- I know this is a difficult question . . . what would you do if you were in my/our position? This too can be a very powerful and fair question to ask.
- Is focusing just on comfort a reasonable option to consider here?
- I know your time is limited and valuable. This decision is so important. Might a *family meeting* be appropriate to discuss it in more detail?

I hope this brief overview provides a framework that will allow the process of making difficult medical decisions to be as effective as it can be. It is your right and obligation to be as informed as possible. It is your responsibility to make as clear as you can your preferences, values, and wishes to those providing your care. For health-care professionals to best help you and your family it is essential that they have as clear a picture as possible of life as seen through your lens. It is a terrible feeling to be in a place where, regardless of the decision made, you feel "damned if you do, damned if you don't." I have been in this place with countless individuals and their families. I have spent many a sleepless night in the process of confronting difficult medical decisions and circumstances as they related to my parents' health and livelihood. I have lain awake contemplating the "what-ifs," the unfairness of bad things happening to good people, and the common and seemingly random injustices that life hands us. Despite our best intentions, bad things happen. If there is any peace eventually to be had, and if there is any basis for eventual healing, it is in knowing that all that could be done was done, to make the most informed decision possible within the context of what your heart and mind were telling you. Ultimately, this is what defines a good decision. No human being could do more.

DO NOT MISS TAKE HOME POINTS

1. It is important to view every decision-making process as a negotiation process.
2. Be sure that you understand your options.
3. Be clear on the role you wish to have in this process—for example, active and fully engaged or passively accepting of the best advice possible.
4. Be clear on your values and preferences as they relate to the options before you.
5. Remember the key ingredients of a good decision-making process: communication, relationships, content, and expectations.
6. When in doubt, seek another opinion.

CHAPTER 10

PREPARING FOR DISCHARGE FROM THE HOSPITAL
It's Not Always the Finish Line

"A wise man should consider that health is the greatest of human blessings, and learn how by his own thought to derive benefit from his illnesses."

—Hippocrates

THE OBJECTIVES of this chapter are:

- To help you appreciate the factors in our health-care system that necessitate faster discharge from the hospital than in the past.
- To provide advice that will help you or a family member prepare a smoother, safer discharge from the hospital.
- To offer considerations that may need to be examined with your physician to minimize the likelihood of a serious problem occurring after hospital discharge.
- To review the general categories of hospital discharge disposition or next steps that you may need to consider.

Discharge planning, as the end of a hospitalization draws near, has never been more complicated for those providing the care as well as for those being sent home. There are several reasons for this:

- People often enter the hospital with a more complicated range of issues—physical, cognitive, emotional, functional independence,

and safety—having received little attention prior to the hospitalization.

- The economic pressures of our health-care system result in much
  shorter lengths of stay in the hospital.
- More "active" treatment continues in the home or outpatient setting, as people are discharged after a shorter stay.
- Treatments, once given only in the hospital setting, such as intravenous medications, blood thinners, pain medications, and nutrition, are now routinely available in the home setting.
- "Ancillary" services—physical or occupational therapy, visiting
  nurses, home health aides—are increasingly necessary to make the
  transition to home safe and effective. More people need assistance
  with their "ADLs" or activities of daily living such as bathing, meal
  preparation, and housekeeping.
- The number of medications prescribed per patient has tripled
  over the last twenty years! There is a finer line between benefit
  and risk with medications these days (see chapter 11, Taking Medications).
- There is a greater need for follow-up testing after discharge from the
  hospital and there are often multiple physicians to see in follow-up.
- Transportation is frequently a challenge in meeting the needs of
  patients after discharge from the hospital.

As is true for many subjects in *The Savvy Patient*, greater awareness
of the potential for issues to arise, before they actually do arise, is essential to achieve smoother sailing. While it is not commonplace or necessarily natural for us to contemplate the "what-ifs" as they relate to the
need for hospitalization, you or a loved one may be walking a very fine
line between safe and unsafe, self-sufficient and dependent, manageable
and unmanageable. The extent to which you contemplate these possible
scenarios, and how you might deal with them if they occur, will go a
long way to diminish the expectation-reality gap as it relates to hospital
discharge planning. I find this gap increasing as patients and families
confront complex management issues and decisions within what can be
a very limited time frame.

In this light, there have been some dramatic shifts in the way health
care is provided that are important for you to understand. Because acute
care or hospital care is much more expensive than provision of care outside the hospital, there is tremendous pressure to limit hospitalization to
problems that cannot be safely treated otherwise and to limit, to the extent possible, the time spent in the hospital treating the underlying prob-

lems. The days of being admitted to a hospital "to run a few tests" and of staying in the hospital until all is perfectly well are gone forever. The positive side to this is that many problems can be safely treated in this manner and for most people, there is no place like home.

Hospitals are not risk-free. For example, despite growing awareness and emphasis on patient safety, medical errors do occur and can be serious. Hospitals are actively engaged in developing better systems and process improvements to further minimize these risks to patient safety. There are also nastier microbes or bacteria that exist in the acute care or hospital setting. This is because of the nature of the problems treated there and the widespread use of more potent antibiotics. Repeated exposure to these antibiotics enhances the development of bacteria that adapt in a way that renders them more resistant to treatment. Exposure to these nastier germs is clearly a greater risk in this setting.

Ironically, hospitals can be anything but healing, peaceful settings. Most individuals who find themselves hospitalized, quickly realize noise, frequent disruptions, limitations on visitation, and a conspicuous lack of the "comforts of home." So while sometimes necessary and indeed potentially life-saving, time spent in the hospital will continue to be more limited as our system adapts to better provision of home care.

These trends in health care are necessary and will continue. As a consequence, there is greater responsibility and pressure to prepare for the challenges of how to make discharge planning and home care as safe and effective as it can be. These are challenges of medical progress. The growing "demand" of medical needs outside the hospital setting is not being currently met by a sufficient "supply" of available human resources and financing. Medical costs are now shifting from the acute care setting to the outpatient setting, and with that shift is a rapidly growing need for outpatient resources.

An *enormous* number of people out there are getting by independently and satisfactorily, *and with a narrow margin of safety*. We are an aging society, "programmed" for autonomy and independence. Medical progress has allowed that to be possible in a way hitherto unimaginable. Since the turn of the twentieth century, our life expectancy has almost doubled! It is increasingly common to develop medical problems as we age—high blood pressure, diabetes, high cholesterol, heart disease, stroke, changes in cognition (diminished memory), changes in vision and hearing, and the need to take more prescription medications. When you superimpose an acute medical illness requiring hospitalization and add a shorter length of stay and greater medical complexity, you are likely to confront a more tenuous and challenging discharge scenario. That modest and acceptable pre-hospitalization status of home safety and self-sufficiency can quickly become a more risky and precarious challenge after discharge from the hospital.

As these trends in the organization, finance, and delivery of health care have evolved, the extended family network of support has also been stretched more thinly over the years. More children and siblings are scattered over large geographic areas. Work and educational opportunities draw people farther from home. More commonly, couples are not from the same hometown. Even when there are family members close to home, usually both partners are working or caring for children. The capacity to mobilize family support around hospital-to-home transition is therefore harder to facilitate. For so many families the angst of not being able to arrange appropriate time and resources to support a loved one in the home setting is on the rise.

Recovering from an acute illness, you or your loved one may find it very difficult to grasp the complexities of a discharge plan. People frequently are far from functioning at 100 percent when they are ready to be discharged. Your memory may not be as sharp. Your ability to concentrate may be more limited. You may feel overwhelmed, anxious, and depressed about the circumstances. These are not the best of conditions to be digesting and understanding what can be many very important issues, shared over a very short period of time (see chapter 15, Health-Care Literacy). The natural desire to get home as soon as possible is often reflected in the unspoken "get me home, I'll figure this out later" mindset.

If you or a loved one are confronting or about to confront a hospital discharge, here is some advice for how to make the process as smooth, clear, and safe as possible.

1. **Try to determine as early as possible in the course of the hospitalization when tentative plans for discharge will occur.**

   This, of course, is not always easy as unforeseen issues might arise, or a quicker than expected resolution and recovery might occur (we always hope for this). Usually it is possible to get a sense a day or two in advance of an anticipated discharge. Ask your primary care physician if he or she can predict the "D/C" date. A medical student, resident, or your nurse may have an idea if your physician has told them. Ultimately, under any circumstances, it will be the decision of your treating physician to send you home.

2. **Ask to meet with your physician prior to discharge.**

Though this should happen as a matter of routine, occasionally your physician may write an order for hospital discharge with residents, nurses, and case managers taking care of the details. If you were not seen by your treating physician prior to discharge, ask your nurse to page him or her so you can talk before going home. Your treatment team will not necessarily appreciate your needs and concerns.

3. **Try to determine a "ballpark" time when your physician will be coming by on the day before or the day of discharge.**

It can be virtually impossible for physicians to predict their whereabouts, given the capricious nature of their work, even when scheduled to be in the office. That's okay. You do not need a specific time. Often, I will tell patients "it will be in the morning between 8:00 and 10:00 or late afternoon between 3:00 and 5:30, or some time after 5:00." Knowing the "ballpark" will allow you to plan accordingly for transportation, having someone at home waiting, and most importantly, having someone come to the hospital to share in the discharge process.

4. **Whenever possible, arrange for a family member or friend to be present for the discharge instructions.**

This is very important. As I mentioned earlier, you or your loved one may not be in the best state of mind to assimilate what can be confusing and overwhelming information. This is important information! It may involve instructions for follow-up tests, treatments, new medications, side effects, and danger signs. A clear, focused understanding, even if not yours, is critical here. Write down everything that seems important.

5. **Write down questions in advance, or have someone help you to make the most of your discharge planning with the treatment team.** Here are some suggestions that may help as you prepare for discharge. These are questions for your nurse and physician

- What are the most important symptoms I or my family need to watch out for?
- What can I expect over the course of my recovery?
- What should prompt me to call you before my follow-up appointment?
- Is there anything that should prompt a visit to the emergency department?

- Which of the medications are new?
- What are some of the common side effects of these new medications that I may experience?
- Are you able to tell me how much these new medications might cost?
- Will any of these new medications interfere with what I was previously taking?
- Are there written instructions for these medications and for the important dietary changes? (There should be.)
- Are there any important interactions between my medications and things that I might eat?
- Could you please list the names of the physicians involved in my care and their phone numbers?
- What is the best way to reach you if I have a question or concern?
- Who can I expect to come to my home for follow-up care?
- Are my follow-up appointments clearly documented?
- Is there anything else that is important for me to know about that we have not touched on?

Here are some possible scenarios you could confront as you prepare for hospital discharge.

What if my loved one or I do not agree with the timing of the discharge? It seems increasingly common for patients and family to be uneasy about an anticipated hospital discharge. As mentioned, there are greater pressures to limit length of stay in the hospital. There is often an uneasiness around lack of a full recovery prior to discharge and general concerns about the "what ifs" that may or may not have been clearly addressed. Reassurance can go a long way and may require a brief review of the big picture and the overall plan. The reality of acute care, that is, the treatment of a problem that has developed over days to a few weeks is such that any time the level of treatment reaches a point that it can be managed outside the hospital setting, discharge will be contemplated. Most hospitals have *case managers*. These are professionals who work with your providers to facilitate timely discharge from the hospital and to ensure that adequate resources are in place to best meet your needs after discharge. This is a process that starts soon after a hospital admission.

In my experience, *concern around the timing and appropriateness of a discharge from the hospital comes more frequently from family than from patients themselves.* One reason for this, as I mentioned, is that patients are anxious to be home and are less likely to resist that decision. Patients, as they are recovering from an acute illness, may not clearly appreciate the realistic challenges of safely managing at home. I cannot tell you how often I have looked into the eyes of a patient who was quick to comment, "Dr. Pettus, I'm feeling better and ready to go home. I can manage fine." I then look into the eyes of their spouse or children and receive a very different non-verbal message. I must emphasize that it is very uncommon for an individual who is medically unstable to be considered for discharge from the hospital. This should never happen. There are, however, a growing number of individuals who come through our hospital systems whose margin of stability is tenuously slim. There may be a fine line, for example, between a stable gait and the possibility of a fall. The ability to maintain understanding and control over a complex prescription regimen can be undermined easily by transient confusion, forgetfulness, excessive fatigue, or prolonged malaise. These are obviously important issues that I find most families concerned about. There may be a critical disparity between the perceptions of safety and timeliness of a discharge plan by the health-care team and the more precarious reality that is not clearly communicated by the patient as they "deny" the potential for problems and the need for more help. It is a mutual lack of clarity in communicating current health concerns, expectations, limitations, and the need for the all-important *reality check* that perpetuates this disconnect. This is where families play an important role, in person or over the telephone, in painting a more realistic picture of the home environment.

As noted earlier, the pressures for families to organize resources for home care are becoming more challenging. Medical progress, worthy and remarkable though it is, has culminated in a growing prevalence of chronic, often progressive problems that over time, or after an acute illness, will require a much greater level of attention and care. While there may not always be an easy way to defer a hospital discharge, there are many things to consider that can diminish the likelihood that you will find yourself at odds with the system. Here are some suggestions for you and your family to consider in preparation for the next steps of care.

- **It is key to openly share thoughts and concerns with other family members.** Do not wait until there is a serious problem or crisis to discuss these matters. It is human nature to avoid contemplating the unsettling "what ifs." It is extremely difficult to confront the growing fragility of a loved one whose independence is threatened, even if for a short time. Unpredictable though these circumstances can be, we do often see the potential writing on the wall. Consider these important and often unspoken thoughts:

❖ Who would take time out of work, if necessary and if at all possible, to care for your family member?

❖ Where will you/your loved one live if not at home?

❖ What resources are available to assist in the home, if necessary?

❖ What would my mother or father want under these circumstances?

❖ Are the individual and family aware of the potential danger of living alone, unassisted?

❖ Is the individual aware of my loving concern for his or her safety and wellness? How clearly have I expressed these concerns?

❖ How will we address transportation needs, administration of medications, home care, and other issues?

• **If your loved one or you is hospitalized and has concerns about what the circumstances will be upon discharge, see if you have a case manager involved in your care planning.** Discuss your circumstances with the case manager. It is very important to advocate for your loved one by sharing your perspective with a case manager in a way that your loved one may not. Start this process as early into the hospitalization as possible.

• **Do your best to discuss your concerns with the supervising physician.** This is a dialogue that should start promptly after the decision to admit to the hospital is made. Physicians are busy people who receive many calls, and it will sometimes require perseverance on your end to connect. You can leave your name, phone number, pager number, etc. with the nurse caring for your loved one to call back. You can do the same at the physician's office. There simply is no excuse for an important call not to be returned.

• **Consider a family meeting if discharge planning might require a major step like transferring to a nursing home or skilled nursing facility (SNF).** (See chapter 7, The Family Meeting.)

• **If you learn about a discharge and are surprised because the timing and planning were not as originally discussed, find out from the nurse caring for you or your loved one who the discharging physician is.** Frequently, a covering physician will make what he or she feels is a safe and reasonable decision to discharge without knowledge of a particular issue that was not communicated. If your primary care provider laid out a clear plan on Friday, and his/her covering colleague lays out a different plan on Saturday, make this discrepancy clear. It may be, and often is, a simple misunderstanding. Covering physicians, particularly on weekends, are bombarded with patient care issues and may not be aware of the finer details of something you or your family discussed with your main provider a day or two ago.

Occasionally, you may feel you are being discharged against your best interest, particularly around legitimate issues of safety.

1. Make sure you and your family discuss this directly with the physician responsible for discharge to clear any misunderstanding or miscommunication (this is usually all that is necessary). You may feel angry, perhaps appropriately so, and constructive, effective reconciliation is more likely with calm collaboration than it is with angry polarization. (See chapter 16, Managing Conflict.)

2. It is not inappropriate, in my opinion, to ask that a covering physician on call for the group call your usual primary care provider if there is a significant difference of opinion around discharge planning. A quick phone call, if your primary provider can be reached, may save both parties unnecessary confusion, anger, time, and energy.

3. Last but not least, hospitals should have a patient relations professional, whose job it is to mediate and facilitate a more clear understanding of these issues. This, when done well, usually reconciles the circumstances. Please keep in mind that physicians should be advocates for you in addition to providing expert care. They also need to understand as much as possible about your circumstances to avoid the all too common gap between expectation and reality. They will need your help in narrowing that gap. Conflict around discharge planning should not become a singles tennis match with you or your family competing against your opponent . . . the physician or the hospital. It should instead be a doubles match . . . you or your family and the physician/hospital playing against the obstacles that stand in the way of safe and effective care planning. As is true in all aspects of one's relationships with a physician and all issues of health and wellness, the responsibility should and must be shared.

DO NOT MISS TAKE HOME POINTS

1. Be as clear as you can in your understanding of the main problems that were present during the hospitalization.
2. Be as clear as you can in your understanding of what to expect after discharge.
3. Have any new medications been added? What and why?
4. What are the most important things to look for after discharge; for example, signs of improvement or of a setback?
5. What are the next steps for follow-up, such as appointments, testing, and the like?
6. If possible, have someone with you when you receive your discharge instructions.
7. Be honest and realistic about any additional help you may need after discharge.

CHAPTER 11

TAKING MEDICATIONS
To Heal, Not to Harm . . . and
Less Expensive, Please

"A desire to take medications is, perhaps, the greatest feature which distinguishes man from other animals."

—Sir William Osler

THE OBJECTIVES of this chapter are:

- To lower your risk of potential medication-related complications
- To lower your risk of non-compliance or an inability to take your medication in the manner it was prescribed
- To reduce your costs for prescription and non-prescription medications
- To reduce the number of pills you take over the course of the day

The pharmaceutical industry has profoundly altered the potential for effective medical treatment by virtue of its prolific research and development of new medications and applied insights. The number of pharmaceuticals out there for treatment of a wide range of medical problems has never been greater. It is challenging even for physicians to keep track of all the various medications reaching the market. The enormous potential for medications to promote improved health outcomes is accompanied by their potential to harm, particularly if not taken appropriately.

Never has a society consumed as much medication as we do here in America. There is something one can take in the form of powder, tablet, caplet, capsule, syrup, chew, into the vein, into the muscle, into the joint, under the skin, or rubbed onto the skin, for just about anything. Some of these pharmaceuticals are unproven and, even if proven, when taken incorrectly, potentially unsafe. Sophisticated research and development, direct to consumer marketing, aggressive promotion, potential for lucrative market share, and a "needier" medication-taking oriented society, have converged to create a vast marketplace for pharmaceuticals.

In the year 2001, Americans spent over $150 billion on prescription medications. This does not include nonprescription medications, nutritional supplements, or herbal remedies. Over three times as many medications are available today as there were twenty years ago! Sir William Osler's quote from 1891, at the introduction of this chapter, could not be truer today, over 110 years later! The escalating costs of research and development, federal regulatory processes, marketing and advertisement, combined with skyrocketing consumer demand, have generated enormous expenditures in health care from prescription medications.

Costs can get in the way of the best intentions of the physician and the patient.

In addition, there have been enormous societal benefits. Newer, more expensive medications not only increase the costs of care, they can be prohibitively expensive for many patients, a common source of noncompliance, the inability to take the medication as prescribed.

This can be particularly challenging for our "maturing" population, often on multiple medications and on a limited fixed income. A recent survey published in the *Journal of the American Medical Association* of prescription drug use among the ambulatory, that is, non-institutionalized adult population, indicated that more than 90 percent of persons over the age of sixty-five used at least one medication per week. More than 40 percent used five or more different medications per week, and 12 percent used ten or more different medications per week! Adults over the age of sixty-five buy 30 percent of all prescription drugs and 40 percent of all over the counter (OTC) drugs in the United States. Greater prescription drug, OTC drug, and herbal/botanical use have resulted in a far greater number of potential medication side effects, adverse drug reactions (significant problems related to the use of a drug or combination of drugs that exceeds common side effects and results in some type of injury), drug-drug interactions, drug-nutrient interactions, and a growing number of patient safety concerns.

There are substantial costs in potential lives lost, need for hospitalization, emergency department visits, tests, and further treatments as a consequence of medication-related problems. Approximately $100 billion per year is spent as a direct/indirect consequence of these complications! The National Pharmaceutical Council estimates that more than 100,000 people die each year from noncompliance or an inability to take medications as prescribed. This is almost twice the number of deaths from automobile accidents. It is estimated that medication errors are responsible for one out of twelve hospital admissions and one out of eight emergency department visits. It is also estimated that in one in every one hundred times a medication is administered in the hospital setting, an error occurs.

When people are asked what they worry about most when it comes to their medications, they respond as shown:

Concern	Percent of Respondents
Receiving the wrong medicine	61
Drug interactions	58
Costs	58
Complications	56
Inadequate information	53
Side effects	49
Taking too many medications	49

Lowering Your Risk of a Medication-Related Complication or Compliance Problem

Figure 11-1 that follows summarizes the common sources of medication errors. As you can see, there are many potential sources of error introduction in the process of prescribing, transcribing, dispensing, administering, and educating in this costly and complex world of taking medications.

What Can You Do to Avoid Medical Errors? Be Informed.

As is true in every aspect of the health-care encounter, your greatest asset for success and maximal effectiveness is your knowledge and understanding of the what, when, and why of taking medications. Nonprescription does not always mean safe. Herbal or "natural" does not always mean safe (see chapter 14, Complementary and Alternative Medicine). The more you or someone who cares for you knows about your medications, the less likely it is that you will encounter an error or adverse effect.

Figure 11-1.   What are the sources of medication errors?

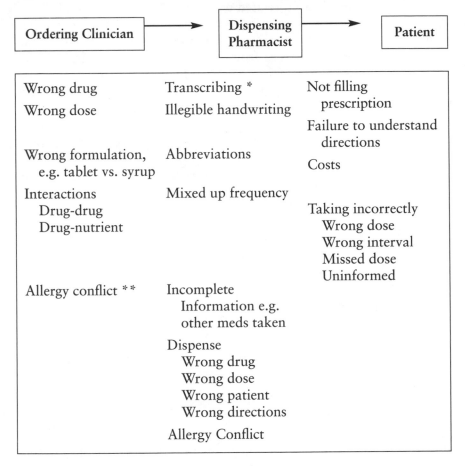

*Problems with transcription refer to the process of transferring information from the prescribing physician to the pharmacist e.g. from a telephoned prescription.
**Allergy conflicts occur if a medication is prescribed that is a known allergy or if it is in the same family of medications you are known to be allergic to.

Pharmacists: The Essential and Forgotten Player on the Health-Care Team

Pharmacists are an essential link in the chain of health care. You need to assume an active role in partnering with them. Pharmacists are medication experts! The role of the pharmacist has shifted from preparation and dispensing to provision of patient-oriented services, education, awareness, and monitoring. Pharmacists train in a five-year Bachelor of Science (B.S.Pharm) or a six-year Doctor of Pharmacy (Pharm.D.) program. For the tenth consecutive year, America's pharmacists topped the Gallup Poll list of business and professional people for "honesty and ethical" standards.

Pharmacists are under-recognized, under-utilized and under-appreciated members of the health-care team!
It is wise to choose a pharmacist as you would choose any professional. Establishing a relationship with a pharmacist by having all of your prescriptions filled in one place will allow knowledge of you, your medications, and your health needs/concerns to be concentrated in one place, with a familiar group of professionals. Many potential sources of error, referred to earlier, can be dramatically reduced via such a partnership. Your pharmacist serves as an important source of information for any questions you may have regarding medication you are taking or prescribed. As you are likely to receive prescriptions from more than one source, consistency with prescription service, the pharmacy, and pharmacist, will make more likely recognition of duplication, potential for drug-drug interactions, and possible allergy conflicts. For example, two different physicians might prescribe a medication that has a different name but are in the same family. As you or the prescribing physicians may not be aware of this, your pharmacist will quickly be able to pick this up as a potential problem, having filled these prescriptions and having a computerized record of your medication history. Potentially serious medication-related errors and adverse effects are more likely to be identified.

Think of your physician and your pharmacist as a powerful team.
Your pharmacist can also monitor your therapy, including non-prescription medications such as vitamins, nutritional supplements, and herbal products. Your pharmacist can provide you with excellent printed materials, as he or she will have access to a large, comprehensive database of information. Here are some examples of questions to consider asking your physician and pharmacist to become better informed:

- What are the brand *and* generic names of this medication, if available? Not all medications are available in a generic form.
- What is this medication for?
- How much should I take and how often?
- When is the best time to take it?

- Should I take it with an empty stomach or with food?
- Is it safe to drink alcohol while I am taking this medication?
- How long will I need to be on it?
- What side effects do I need to look out for?
- What should I do if I miss a dose?
- Will this interact with any of my other medications?
- Where should I store it? Will it be affected by exposure to sunlight, humidity, or extreme temperatures?
- Are there less expensive generic equivalents of this medication? This is very important as it could save you significant sums of money.
- Are there longer-acting forms of this medication that would allow me to take it less frequently, for example once or twice daily instead of three to four times daily?
- Will my allergies be affected by this medication?

Avoiding Medication Errors at Home

Approximately 30 to 50 percent of people who use medications do not use them as directed. This is a staggering statistic! Much can be done, in addition to acquiring knowledge and understanding, to reduce your risk of a medication error.

- Make a list of your medications, including non-prescription medications.
- Include the dose, description of the tablet (shape and color), how often you take it, and what you are taking it for.
- Keep this list up-to-date with any changes that are likely to occur.
- Document any allergy you may have on this list.
- Include your physicians' and pharmacist's names and telephone numbers on your medication list.
- Keep a copy in plain view at home and a second in your wallet or pocketbook.
- Keep pills in their original container except for those you are placing in a special organizer such as a weekly pillbox.
- Read all prescription bottle labels carefully to make sure the person, drug, dose, and frequency are clear and understood. Also, keep a watchful eye on any special precautions that are "flagged" on the label.
- If you have trouble with your vision, have important instructions printed in large print or have someone you know read the labels for you.

- Make sure you know the expiration date, as the effectiveness of the medication may diminish considerably if the date has expired.
- Try your best not to skip any prescribed doses and understand what you should do if a dose is inadvertently missed.
- Shake liquid medication vigorously to assure thorough mixing prior to taking.
- Keep medications safely away from children.
- Make sure the room is well lit when you take your medication to ensure what you are taking is indeed what you intend to take.
- Never take another person's medications. You may be tempted if it is a medication that has worked for someone else under similar circumstances. We are all different, even if our diagnosis might be the same. You may experience allergic symptoms or other side effects that could be potentially dangerous even if someone you know has not had a problem taking the medication.
- Let your prescribing physician and pharmacist know if you are pregnant or are breastfeeding, as some medications can affect the fetus or be transmitted through breast milk.
- Be careful *not* to chew or crush a capsule or enteric-coated medication intended to be swallowed.
- For liquid medication, use a precise, pre-measured syringe or spoon for more accurate dosing administration. Your silverware teaspoon or tablespoon may not be accurate.

If you go to the emergency department or hospital, it is very important to bring a list of your current medications with you. Take this list with you if you are traveling out of town. It is also good practice, when seeing your primary care provider, once or twice per year, to brown-bag your medications in their prescription bottles for review, confirmation, and clarification. *If you are in the hospital, you should feel certain and comfortable that all of the medications being dispensed are accurate and consistent with what you have been taking at home.* You should be informed or inquire about any medication that is new or different. If you have allergies, make sure they are well documented by letting your nurses and physicians know, as well as having this on a written list that should accompany you at all times. Frequently, when in the hospital, the dispensing routine for medications and dietary restrictions may vary from what you are used to at home. Any departure from what you are accustomed to, particularly if it is causing problems, such as a low blood sugar reaction because of a different dose of insulin or dosing schedule, should be addressed with your treatment team. This is particularly important in the hospital management of diabetes. If you are able, assume as much control over this aspect of your management as you feel comfortable with. People taking insulin for many years have good instincts about the regimen that works best for them.

Food-Drug Interactions

Fortunately, most food-drug interactions are mild and do not cause serious harm. Any time, however, that a food or beverage has the potential to alter the effect of a medication, a food-drug interaction is possible. As people take larger varieties of pharmaceuticals and supplements, the potential for interaction with food is on the rise and being recognized with greater frequency. Most medications are not at all influenced by nutrients, and if they are, it is by specific nutrients such as calcium or iron. Food-drug interactions can occur with OTC, prescription, herbal, and dietary supplements.

While foods may affect drug activity by how they are prepared or how much you ingest, most have an effect on the absorption of medications due to the timing, for example, one or two hours between ingestion of the food and ingestion of the medication. Occasionally, nutrients can affect the metabolism of the drug once it is absorbed. An example of a food-drug interaction is the effect that vegetables high in Vitamin K, such as spinach and broccoli, have on the blood-thinning effects of warfarin or coumadin. Foods with high Vitamin K content inhibit this blood thinning effect that has important implications in preventing blood clots from forming or progressing. Ginkgo, Vitamin E supplements, onions, and garlic may increase the effects of blood thinners and increase the risk of bleeding. Dairy products high in calcium or calcium supplements, commonly used in the prevention and management of osteoporosis, can interfere with the absorption of some antibiotics such as tetracycline or similar antibiotics. Citrus, high in Vitamin C, enhances iron absorption. Iron supplements, if taken within a few hours of thyroid hormone replacement therapy such as Synthroid or levothyroxine, can inhibit the absorption of the thyroid medication. This is particularly important as your treating physician may feel you need more medication because blood tests suggest you are not getting enough. The problem may be that you are getting enough and it is not being absorbed.

Foods high in tyramine, an amino acid found in beer, wine, avocados, some cheeses, and processed meats, slow down the metabolism of an antidepressant medication family called MAO inhibitors. This interaction can lead to high blood pressure, a potentially dangerous interaction.

Grapefruit juice has been receiving a lot of attention because of its potential to interfere with some important prescription medications. A substance in grapefruit juice increases the absorption of some medications and can interfere with the liver's metabolism or breakdown of the medication. An example is in the use of cyclosporin, an important medication used in organ transplantation to prevent rejection. Another example is in the use of medications in a class called "statins," used to treat high cholesterol.

If you have any questions about food-drug interactions, talk to your pharmacist and discuss how best to navigate with respect to your medications. PPSI, Pharmacy Planning Services, Inc., is a California non-profit corporation offering a large number of programs to promote public health and awareness. More information on food-drug interactions can be found on their Web site in addition to other useful information on medication safety: www.ppsinc.org/fooddrug.htm.

Drug-Drug Interactions

Among the most frequent sources of medication errors, side effects, adverse reactions, and costs of treatment are the drug-drug interactions. It is commonplace to see individuals taking three or more medications at the same time. So common is this circumstance that medical students, residents in training, and I often view the "over sixty-five" individual taking less than two or three medications as noteworthy. This has become the exception, not the rule. While this phenomenon is more common in general, it is particularly problematic in the elderly. Chronic medical conditions, alteration in metabolism from changes in liver or kidney function, changes in diet, changes in body distribution of fat and muscle, and a lower threshold for side effects, put our elderly population at greater risk for drug-drug interactions. There are too many published drug-drug interactions for me to discuss in detail here.

The greater potential for these sometimes-dangerous interactions requires your being mission-oriented in having your physician and pharmacist assess this specifically. Some drug-drug interactions will be so mild as to leave you unaware. Other interactions may have the effect of:

1. Enhanced effect of one or both medications
2. Diminished effect of one or both medications

This might manifest itself by new signs; for example, easy bruising because of the enhanced blood thinning effects of coumadin or warfarin when taken with antibiotics. It may be found by routine blood work, for example, increased prothrombin time or INR in a person on coumadin or warfarin and antibiotics. It may express itself with symptoms of diminished appetite, nausea, or fatigue related to recent changes in your medications or doses of medications.

Drug-drug interactions are also possible with non-prescription medications:

- NSAIDs or anti-inflammatory medications such as Ibuprofen and Naproxen can interfere with the blood pressure lowering effects of diuretics such as hydrochlorothiazide (HCTZ).
- Decongestants such as pseudoephedrine can raise blood pressure, particularly in people taking MAO inhibitors, a class of antidepressants.
- Easy bruising can occur in people taking aspirin or other blood thinners and ginseng or Vitamin E.

To assist consumers with OTC use and safety, the American Pharmaceutical Association and McNeil Consumer Healthcare (makers of Tylenol) have joined efforts to form the Partnership for Self-Care, a three-year educational program to diminish the risks of OTC drug interactions.

Additional information can be obtained at:

- www.pharmacyandyou.org
- www.safemedication.com
- www.drkoop.com (hit link to "drug information")

Strategies to Assure Compliance

Noncompliance, as noted, is the failure to take the prescribed medication as intended. Noncompliance can vary from not taking the medication at all, missing doses, taking doses at incorrect times, taking too much, taking too little, or not following directions. Noncompliance leads to excessive costs—more than $100 billion per year estimated by the National Pharmaceutical Council; emergency department visits; hospitalizations; delays in clinical improvement; lost school/work productivity; and absenteeism. Evidence supports several common causes for failure to comply (see figure 11-1 on page 142).

- Lack of understanding, for example, importance, dose, time, directions
- Costs are a major reason people are unable to comply. In my experience, many people are reluctant to mention costs as an issue due to awkwardness, pride, shame, or embarrassment.
- Discomfort about taking medications in front of others at work, school, or when out socially
- Forgetfulness
- Concern about potential side effects or the actual experience of side effects
- Feeling better before the prescription is finished
- Medication regimen is too complicated, for example, too many pills taken at too many times per day

What Can You Do to Protect Yourself?

The best place to start is by having your physician or an office staff R.N. and pharmacist assist you with your understanding of all aspects of the prescribed medication. They can also assist with strategies to organize and simplify administration of your pills. Some examples might include:

- Keep a calendar to mark each time you take your medications.
- Have a family member or friend assist you with your medications.
- Use a weekly pillbox.
- Use a timer or watch alarm for reminders.
- Keep your medication with you if you anticipate having to take it while away from your home.
- If you think you are experiencing side effects, discuss this with your physician/pharmacist. What you are experiencing may be unrelated to your medication. If it is a side effect there may be better alternatives than just stopping the medication on your own.
- Consider ways to assist with keeping track of medications—keep a check-off chart or a color-coded chart, or color code medication vials with those on your medication list.

Costs

Costs are a major concern for many people who are prescribed medications. Many insurers, like Medicare, have not historically covered prescription medications. Congress is currently examining options to include some form of prescription drug coverage. At the time of this writing, Congress has passed a prescription coverage plan for Medicare recipients that will likely be modified with time. Congress has voted to allocate $400 billion in drug assistance over the next decade. This is estimated to represent approximately 25 percent of the amount seniors are expected to pay for prescription medications. This is clearly a legislative priority and a necessity. It is estimated that the average senior will have $3,160 in prescription drug costs per year in 2006. Starting in April 2004, all Medicare beneficiaries would be eligible to purchase a discount card for buying prescription drugs. Some Medicare recipients would see an immediate 10 percent to 15 percent cut in their prescription drug costs when filling prescriptions at their retail pharmacy. The cost for the card is thirty dollars. The full entitlement plan would take effect in 2006. Participation is voluntary, though a penalty surcharge may be imposed if a senior defers the decision to participate. Once the new benefit takes effect in 2006, the law will prohibit sale of Medigap policies that seniors can currently purchase to supplement coverage and reduce out-of-pocket drug expenses. This new policy may be difficult to understand. Private insurers and HMOs will be encouraged to offer competitive plans that may create confusion as to what is covered and for how much. At the time of this writing, coverage would break down as follows:

- Medicare recipients pay the first $250 as a deductible.
- They then share 25 percent of the costs between $250 and $2,250.
- They are responsible for all costs between $2,250 and $5,100.
- For catastrophic costs (greater than $5,100) they share 5 percent of the costs.

Individuals with incomes below $13,055 and couples with incomes below $17,619 and with assets no greater than $6,000 per individual and $9,000 per couple would pay no deductible and no monthly premium for their new drug benefit. Retirees with incomes above $80,000 for a single person and $100,000 for a couple would be required to pay more for their Part B benefits. Average premium costs will be $420 per year.

Many people without insurance are without jobs or struggling to make ends meet. The sad truth is that many medications are prohibitively expensive and as a consequence are not taken, even with an understanding of the potential health risks of doing so. The best intentions cannot ensure compliance under these circumstances. Many pharmaceutical companies have financial assistance programs. Ask your physician and your pharmacist for some suggestions. It is important to know what your insurer will cover. Some health plans cover specific generic or trade brands that may be similar to what you were prescribed, if not covered by your plan.

A new Web site offers a free service to assist older patients in finding out if they are eligible for prescription drug assistance. This was developed by The National Council on the Aging and will require filling out a short questionnaire. This is a nonprofit site also supported by AARP, the Pharmaceutical Research and Manufacturers of America, and endorsed by the Centers for Medicare and Medicaid Services (CMS). Drug discount card programs and government plans for which you are eligible will be listed. You can determine whether you are eligible for Medicaid or any of some 30 state-funded pharmacy programs or 116 company-sponsored patient assistance programs. This very good Web site called *Benefits CheckUp* can be accessed at: www.benefitscheckuprx.com.

Another Web site that may be of assistance is www.helpingpatients .org. This is designed to help health-care professionals with resources for their neediest patients. For over ten years members of the Association of Pharmaceutical Research Companies (PhRMA) have been providing free drugs for patients in need. In 2002 free medications were provided to over five million Americans. This would be a good Web site to give to your providers if they are not already familiar with it.

Obtaining larger quantities, particularly if it is a medication you have been taking for awhile, anticipate needing indefinitely, and at a stable dose, will be cheaper per dose. If that is not an option and you are strapped for cash, ask your doctor if he or she has any samples at the time you are given the prescription. Samples, in addition to being free, have the added advantage of allowing you to see how well you respond before filling a more expensive prescription. The pharmacist can also give you fewer tablets until you are able to afford more. For long-term medication use in stable doses, mail-order pharmacies can provide bulk medication at discount prices, for example in three-month supplies. Many pharmaceutical companies also offer discount cards for people who meet financial eligibility.

Generic Medications

When pharmaceutical companies develop new medications, they apply for a patent that prevents other drug manufacturers from producing similar drugs. These medications are more expensive given the costs to research, develop, and promote. The high demand for them adds to the costs. The lack of alternative manufacturers who can leverage costs through competition and increased supply also contributes to the high costs. When a patent runs out, usually after several years, other manufacturers can produce the exact equivalent medication. This is what generics are. Congress is soon going to pass legislation to allow generic medications to enter the marketplace more quickly. Generics also exist for nonprescription medications, usually found under the "store brand."

You will definitely save a signifi-
cant amount of money by com-
paring a name brand with a
store brand. As a random exam-
ple, take Tylenol™ and compare
to store brand acetaminophen,
or MotrinIB™ with ibuprofen.

Generic drug availability can significantly reduce medication costs, according to the Congressional Budget Office. Consumers could save eight to ten billion dollars per year! There is very little, if any, difference between generic and brand name drugs except for the costs. FDA-approved generic drugs meet the same rigid standards as the original drug.

Not all drugs are available in generic form. Most states have laws that allow pharmacists to substitute generic for brand names if the physician does not sign the "No Substitution" line on the prescription. One survey, published in 2001 in the _Journal of the American Pharmaceutical Association,_ found that 52 percent of physicians chose to allow pharmacists to substitute generic drugs rather than to write a prescription for the generic themselves. The bottom line is to ask your prescribing physician and dispensing pharmacist whether a generic equivalent is available.

In a recent study: AARP RXHEALTHVALUE and the COALITION for a COMPETITIVE PHARMACEUTICAL MARKET, one thousand people over the age of forty-five were surveyed:

- Ninety percent said they would accept generic versions of drugs in order to reduce out-of-pocket costs.
- Eighty-four percent believe greater access to generic drugs is an important way to control rising costs.
- Seventy percent said that pharmaceutical companies exert too much power over Congress.
- Sixty-six percent said they usually choose generics over brand-name drugs when given a choice.
- Sixty-six percent said they favor legislation to close the loopholes used to keep generic drugs off the market.
- Twenty-four percent said they have not been able to afford a prescription when no generic was available.
- For more information on generic medications, access www.fda.gov/cder/ogd.

Tablet Splitting

The economic burden on people struggling to reduce prescription medication costs has fostered the practice of tablet splitting. The reason for this is that if higher doses can be split into twice as many equivalent lower doses, similar to what you are prescribed (one 40 mg tablet split into two 20 mg tablets), you can get two tabs for the price of one. This is obviously true only if the cost of the higher dose is the same as the cost of the lower dose. This is indeed often the case. The American Pharmaceutical Association strongly recommends that individuals discuss this practice with their physician and pharmacist prior to splitting tablets. Economically appealing and perhaps necessary, tablet splitting should not be viewed as safe under some circumstances. Simple criteria for safer consideration of tablet splitting would include:

- Tablets are uncoated and scored with a clearly defined groove in the center of the tablet.
- Tablet breaks easily into two equivalent pieces without crumbling or fragmentation.
- There should be one clean break.
- The patient or the caregivers are able to split the tablet, using a knife or special pill-cutting device if necessary. Pill-splitting devices vary in price; you can probably find one for less than twenty dollars.
- Splitting a coated, sustained release capsule or fragmenting a pill into uneven pieces will clearly alter the dose. Capsules should not be opened or split.

Preventing Medication Errors in Children

As is true for minimizing the risk of any error with respect to your care, being informed, educated, and having a watchful eye make all the difference. Here are some tips developed by the Agency of Health-Care Research and Quality (AHRQ) and the American Academy of Pediatrics (AAP) for preventing medication errors in children.

- Be an active member of your child's health-care team. No one can advocate for a child more passionately than his or her parent. *Educate yourself to better advocate for your child.*
- Maintain accurate documentation of your child's weight, as medication doses are based on weight.
- Make sure that all providers have an updated list of allergies and prescription and nonprescription medications.

- When given a prescription, make sure you have documented your child's name, the drug name, dose, frequency, duration, and special precautions.
- Give your child the entire amount prescribed even though your child is likely to feel better before the medication is finished.
- Clarify expectations for side effects, anticipated time for improvement, and "what to look for."
- Know and write down on your list of *emergency phone numbers*, the number of your state Poison Control Center. You can find this at: www.pharmacyandyou.org/poisoncontrol/poisoncenters.html.

Your children will have questions when they take medications, as mine usually do. You and your child can learn together by asking questions of concern. What will the medicine taste like? Does this medication come as a pill to swallow, a chewable, or a syrup? When do I take it? Will I need to take it at school or at work? Do I need to limit my activity in any way while on this medication?

Internet Pharmacies
It is safest to have one source for obtaining your medications. If a person receives some medications locally and some via the Internet, there is a greater risk of not knowing about a potential allergy or drug-drug interaction. It can also be advantageous to have access to a pharmacist, as there is no substitute to talking with someone face to face. Community pharmacies also sometimes offer other health-related services such as blood pressure screening and cholesterol checks, and they can help monitor your progress as they establish a relationship with you.

DO NOT MISS TAKE HOME POINTS

1. Understand as much as possible about the medications you are taking (prescription and nonprescription), such as what they are for, common side effects, and how often you should take them.
2. Nonprescription or natural does not necessarily mean safe.
3. Are there any important interactions, such as between medications or medication-food that you need to know about?
4. Do effective and less expensive generic substitutes exist for what you are taking (prescription and nonprescription)?
5. Keep a list of your medications in your wallet.

CHAPTER 12

CONTEMPLATING NURSING HOME PLACEMENT

When Home May Not Be the Best Option

*"Where duty is plain, delay is both foolish and hazardous;
where it is not, delay may provide both wisdom and safety."*

—Tryon Edwards

THE OBJECTIVES of this chapter are:

- To review the common conditions that lead to consideration of nursing home placement or extended care
- To review the options for living outside the home
- To provide a Medicare-based checklist of necessary features to look for in choosing a quality nursing home or extended-care facility

Over ten years ago, my mother was discharged from the hospital after a prolonged and complex medical course, marked by many complications. She was a young woman, in her early sixties, with numerous medical issues. She had suffered a stroke that left one side of her body weakened and made her unsteady on her feet. She had chronic progressive failure of her kidney function and was confronting the need to start hemodialysis. She had depression, a lifelong problem intermittent in severity, which had worsened over the previous months. On top of all of this, she had suffered a heart attack that had left her heart weaker. A once vibrant, energetic, very funny, and determined soul was now weak, debilitated, and dependent on others to safely navigate tasks most would take for granted. She was devoid of the very spirit of life that characterized her loving, remarkable, and outgoing nature. It was, to say the least, a heartbreaking transformation of a life marked by zeal and deep faith, to one deeply wounded and broken. My father's health had deteriorated as well over this same period of time. He lost his vision from a stroke and remarkably did all he could to adequately care for himself. He could do some things to assist my mother; however, the scope of her needs far exceeded his capacity to deliver what he could have had he been healthier. My sister, whose work was extremely demanding and consuming, took on the role as primary caregiver. Her unrelenting love, purpose, courage, and boundless strength made it possible for my mother to be at home, the dream of a lifetime she and my father had worked so hard to reach.

I had just finished my renal fellowship at The Massachusetts General Hospital and had moved to the Berkshires in western Massachusetts, about 150 miles from Boston, Massachusetts where I grew up. It was impossible for me to work, raise a family, and be with my mother as much as she required from the standpoint of daily needs and safety. Uncertain of the future, my father, sister, and I realized sadly that she might one day soon need to be placed in a nursing home or skilled nursing facility. This was an unthinkable reality at her young age. It would be a last resort. We had visited a few nursing homes in our area. My mother had improved some, and with the tireless devotion of my father and sister, she was able to remain in her home until she died four years later. This was made possible by exceptional commitment and sacrifice, often not possible by virtue of the demands on people's lives.

There is no place like home. For most people, home is an extension of who they are. Our homes silently embrace our most meaningful experiences and surround us with a comforting familiarity. Our homes are a constant in an ever-changing world. Our homes are where our deepest thoughts, concerns, joys, fears, and privacy dwell. In my experience as a physician, there are few decisions more painful to contemplate than the need to place a loved one in a nursing home. Reaching this difficult crossroad implies that the circumstances you are confronting are not likely to turn around. It also implies that all options to allow safe and acceptable living in the home setting have been exhausted.

The need to consider alternative living settings for those we love dearly is an increasingly common scenario. Examples of such alternative settings include:

- **Independent living:** These are often apartments in a community-oriented complex. Community meals and other resources such as transportation, housekeeping, and other conveniences may be available. People choosing this option are well enough to function safely and independently. Being in a community setting offers additional security for support resources if needed and very importantly, the social support of community inclusion, stimulation, and participation.

- **Assisted living facilities:** These resident settings are also for independent living with available resources for meal preparation and assistance with activities of daily living such as shopping, cleaning, bathing, and dressing. They also offer nursing support for health maintenance and emergency needs.
- **Skilled nursing facilities:** SNF or nursing homes offer more complete twenty-four-hour available nursing and skilled care.

The need for skilled nursing facilities has grown remarkably in the last ten years. There are many reasons for this. We are an aging society, and the odds are that we will one day confront an acute illness, or more likely a chronic, progressive illness that will challenge our ability or a loved one's ability to safely and effectively live independently. As our ability to treat acute and serious illness improves, we are seeing many "survivors," who over time develop problems such as chronic emphysema or other lung diseases; chronic kidney diseases eventually requiring dialysis; cardiovascular diseases; chronic arthritis; Alzheimer's; Parkinson's; and others. These are in some respects "diseases of medical progress." The effects that many of these chronic progressive problems have on physical, emotional, and spiritual wellness can, over time, overwhelm the available resources necessary for safely remaining in the home setting.

Federal and state funding for home care has seen dramatic cuts over the last five years. The Balanced Budget Act, in an effort to rein in escalating Medicare expenditures, redefined criteria for receiving reimbursement for home care. Medicaid coverage and reimbursement have also been significantly reduced as states struggle to balance their budgets in the midst of "the perfect storm" of fiscal uncertainty and budget deficits. As a consequence, it is becoming increasingly difficult to receive skilled care except for an hour here and an hour there. This is simply not enough to allow many people to remain at home.

In addition, the network of family support, that years ago might have been readily available to share in the care of a loved one, has become destabilized. For example, it is now uncommon for many siblings to remain in the same town they grew up in. Educational and occupational opportunities have scattered many families, often to great distances from a needy loved one. The significant others we meet in our lives are more often not from the area we grew up in. Siblings, even if nearby, are usually fully immersed in situations where they and their spouses must work to get by. In addition, they are more likely to have younger children to care for. Many baby boomers, like me, find themselves part of the "sandwich" generation. There is a strong likelihood that we may become responsible for the safety and wellness of our parents in addition to the needs of our children, while at the same time having to work one or more jobs to make ends meet. This is a very difficult and exhausting place to be. It is also a rapidly escalating social dilemma and a major problem for home health-care support these days.

While I discuss long-term-care insurance in chapter 17, it is worth mentioning here. If you are confronting an imminent need for nursing home placement this will not help you at this time. However, if you or a loved one have a chronic medical disease that may progress over time, making it impossible to be at home, long-term-care insurance is definitely worth thinking about.

Long-Term Care Insurance

Since the start of the twentieth century, our life expectancy has almost doubled. When I finished my training twenty years ago, it was uncommon to be treating a person over the age of ninety in the hospital. It is now common to be treating people in their late eighties, nineties, and with greater frequency, at one hundred years of age!

Most people, as they age, will confront a debilitating illness such as stroke or heart disease, or a chronic progressive illness such as Alzheimer's that limits their ability to care for themselves safely and independently. Long-term insurance (LTI) was conceived as a consequence of this reality. LTI provides coverage for care received at home as well as in a skilled nursing facility. Examples of covered services include:

- Home health aides assisting with bathing, dressing, and other everyday activities
- Homemakers who assist with chores such as cleaning, shopping, or meal preparation
- Long-term skilled nursing care
- Rehabilitative therapy

Most traditional insurance plans cover these services minimally or not at all. Medicare pays for home health care with time limitations and only under certain conditions. Medicaid covers skilled nursing in nursing homes. There are stringent financial criteria with respect to income; for example, your income must be less than twice the official poverty level and your assets must total less than $2,000. To become eligible, people often have to "spend down" their assets to meet the criteria. My father was forced to do this for transportation! Transportation is a real problem for many people who are unable to drive. My father needed dialysis treatments that required transportation three times per week. As he was legally blind, he was unable to drive. The nearest dialysis center was twenty-five miles away. He had Medicare and for many years paid expensive premiums for Blue Cross/Blue Shield, an excellent insurance plan. Transportation, however, was not covered. Taxi fare would have cost fifty dollars per round trip, three days per week, fifty-two weeks per year. You can do the math. On a fixed income with a meager pension and social security, this simply was not possible. As a consequence, he had to "spend down" to become eligible for Medicaid, as this was the only means of covering his transportation. It was a nightmare.

Long-term care is expensive, as average annual nursing home costs are now in excess of $55,000 per year! Skilled nursing at home can cost approximately twenty-five dollars an hour and home health aides ten to twenty dollars an hour. This can add up quickly, depending on the nature of the underlying medical problem, the overall need for home support, and the available additional resources such as spouse and family to assist with care.

Premiums for long-term care are variable, depending on the range of benefits needed, the age of the insured, and other factors. One consideration is the benefit period, such as three years to lifetime; daily benefit, for example, $150/day in a nursing home, plus $100/day for home care; "inflation protection"—if nursing home costs rise, your benefits will rise as well. Expect your premiums to increase as you get older. As of this writing, LTI premiums average approximately $2,200 per year.

In general, long-term-care insurance is a good idea if you can afford it. It can be a comforting safety net, particularly as chronic progressive health-care problems are increasingly common and not adequately addressed by most types of health insurance.

Despite our most loving intentions and efforts, the needs of a loved one can exceed our resources. It simply becomes untenable to allow a loved one to stay at home. There is tremendous guilt attached to the contemplation of a nursing home placement. This feeling of guilt emerges, as our desire and need to do more cannot always be met by the perpetual and certain demands on our lives. In addition to feelings of guilt people often experience *shame*—embarrassment, dishonor, or a feeling of disgrace, as expectations for reciprocating loving support for our parents, as we get older, are overwhelmed by the complex demands of our circumstances. Compounding this, a loved one, such as a parent, may bitterly resist nursing home placement. After all, who wouldn't? An aging, proud, and sometimes stubborn parent or grandparent may not recognize the risk they are to themselves and the deep pain their families are confronting as these circumstances unfold. The paradox here is that people who are at the greatest risk when at home are least likely to be aware of the risk. It can be exceedingly difficult to get a loved one to see and understand the tenuous and potentially dangerous nature of his or her circumstances, particularly if the alternative is to be placed in another setting for daily living.

The recognition of needing nursing home placement may be seen as the ultimate threat. It can represent a threat to that last precious vestige of independence and privacy; a threat of being displaced from one's precious "space" and all that it represents; a threat to the "only way of life I know."

I have found there is no easy way to reconcile these feelings. It may require a meeting of family and friends. This has to be done sensitively and delicately so as not to be perceived as a threat or collusion. Sometimes having *trusted* individuals such as friends, family, physician, or pastor lovingly share their concerns, helps bring a harsh and necessary reality into proper focus. The one sentiment I hear most often expressed by patients as they see their independence slipping away is "I would never want to be a burden on my family."

If you are struggling with the need to have a loved one placed in a skilled nursing facility and the individual is persistent in his or her struggle to remain at home, you might rephrase your concerns. "Mom, I know how much your home means to you. It is where your dreams became reality and where your life has journeyed for many years. Are you fearful that you cannot find happiness and joy elsewhere? Do you feel abandoned? Do you feel that your relationships with friends and family will change? You mentioned you would never want to be a burden on us. There is no burden so great that our love cannot handle. The only burden I could not bear is the burden of having something happen to you while you are alone at home. This is a burden that I am currently confronting. It is a burden we all are confronting. At times it seems it is too much to bear."

Though no one template or formula can easily reconcile the dilemma that nursing home placement creates, a person's perspective may shift when he or she understands that the "burden to bear" for loved ones can be substantial under the current circumstances. Framing your concerns in this manner addresses the specific values of your family member, for example, "not to be a burden." This addresses the fundamental issue that many people needing nursing home placement confront—that as long as I am home and as independent as possible, I am less of a burden to my family, even if the risks of being at home are unacceptable. For the individual confronting nursing home placement, the burden is that of increasing dependence on others. For loving family, the burden is one of safety and wellness. The shared burden is one of uncertain and profound change and grasping the reality of a major turn in one's life. Some individuals may not see the reality until repeated hospitalizations or emergency department visits for situations such as progressive weakness, repeated falls, or worsening nutrition brings home the tenuous nature of the current situation. I should add that nursing homes can on occasion be used for a short stay to bridge an acute care hospitalization, such as for a stroke, to eventually returning home. Some problems may require several weeks of intermediate care such as physical, occupational, or speech therapy; nutritional support; or ongoing skilled nursing for wounds, medications, and IVs, with anticipated improvement over time. This support can best be provided in a skilled nursing facility. Contingent on the level of improvement, returning home may then become a safe and feasible option. Rehabilitation hospitals and transitional skilled nursing programs are a superb alternative for the more intensive care that some health problems may require. They can be viewed as a bridge from the acute care hospital setting to home over a period, usually of several weeks.

Long-term skilled nursing is considered when intermediate transitional care will not result in a significant enough improvement to allow a person to return home, within the limits of resource availability, safely and effectively. There may be some alternatives to nursing home placement, though these are usually contingent on available human and financial resources such as long-term-care insurance to cover some home services; or financial resources/insurance to provide nursing, PT/OT, home health aides, and personal care attendants, or PCAs. The Family and Medical Leave Act (FMLA—see chapter 17, Health-Care Coverage) may allow you to assist a loved one, without jeopardizing your job, particularly if the nature of the underlying health problems is such that some improvement is possible and expected. Elder services and community-based day programs may provide a *social day-habilitation* environment if the circumstances are appropriate. My mother participated in such a program in our community. It was a godsend! It provided her with a nurturing and caring network of friends and support staff. It was an essential socially stimulating environment that would not have been possible at home. It provided much-needed respite for my father, as my sister worked long hours during the day. Consider a "meals on wheels" program to assist with meal preparation and provision. A social worker or caseworker in your local hospital or through elder services can assist with identifying as many community resources as possible to assist with the care of an individual, short of nursing home placement.

For more specific information on over 17,000 Medicare and Medicaid-certified nursing homes in the United States, go to the government site for people with Medicare, www.medicare.gov/nursing/overview.asp.

The Web site contains useful information on alternatives to nursing home care, inspections, paying for care, patient rights, and a nursing home checklist (see page 163). A section entitled Nursing Home Compare is a tool to access comparison information about nursing homes, including:

- Nursing home characteristics such as number of beds, ownership, Medicare or Medicaid participation
- Resident characteristics
- Comparison data on some quality measurements such as percent of pressure sores, urinary tract infections, etc.
- Summary information about nursing homes during their last inspections
- Information on the number of R.N.s, licensed practical nurses, nursing assistants, and other staff in each nursing home. Information about nursing home inspections including health deficiencies and complaint investigations is available. In addition, a detailed information guide (64 pages) entitled "Guide to Choosing a Nursing Home" can be downloaded and viewed in Adobe PDF format.

Like many profound life changes, the anticipation of what is to happen is often much worse than the eventual experience. It is natural for our worst fears to become the implicit assumptions of what the future will hold. My mother was adamant about not attending our local community social day-habilitation program. I believe she was sensitive to being out of the house, cognizant of her disabilities, and insecure in a new environment. This is a natural and anticipated response to such circumstances. In the end, it was one of the great sources of joy in her life. Many people, as they struggle with profound physical, emotional, and spiritual wounds, see themselves as "incomplete," unable to contribute as they once could. I am convinced there is no such thing as a disabled spirit. The essence of our humanity is capable of transcending the most trying of circumstances.

What my mother did not anticipate was how much she was able to give to others, under any circumstance. In receiving she was able to joyously give. And by giving she was able to joyously receive. The experience was profoundly more positive than she or my family could ever have anticipated.

As you contemplate nursing home placement, consider, if possible, taking your parent or grandparent to visit nursing homes you are considering. With advance planning, the staff should be happy to provide a tour and to allow observation and participation in some community social activities. Consider opportunities to talk to some of the residents. The staff can consider in advance who could best share experiences in a way that might comfortably relate to your loved one. In the end, difficult though it will be, you do what you know in your heart is best.

Nursing Home Checklist			
	Yes	No	Comments
Basic Information The nursing home			
Is Medicaid-certified.			
Is Medicare-certified.			
Has the level of care needed (e.g., skilled, custodial).			
Has special services, if needed, in a separate unit (e.g. Alzheimer's or dementia, ventilator, or rehabilitation).			
Is close enough to allow family and friends to visit.			
Has a bed available in the appropriate unit.			
Resident Appearance			
Residents are clean, appropriately dressed for the season or time of day, and well groomed.			

	Yes	No	Comments
Living Spaces			
Free from overwhelming unpleasant odors.			
Clean and well kept.			
Temperature is comfortable.			
Has good lighting.			
Noise levels in dining room and other common spaces are acceptable.			
Smoking is not allowed or is restricted to specific areas.			
Furnishings are sturdy, comfortable, and attractive.			
Staff			
Relationship between staff and residents appears warm, polite, and respectful.			
All staff members wear nametags.			
Staff knock on the door before entering residents' rooms.			
Staff refers to residents by name.			
Nursing home offers training and continuing education for staff.			
Nursing home does background checks on all staff.			
Your tour guide knows residents by name and is recognized by them.			
A Registered Nurse (R.N.), other than the Administrator or Director of nursing, is in the nursing home at all times.			

	Yes	No	Comments
The same team of nurses and Certified Nursing Assistants (C.N.A.s) works with the same residents 4 to 5 days a week.			
C.N.A.s work with a reasonable number of patients.			
C.N.A.s are involved in care planning meetings.			
A full-time social worker is on staff.			
A licensed doctor is on staff. Is he or she there daily? Can he or she be reached at all times?			
The management team has worked together for at least one year.			
Residents' Rooms			
Residents may have personal belongings and/or furniture in their rooms.			
Each resident has storage space (closet and drawers) in his or her room.			
Each resident room has a window.			
Residents have access to personal telephone and television.			
Residents can reach water pitchers.			
There are quiet areas where residents can visit with friends and family. Residents have a choice of roommates.			

	Yes	No	Comments
There are policies and procedures to protect residents' possessions.			
Hallways, stairs, lounges, bathrooms, and exits are clearly marked.			
The nursing home has smoke detectors and sprinklers.			
All common areas, resident rooms, and doorways are designed for wheelchair use.			
There are handrails in the hallways and grab bars in the bathrooms.			
Menus and Food			
Residents have a choice of food items at each meal (ask if favorite foods are served).			
Nutritious snacks are available upon request.			
Staff members help residents eat and drink if necessary.			
Activities			
Residents, including those who are unable to leave their rooms, may choose to take part in a variety of activities.			
There are outdoor areas for residents' use; staff helps residents go outside.			

	Yes	No	Comments
Safety and Care			
The nursing home has an emergency evacuation plan and holds regular fire drills.			
Residents get preventive care, such as flu shots.			
Residents may see their personal doctors.			
The nursing home has an arrangement with a nearby hospital for emergencies.			
Care plan meetings are held at times that are convenient for residents and family members whenever possible.			
The nursing home has corrected all deficiencies (failure to meet one or more federal or state requirements) on its last state inspection report.			
Additional Comments:			

DO NOT MISS TAKE HOME POINTS

1. Making the decision for yourself or for a loved one to relocate to a nursing home or long-term care facility is one of the toughest you will ever face.
2. It is essential to be aware of limitations in the home that simply cannot ensure a safe and supported quality of life.
3. Consider a family meeting with your physician if you or a loved one are uncertain about the best course to take.
4. Engage the services of a case manager who can help you explore your home care and nursing home care options and the financial/insurance implications.
5. Visit a few long-term care facilities with family members. Be mindful of what your "gut" tells you as to the best fit.
6. Use the nursing home checklist as a guide for questions when you examine nursing home options.

CHAPTER 13

PREPARING FOR SURGERY
Staying a Cut Above

"Surgeons must be very careful
When they take the knife!
Underneath their fine incisions
Stirs the culprit—life!"

—Emily Dickinson

THE OBJECTIVES of this chapter are:

- To help you understand what you need to know to be best prepared for upcoming surgery.
- To review the basic types of available anesthesia.
- To emphasize the importance of minimally invasive procedures.
- To review current guidelines with respect to medication use just before and after surgery. Emphasis is placed on blood thinners and diabetic management.

Most people will confront the need for surgery during their lives. It may come suddenly and unexpectedly in the form of acute appendicitis or it may be electively planned in advance in the form of gallbladder removal, for example (in medical terms known as a cholecystectomy). It may be a minor procedure requiring local anesthesia such as cataract removal or a major procedure requiring general anesthesia such as the removal of an aneurysm (also known as AAA or abdominal aortic aneurysm—not to be confused with the Automobile Association of America).

Obviously, it is hard to prepare for an unexpected problem like a rup-

tured appendix. The best advice our parents gave us, in the event of an unexpected trip to the hospital, was to wear clean underwear. I must say, as a
physician, this is something I have never, ever, paid any attention to, not to
discourage its importance. To a large extent, the degree to which a patient
does well during and after an operation is determined by the shape they are
in as they go to the operating room (O.R.). To that end (see chapter 20 on
the best medical advice possible), there are many important aspects to the
preparation for surgery, whether expected or unexpected, that you need to
be aware of. Some are healthy habits for daily living that can leave you
holding better cards in preparation for an operation. For example:

- Exercise regularly—at the minimum, walk for thirty to forty-five
  minutes four to five times a week.
- Stop smoking! This can make a huge difference even if stopped
  within weeks of your planned operation. It is both very, very tough
  and very doable. Anticipated surgery can serve as a potent motivator to reexamine the habit.
- Maintain a balanced diet with respect to fruits, vegetables, grains
  and moderate fats and carbohydrates. Remember, "Color on the
  plate adds color to your life."
- If you are prescribed medications, take them faithfully, unless told
  otherwise by your treating physicians.

If your surgery is planned electively, there are several important issues
to consider as you prepare.

How Informed Are You?

**Do you have a clear understanding of the reasons for the operation,
including the risks and the benefits?**
This may be quite clear in the case of removing a ruptured appendix or
less clear in the timing of removing a gallbladder with gallstones or the
surgical removal of an aneurysm in the abdomen. Indications for proceeding with surgery may be heavily influenced by the presence of other medical problems such as heart disease, diabetes, chronic lung disease, and
advanced age. "Advanced" is a subjective determination. Physicians often
look less at chronological age and more at physiologic age, the state of
health, performance capacity, or functional status of an individual. For example, an eighty-five-year-old with few underlying medical problems who
can easily carry a bag of groceries in each arm up a flight of stairs is likely

to be in much better physiologic shape than a fifty-year-old with diabetes and heart disease who is short-winded and laboring after walking fifty feet. Age is a relative factor only. On the other hand, an indication to proceed with an aneurysm repair in a sixty-year-old with high blood pressure will be met with much greater caution in an eighty-year-old with heart disease, diabetes, and kidney failure. A careful review and understanding with your physicians of your *individualized* risks and benefits is very important. It is also very important to bear in mind that what may be an *unacceptable* risk or an *acceptable* benefit will vary between individual patients and physicians.

Are there options other than surgery that may change the risk-benefit analysis?

For example, as techniques and outcomes improve, some problems may have reasonable treatment alternatives to surgery. The results, for example, with balloon angioplasty and aggressive treatment with medications for selected individuals will provide results comparable to coronary artery bypass surgery for narrowed or blocked coronary arteries. This is not to say that CABG ("CABBAGE" or bypass surgery) is not effective. People do marvelously well with this procedure, but there may be less invasive options. Many people are referred to surgeons after "failing" medical management such as use of medications, behavioral/lifestyle modifications, or less invasive procedures. It never hurts to ask your primary care physician if all non-surgical options have been considered. Here are some common examples of surgery being necessary because "less invasive" alternative medical therapies have failed.

- G.E.R.D.—Gastroesophageal Reflux Disease, though usually responsive to medications, can sometimes be resistant, prompting consideration of surgery.
- Diverticulitis—this is inflammation of the colon, usually on the left, lower side of the abdomen, where an out-pocketing (common as we age) bursts. This causes pain and usually fever.
- Amputation of a toe, foot, or leg because of a severe infection, unresponsive to intravenous antibiotics, wound care, and analgesia (pain control). This is a problem more common in diabetics.

Are there different techniques for performing this necessary surgery and how might they differ in outcomes and recovery?

Many interventions that once required more extensive surgical incisions can be done with minimally invasive techniques, using fiber optics or endoscopy. These small scopes require much smaller incisions, often less than an inch long. Through fiber optic visualization and use of ultra small "microsurgical instruments," a procedure that historically required a several-inch incision can be done just as effectively. Surgeons who perform these techniques have special training in "laparoscopic surgery." Examples where these techniques (a list that is growing) are being used successfully include:

- Removal of a gallbladder with gallstones—laparoscopic cholecystectomy
- Hernia repair
- Gynecologic procedures such as treatment or removal of an ovarian cyst
- Breaking up or "lysis" of adhesions or scar tissue that occurs after previous surgical procedures. These adhesions can, over time, block or partially block the intestinal tract, causing nausea, vomiting, abdominal pain, and distention. Distention refers to a growth in size of the abdomen due to increased buildup of gas behind the blockage.
- Laparoscopic removal of the appendix
- Weight-reducing surgery, also known as bariatric surgery

There is a growing list of accepted indications for minimally invasive surgical procedures. If laparoscopic, less invasive surgical alternatives exist and are appropriate for your particular circumstances, look into this. Advantages include smaller scars, diminished pain, less time in the hospital, and faster recovery time.

Another example of a less invasive intervention for which experience is still growing is in the treatment of aneurysms in the abdomen. Aneurysms are a balloon-like effect in the aorta, the large blood vessel that connects the heart with other organs. We know that aneurysms beyond a certain size have a greater risk of rupturing. This is a catastrophic event that is often fatal. Historically, the only way to repair these was to have a vascular surgeon remove them. This can be a big operation with many risks involved. In recent years, there has been interest in using stents, artificial, synthetic mesh-like material that opens as a sleeve, placed into the aneurysm to secure it in the hope that a more involved and risky operation can be avoided. Though not appropriate for everyone and still being studied as an alternative to conventional surgery, this is an example of the growing number of alternatives to riskier operations currently under study.

Should I get a second opinion?

This is an important consideration whether or not you are having surgery, if the diagnosis, treatment, or both leave you with any uncertainty. With many medical problems, diagnosis and treatment are very straightforward and leave little room for doubt. Here a second opinion will not add anything and could possibly result in a delay of important time-sensitive treatment such as unblocking a coronary artery or removing an aneurysm. It is also possible that having more of your questions and concerns addressed by your care providers can clear up any lingering uncertainty you have.

Some health insurers may require a second opinion before an elective surgical intervention is scheduled. This is their way of making sure there is no other, usually less expensive, alternative and that the surgery is clearly indicated. Though the insurer's interests may be in part financial, the options resulting from another opinion may be in your best interest. I've given many second opinions, and in my experience the greatest benefit is *reassurance* that the diagnostic and treatment options are the best available for your specific circumstances.

People may desire a second opinion but feel awkward or uncomfortable asking this of their treating physician. This uneasiness usually results from concerns that the treating physician will be angry, or that a feeling of distrust will ensue. You may be concerned that your physician will respond defensively, as if his or her credibility is being challenged. Physicians sometimes have large egos—for example, the kind of egos that years of hard work, deep pride, practice success, and meaningful values cultivate. The ego can occasionally get in the way of more meaningful understanding. Some physicians may react defensively to the suggestion of a second opinion. In my experience this is very uncommon, though it can occur. The bottom line is this: if delaying a test or intervention by obtaining a second opinion will not put you at greater risk *and* if it will leave you with a greater sense of peace, comfort and trust, *go for it*. You may or may not confront out-of-pocket costs, however, depending on your insurer and your individual circumstances.

Here are some thoughts on how you can share your interest in a second opinion with your treating physician, in a way that will meet your needs and be perceived as minimally threatening:

"Dr. _____, I appreciate all you have done for me to this point. I understand that you feel the best next step is this _____ treatment (or this _____ surgery). You might imagine how the thought of this operation is making me somewhat apprehensive and even a little scared. I feel I would be reassured by seeking a second opinion. This is in no way a judgment about your competency or about my trust in you. Again, I appreciate all you are doing and will probably soon realize that the advice you have given is indeed the best advice for me (if not, the second opinion was indeed a good idea). I hope you appreciate that my intent is to be as informed as possible before moving forward to this next big step. I'll be in touch soon thereafter. Thanks again for your help."

You may be thinking that this is unnecessarily delicate toward the physician's feelings. After all, any physician who reacts negatively and defensively in response to a request for a second opinion may not be worthy of your trust. I would hardly disagree. The main issue here is influence and how best to serve your needs and values.

A surgeon, for example, may have the best experience and outcomes for a particular procedure, such as bariatric surgery for weight reduction. His or her ego may not allow the request for a second opinion to be received without a sarcastic, defensive response and possible refusal to consider your case. It is also rare in my experience. Your needs and values here may be more technical than interpersonal, particularly if this is a physician with whom you will have a limited term of care.

Any treating physician who doesn't react favorably to these concerns would, unfortunately, be missing the point. Quite frankly, a negative response might indicate that the physician does not understand where you are coming from.

What are my options for anesthesia?

You should meet with the anesthesiologist before your surgery to review this. The anesthesiologist will review all available options and recommend the one he or she feels will best allow smooth sailing and post-operative comfort. Options include:

- **General Anesthesia:** This implies being put to sleep. This may require a tube temporarily placed into your windpipe (trachea) to allow adequate breathing while asleep. You are put to sleep prior to placement of the tube. The tube is removed as promptly as the clinical circumstances allow. Some operations must be done with general anesthesia, for example neurosurgery involving the neck or brain, chest surgery involving the heart or lungs, major procedures in the abdomen, and others.
- **Spinal or epidural:** This type of anesthesia can be very effective for surgery in the lower abdomen, pelvis, or legs, such as for repair of a broken hip, hysterectomy, or hernia repair. Here a small tube

(smaller than an IV) is placed into the lower back after a local anesthetic has been applied. Once the tube is in the space around the spinal cord, anesthesia can be given. In addition, pain medications can be given through this route and can provide an excellent means for pain control after surgery.

- **Regional anesthesia:** This is used when operating at a more distant area on the arms or legs, where only that extremity is anesthetized.
- **Local anesthesia:** A "local" is used to "numb" just the area involved in the procedure, such as removal of a skin growth or suture of a wound.

The risks of anesthesia are reduced, in general terms, as less of the body is anesthetized. Anesthesiologists will also often use "conscious sedation" in addition to a spinal or regional strategy. This is a process in which medications are used to produce a sedated, relaxed state, sometimes affecting the short-term memory after the procedure. A common example of conscious sedation is that which is used during a colonoscopy procedure. These are short-acting agents that leave you feeling pleasantly drowsy. Your memory for recent events will usually be impaired as the sedation wears off.

Anesthesiologists are the experts here. They will explore the best options with you.

What are the potential complications from and after surgery, and how likely are they to occur?

This is much too broad a topic to review in detail here. You should have a clear understanding of this, however, before going ahead with surgery or any special procedure. Complications can occur from the underlying problem for which you are having surgery, such as a stroke if you are having a carotid endartectomy (cleaning out a narrowed or blocked artery in the neck), or from the surgery itself, for example, a wound infection or bleeding. The risk of complications goes up considerably if the nature of the underlying problem you are having surgery for is serious, as in removal of a lung tumor or if you have other medical problems such as heart disease or diabetes. For example, you may be having surgery to improve the circulation in your legs and are at greatest risk from your heart. No surgical intervention is without risk. It is certainly fair to ask your surgeon what his or her most common complications are and how often they occur, particularly in people like yourself. Generalizations may not apply if you have many other medical problems.

How long can I expect to be in the hospital, and what can I expect during the recovery period?
You will again be given "ballpark" figures that may vary considerably if you have other medical problems. LOS, or length of stay in the hospital, has diminished remarkably over the last twenty years. I cannot believe how much this has changed since I started in practice over fifteen years ago. Many factors will determine how quickly you recover after an operation. Depending on your circumstances, the nature of the surgery, experience with post-operative pain, complications, and mobility, the time it will take for you to function safely, comfortably, and independently at home will vary. It may take some time after your discharge from the hospital. Having a clear sense of what to expect will allow you to plan ahead. This planning may include arrangements for your spouse or other family members to be more available until you have recovered or planning home services such as nursing care or housekeeping to assist your convalescence and recovery. You or your family member may need to plan time out of work with an eventual "step up" return based on the type of work you do, the nature of your operation, and your level of improvement. Many people require transitional care between the acute care hospitalization and returning home. This might include a rehabilitation stay in an inpatient facility. Here there would be a focused multidisciplinary (team) approach to strengthen, condition, and stabilize your general ability to walk and get around, and to improve any activity of daily living (ADL) that will be necessary to improve your independence and safety. A transient skilled nursing stay (SNF) may be necessary to allow less acute care or intermediate care to more safely bridge you from hospital to home. Intermediate care, depending on the circumstance, might last anywhere from two to four weeks.

I have, on occasion, cared for patients who were surprised and disappointed that they could not return home immediately after surgery. Often, these "surprises" are hard to see coming. If for example, an unexpected complication occurs or if other underlying medical problems exist, the pace of improvement can be slower than expected. Anticipating and planning for intermediate care, when possible, will diminish the "expectation-reality gap" that may occur after your surgery. In my opinion, narrowing this gap leaves the individual more positive, emotionally and mentally focused, and with more realistic expectations. These are all key elements to the healing process.

As you recover from surgery, or any significant illness for that matter, discomfort, medication-related side effects, limited mobility, more prolonged than expected healing, altered sleep-wake patterns, and diminished appetite and strength will challenge your *motivation* and *will* to move forward. In my experience, one of the best determinants of how well and how quickly a patient recovers from surgery is how fast the individual begins to mobilize. Motion is the lotion! Movement "lights up the brain" in areas that leave one feeling more confident, in control, and upbeat. Movement, difficult though it may feel early on, actually lessens discomfort and improves mood over time.

You may have to force yourself to move through the pain. You may have to push yourself to transcend the fatigue. You may have to motivate and inspire yourself to rise above the frustration of an uphill climb against obstacles (see chapter 4, Coping in the Midst of Illness).

It's not always enough to just say "I can do it." Try this. Think about the activities and aspects of your life that bring you the greatest joy. Allow these images to fill your mind. See yourself, every dimension of who you are, moving in that direction. Allow the gifted medical personnel to enter your life in the most effective way possible. Take a chance. Allow the "opportunity" of sharing your frustration, fears, and concerns with those whose role it is to move you closer to the door, to bring you nearer to where you want to be. Have faith. Stay focused. Do the best you can. No one could ever ask for more! Ask your nurse or doctor if you can talk with a patient going through a similar experience. This might be an enormous help to you.

What specific testing will I need prior to surgery?
The testing required prior to surgery varies depending on the nature of the surgery and on your underlying medical problems. For example, removal of a skin tumor or cataract may only require routine blood work, if anything at all. More involved surgery, such as a bypass operation in the legs to improve circulation, will involve more testing (see chapter 18 on common medical tests), like blood work to check red blood count (known also as hemoglobin and hematocrit), platelet count (platelets are blood cells that assist with blood clotting), electrolytes (potassium, sodium), kidney function (BUN and creatinine) and blood clotting efficiency (PT/PTT or INR, prothrombin time). A routine electrocardiogram (ECG) may also be done. A person with a more extensive cardiac history, such as a heart attack or angina, may need to see a cardiologist before the surgery to get expert advice on steps to take to lower the risk of a complication. This might require more testing, for example, stress testing, or an echocardiogram, a sound wave test of the heart, depending on how stable your cardiac status is and the degree of risk to your heart from the surgery itself. On the far extreme, individuals preparing for an organ

transplant would require extensive testing to be certain that everything is as "fine tuned" as possible, given the risks of the surgery and medications used to prevent rejection of the organ.

Most operations will only require routine blood work and an ECG (or EKG).

What should I do with my medications before surgery?

Your treating physicians should review medications in detail with you before your surgery. Most medications will be continued until the morning of surgery. If you have diabetes, your medication or insulin will probably be reduced on the day of surgery; in the case of medication by mouth, it may be withheld altogether. Insulin doses are often reduced by 50 percent, as you will not be eating in typical fashion. Your sugar will be monitored closely and adjustments made as necessary to achieve adequate control.

An important observation here is that often people who monitor their blood sugars closely at home and have "tight" control (fingerstick sugar < 110 first thing in the morning and < 160 after eating), will see the numbers go out of whack when in the hospital. Your surgery, underlying medical problems, and change in dietary intake will affect your blood sugar readings; patients are often frustrated that things are "done differently" when in the hospital, compared to at home. If you feel able, suggest that you play a more active role in the management of your blood sugars while in the hospital. The type of insulin and doses you would ordinarily use, and the timing of insulin administration, are extremely important factors in maintaining tight control. Best medical evidence suggests this to be critical in reducing infections, heart complications, and other problems. It is also essential to partner with your care providers to avoid unnecessary low blood sugar reactions. This is a scary thing indeed. Often we make the mistake of using a one-size-fits-all approach to the management of diabetes—what we call a "sliding scale" approach, based on sugars checked at times unrelated to meals, bedtime, or other activities. I have had many patients share with me their concerns and frustrations with how different this management is compared to their home strategies. We often remove management of blood sugar in the hospital setting from the very person who knows himself or herself best—the patient. We are very accustomed to the one-size-fits-all approach in the hospital setting, an approach not proven to be effective at all.

How sensitive a person is to a particular dose and timing of insulin can be quite variable. For example, six units of regular insulin for a blood sugar of 300 may be fine for one individual, and for another may send the sugar through the floor. If you have these concerns, discuss them with your primary nurse or treating physician. Fingerstick sugars should always be checked first thing in the morning, prior to meals, and at bedtime. They may require more readings at other times depending on the clinical circumstances. A one-size-fits-all approach that involves checking sugars three or four times a day without any relationship to fasting state, meals, or bedtime is, in my opinion and that of most endocrinologists (diabetes specialists), unsafe and ineffective. If you are able, recommend the doses and types of insulin that work best for you. Having adjustments made in your oral medications or longer-acting insulin is much better than frequent doses of short-acting insulin during the day. It is preferable to be in as much control as possible. There . . . now I feel better.

A few other generalizations about medications and surgery:

- Be particularly careful not to stop any medications you are taking for your heart unless specifically instructed by your physician.
- If you are on a blood thinner such as Coumadin or Warfarin discuss clearly and in detail what you should do prior to surgery. Your physician will determine this strategy based on the risk of a complication while off the medication, for example, a clot in the heart with an artificial heart valve, possibly causing a stroke or a clot in the heart chamber from atrial fibrillation, with the benefit of reducing bleeding complications from the surgery itself. These can be complex decisions, though they will usually fall into a few categories:

  ❖ **The risk of a clot complication is high and the risk of bleeding from surgery is low;** for example, removal of a small skin tumor in a person with an artificial heart valve. Usually the Coumadin (Warfarin) is continued without significant change.

  ❖ **The risk of a clot complication and the risk of bleeding from surgery is high;** for example, removal of an aneurysm in a person with a mechanical heart valve. Usually the person is admitted to the hospital one or two days before the surgery. Their Coumadin is discontinued and they are placed on heparin (a different kind of blood thinner). The heparin is stopped about twelve hours before surgery and restarted twelve to twenty-four hours after it. Once a person is stable after surgery, usually on the second or third day, the Coumadin is restarted while heparin is continued. Once the Coumadin has the blood adequately thinned (INR or prothrombin time is in a good range), the heparin is stopped.

❖ **The risk of a clot complication is low and the bleeding risk is high;** for example, a person with chronic atrial fibrillation undergoing removal of a lung tumor. The Coumadin may be discontinued five to seven days prior to surgery and restarted two or three days after surgery if all is well. Heparin may be started at that time until the Coumadin has begun to work again (usually five to seven days).

There are other important issues to discuss with your physician. More and more people are on aspirin or another "antiplatelet" medication such as Clopidogrel, Plavix, Aggrenox, or Persantine. Traditional thinking was always to withhold these medications approximately one week before surgery in order to minimize bleeding complications. While the jury is still out on this issue for many surgical procedures, it may be best to continue these medications, particularly if you have a history of heart disease or stroke, or if the surgery you are having is "vascular"; for example, bypass of coronary arteries or for poor circulation in the legs. Cardiovascular complications may be reduced by continuing these important medications with benefits potentially far in excess of the risks for bleeding.

If you are on a statin, a class of medications to lower cholesterol (examples of brand names are Lipitor, Zocor, and Provachol), it is probably best not to stop these before surgery. They may have "vascular protecting effects" independent of their cholesterol lowering effects. A sudden discontinuation of these medications (like aspirin and aspirin-like agents) can cause a "rebound" effect, increasing the risk of cardiovascular complications such as heart attack, angina, stroke, or even death.

Glucophage or metformin, a commonly prescribed medication for diabetes, should be stopped forty-eight hours prior to surgery. It will usually be restarted in forty-eight hours after your operation if all is going smoothly.

And last, but by no means least, if you are anticipating surgery using general anesthesia and you have risk factors for heart disease, such as . . .

- History of heart attack (myocardial infarction)
- Angina, that is, chest discomfort or breathing problems from a narrowed or blocked coronary artery, or if you have more than two of the following:

- History of peripheral (lower leg) circulation problems
- Age >65 years
- High blood pressure
- Diabetes
- High cholesterol
- Family history of heart disease, in a male age <55 or a female age <60

. . . ask your physician about the potential benefits of a medication belonging to a class of drugs called *beta blockers* (e.g. Atenolol, Tenormin, Lopressor, Toprol). There is some evidence in the medical literature that starting these medications, if you are not already on one, for one to four weeks before surgery and continuing for at least one week after surgery, may reduce your risk of having a heart attack or heart-related death after surgery. These medications may not be for everyone, such as people with a history of severe lung disease, asthma, or slow heart rate, but they are certainly worth discussing with your treating physician. This is an inexpensive intervention that could produce dramatically beneficial effects on the cardiovascular system. I am coordinating an effort in our hospital to improve the likelihood that eligible individuals at high risk for heart disease, and in the absence of a slow heart rate (less that sixty beats per minute), who are undergoing surgery under general anesthesia, will be placed on a beta blocker medication before, during, and one week after their operations.

How many operations like mine do you perform each year, and how do your complication rates compare to state/national averages?
This may seem like an awkward question to ask a surgeon. It is like asking about a second opinion. I certainly do not mean to suggest that this is an appropriate question to ask for all operations. There is some evidence, however, to suggest that some operations performed by surgeons in "high volume" centers may have fewer complications associated with them. Recent studies demonstrate an important relationship between surgical volume and patient outcome. While hospitals that perform more complicated operations may have better outcomes, the data suggests this to be more specific to the surgeons and their individual volumes. Individual surgeon volume may trump hospital volume. This is not an issue for procedures like groin hernia repairs and removal of inflamed gallbladders. Studies also suggest that travel time to the nearest high volume surgical centers would not be prohibitive for most individ-

uals. Operations where statistics and results may be available and variable include:

- Organ transplants
- Heart bypass operations
- Aortic valve replacements
- Repairs of aortic aneurysm in the abdomen
- Surgery for weight reduction
- Surgery involving removal of part of the esophagus
- Removal of parts of the lung, most commonly for cancer
- Surgery involving the pancreas, for example, "Whipple's" procedure, or removal of a tumor

It is also true that volume is only one of many factors that might result in variable results from one hospital to another. The skill of the individual surgeon, other involved physicians, hospital systems, and types of patients being served are important factors that play a role in determining outcome. I have always been impressed with the remarkable capacity of surgeons to treat the most complex of problems. The body has remarkable healing capacity, even after very involved interventions.

It is important that your primary care provider and any consultant, such as a cardiologist or pulmonologist (lung specialist), be notified of your date for surgery. Their concurrent input into your care or just "checking in" can play an important role, even when all is smooth sailing. Sometimes, inadvertently, those key players are left out of the loop. You may need to call and remind them yourself. As you probably know, the more reminders a busy physician gets, the better.

DO NOT MISS TAKE HOME POINTS

1. Be as informed as you can be.
2. Make sure you are comfortable with your understanding of the risks and benefits of your operation.
3. Get a second opinion if you feel that one is warranted.
4. Discuss with your treating physicians any reasonable nonsurgical options, if they exist.
5. Discuss the availability of minimally invasive procedures such as laparoscopy, that may be less risky and allow a faster recovery.
6. Be clear on what to do with your medications before surgery.

7. Do not stop any heart medications prior to your surgery unless specifically instructed by your treating physician.

8. If you have diabetes and are able, be an active contributor to your management, for example, timing and dose of insulin, blood sugar testing, and diet.

9. Be clear on the "typical" post-operative course in order to prepare and plan accordingly, by arranging more help at home, planning a transitional return to full work duties, or anticipating the possible need for interim rehabilitative/skilled nursing care between your surgery and your return home.

10. Alert other specialists involved in your care about your scheduled plans for surgery.

CHAPTER 14

COMPLEMENTARY AND ALTERNATIVE MEDICINE

A Primer on "CAM" Therapy

"A human being is part of a whole, called by us the Universe, a part limited in time and space. He experiences himself, his thoughts and feelings, as something separated from the rest—a kind of optical delusion of his consciousness. This delusion is a kind of prison for us, restricting us to our personal desires and to affection for a few persons nearest us. Our task must be to free ourselves from this prison by widening our circles of compassion to embrace all living creatures and the whole of our nature in its beauty."

—Albert Einstein

THE OBJECTIVES of this chapter are:

- To provide a general overview of CAM or integrated therapies.
- To emphasize the importance of these therapies as *best integrated with*, not kept separate from, traditional medical models.
- To provide excellent sources of information that will empower you to make safer, more effective decisions.

There have been considerable shifts in thinking about health, healing, and the inherent limitations of modern medicine in meeting the varied and complex needs of human beings. Western perspectives on health and disease examine how we feel and how we heal in terms of alterations in our normal biologic structure and function. To be sick is to have an alteration of this beautifully fine-tuned biology. To be cured implies restoration of this biologic homeostasis. For millennia, ancient worldviews have seen the project of healing as a natural intersection of the physical and the spiritual. There is a growing and fascinating body of research illustrating the complex connections between our emotions and attitudes and well-defined effects on our biology and physiology. The field of psychoneuroimmunobiology is that which interconnects our feelings with our thinking with our immune function with our general state of health. When one considers the project of health as renewal, restoration, and maintenance of our incredibly integrated amalgamation of mind, body, emotion, and spirit, broader contexts within which we understand and treat emerge.

I have been out of medical school for twenty years. I am amazed at the growing sophistication of modern medicine's scientific insights. These insights have profoundly changed the potential for treatment, cure, and longevity. Current molecular (e.g., genetic or chromosomal) insights will soon enable an understanding of many diseases that hitherto have been beyond our full grasp. These insights, as they grow exponentially, will allow potential cures that will dramatically alter life as we know it. As an example of modern medicine's progress, I will never forget observing a renal (kidney) transplant while doing my fellowship training at Massachusetts General Hospital. An individual whose kidneys had long since failed, requiring dialysis for years, was in the process of receiving a kidney that had been removed from a young man more than one thousand miles from Boston.

The donor had sustained a tragic motor vehicle accident. Because he was without brain function and had no hope for a meaningful survival, his family agreed to allow his organs to be donated. A transplant team flew to the area and harvested his kidneys. His kidneys were "preserved" to maintain their viability. Within hours, this kidney was placed into the abdomen of a woman who would never know the young man from whom it came. Because her kidneys had failed and she had required dialysis for many years, she had not made a drop of urine in some time. Her diet had to be dramatically altered to prevent accumulation of potential toxins in her system. Her quality of life was challenging and marked by fluctuations in energy, mood, and appetite. She acquired a "technologic dependence," that is, chronic hemodialysis, for survival. Within seconds of receiving the kidney transplant, urine began to appear while she was on the operating table. Now it may be hard to appreciate the joy that observing urine production can bring, particularly in someone incapable of kidney function for over ten years! For those present in the operating room, it was indeed a welcome sight.

Consider the things we take for granted. For this and many other reasons, when my children were very young, I was one dad who welcomed the opportunity to change a wet diaper. After the transplant, the patient was placed on sophisticated anti-rejection medications and made a fine recovery. The quality of her life was profoundly changed for the better with the assistance of many sophisticated medication protocols. This is science and modern medicine at its very best, and for many problems people confront in their lives, there is no substitute.

If practicing medicine has taught me anything, it is that human beings are marvelous and complex tapestries, with remarkable healing potential. The construct from which I, and most physicians, have been trained falls short of providing a clear and satisfactory understanding of the many cases we confront. In illness and in health, people are increasingly interested in looking outside our conventional system of care for healing of the mind, body, and spirit. Our wounds are not just physical. Biology is not the only language that expresses our wounds. People are increasingly curious and interested in alternative frameworks or paradigms for understanding disease and health, particularly if they can result in a quality of life that traditional or conventional perspectives and methods might not allow.

Currently, approximately 50 percent of Americans spend billions of dollars on what is referred to as CAM, or Complimentary and Alternative Medicine. I must say, as a "conventionally" trained physician, I am anything but expert in this field. Andrew Weil is a leader in the research, writings, and insights of Integrative Medicine. I highly recommend his books as interesting, balanced, and informative sources of information on CAM. The growing diversity and availability of CAM therapies is beyond the scope of this chapter.

It is intuitive to consider that in a self-sustaining ecosystem, as is this wondrous cosmos, inherent paths to healing can be found from within and from what nature surrounds us with. Some of our most important drugs; for example, digitalis used to treat heart failure or atrial fibrillation and taxol, a cancer-treating medication, are of plant or botanical origin. It is now necessary for physicians to understand how CAM therapies can be effectively applied, understand their potential toxicities, and understand their limitations. So important has this area become that the NIH (National Institutes of Health) recently started a separate division to promote research, understanding, and education in this area, the National Center for Complementary and Alternative Medicine, or NCCAM. In 2000,

Congress provided almost $70 million to support the efforts of this division of the NIH. It reflects a significant, meaningful, and necessary shift in modern medicine and the scientific community's interest and willingness to explore uncharted waters in this important area. NCCAM is a necessary response to a growing social mandate to address other potentially useful healing perspectives and therapies, as well as to serve a vital public health, education, and safety role.

"Alternative" and "natural" do not necessarily mean effective and safe. For example, some herbs like Kava, that may have medicinal benefits in relieving anxiety, are now known to cause, in some instances, potentially life-threatening liver damage and death. I will elaborate on the importance of this example in a moment.

As people are clearly interested and willing to spend enormous sums of money on CAM therapy, there must be some meaningful understanding, to the extent that it exists, of the implications of these therapies. As I noted earlier, I am not an authority on this topic. There are many excellent texts and reviews of this vast and growing area. I will provide some references where excellent information can be obtained in more detail. First, it would help to define some terms.

Traditional or conventional medicine, at least as defined by Western traditions, would encompass an understanding of disease and treatment as learned and applied by most practicing M.D.s (Medical Doctors), D.O.s (Doctors of Osteopathy), and other allied health professionals such as P.A.s (Physician Assistants), N.P.s (Nurse Practitioners), physical therapists, R.N.s (Registered Nurses), psychologists, and others. A growing number of "conventionally" trained practitioners have interest, training, and skills in CAM.

Complementary Medicine examines treatments that are used *in addition* to conventional treatments. These time-honored modalities have many proven medical benefits. Common examples include meditation and its role in reducing blood pressure, anxiety, and cardiovascular "stress," or Hatha Yoga and its benefits for some neurological disorders such as multiple sclerosis.

Alternative medicine implies treatments that may be used *in place of* conventional medicine. An example of this might be the potential benefits of a macrobiotic diet as an alternative to chemotherapy in the treatment of cancer.

I believe experts in this field would prefer the term *integrative medicine*. This would be a thoughtful balance of both conventional and complementary medical strategies that address the diverse mechanisms of health and disease that defy a particular category or "one-dimensional" way of thinking. An example of a common medical problem where integrative therapies can be very helpful is fibromyalgia. This pain syndrome is not well understood, has no diagnostic test, and defies (at this time) a clear scientific understanding. As a consequence, many conventionally trained M.D.s see fibromyalgia as a "head problem." Perhaps this sounds familiar to some of you?

To the extent that fibromyalgia can affect clarity of thought, memory, and sleep, some of its many manifestations, including the pain, might be "in the head." There are many excellent physicians who recognize that absence of proof is not proof of absence. Failure to understand is not failure to exist. Through an effective, balanced, and integrated understanding and therapeutic approval, many patients benefit from conventional medication; for example, for pain and alteration in sleep; myotherapy or massage therapy for deep muscle and tissue pain; yoga for stretching, mobility, and relaxation; prayer; balanced nutrition with a diet high in fruits and vegetables; avoidance of caffeine and alcohol; supplements of vitamins and amino acids; and chiropractic and Reiki therapy. This is a common example that illustrates the potential for applied integrative insights and interventions. Integrative medicine is an inherently multipronged approach to health promotion, disease prevention, and disease management.

An excellent, concise categorization of many diverse therapies, as well as a wealth of other good information, can be found at the NCCAM Web site (http://nccam.nih.gov). In brief, CAM therapies tend to fall into one of the following categories:

Energy therapies. Ancient wisdom and healing practices have long recognized the role of life energy or divine energy that defines the essence of who we are. These energy fields surround and penetrate the human body and connect us with all life. Disease stems from an alteration in this energy or spirit that manifests itself in a biologic way. Hindu wisdom, for example, recognizes seven chakras or divine truths that are energy centers whose imbalance alters biologic function and health.

- **Reiki** ("ray-kee") is of Japanese origin. It too recognizes a universal life energy that is channeled through and around us. A Reiki master and friend demonstrates this energy in the following way. Close your eyes and rub your hands together briskly. Now separate your hands and slowly bring them toward each other, palm toward palm. Before they actually touch, you will sense the energy and heat present in the space between. When this energy or life force is channeled through a Reiki practitioner, the individual's balance and flow of energy is restored and healing is facilitated. This, in turn, heals the physical body. My wife, after returning from a Reiki session for a migraine headache, appeared remarkably asymmetrical. The side of her head where the migraine was causing pain was red, flushed, and very warm to the touch compared to the side of her head that felt fine. Migraines typically cause pain on only one side of the head. This was a physical manifestation of the energy liberated from that source of pain. Her headache indeed had resolved after several traditional pain medications failed. I too have had Reiki for migraines with remarkable success. Like many of these therapies, Reiki is also very relaxing and calming.

- **Qi Gong** (chee-gung) is based on traditional Chinese medicine. It combines meditation with mind-centered breathing to enhance the flow of energy or qi (chee), improving bodily function and allowing one to enter a deeper connection with divine origins and higher consciousness.

- **Therapeutic touch** is an ancient technique of the laying on of hands. The theme again is that of a healing energy force transferred from the therapist to the patient. Balance and unimpeded flow of energy promote healing.

Mind-body interventions. Mind-body techniques enhance awareness of the mind's capacity to affect bodily function and symptoms. Dr. Herb Benson's pioneering work on the relaxation response, for example, where mind-centered relaxation, meditation, and prayer predictably lowered heart rate, blood pressure, and respiratory rate, has been demonstrated in many types of mind-body interventions. In the 1960s, these were radical and hard to accept notions, particularly coming from the laboratory of a successful conventionally trained cardiologist. His courses at Harvard's Mind-Body Institute, in addition to Harvard's courses on Spirituality and Medicine, are among the most popular of Harvard's superb educational offerings for health-care professionals. Fortunately, albeit too slowly, time and events alter perspective and conventional wisdom.

Many techniques such as meditation, biofeedback, and cognitive behavioral therapy have been proven quite effective. Prayer, pet and art therapy, and music and dance are other common expressions of mind-body interventions.

This is an area of active research and interest. No longer do most practitioners view the mind and body as separate constructs. Sorry, Descartes. The fascinating and growing science of "psycho-neuro-immuno-biology" indeed supports the modern view that these historically separate domains are, in fact, beautifully and masterfully integrated as one.

Biologically based therapies. These therapies are perhaps the most widely used and least understood of the CAM therapies. They include "natural" substances, for example, herbs such as St. John's Wort, vitamins, and many varieties of dietary supplements. These supplements may include, in addition to the above, other minerals, amino acids and botanicals, or substances derived from plants. Some dietary supplements are now considered "conventional" in their proven benefits. An example is folic acid, which can reduce the incidence of certain birth defects and can reduce homocysteine levels in the blood. Homocysteine in high levels may be a risk factor for cardiovascular disease.

Manipulative and body-based therapies. These therapies are based on movement or manipulation of the body. Chiropractic techniques have proven successful for many varieties of medical illness and for health maintenance. Chiropractors use manipulation, usually of the spine, to improve balance between body structure and function, a basis for preservation and restoration of health. I have found chiropractic intervention particularly helpful for individuals with acute back strain and lumbo-sacral (lower back) pain in addition to its many other utilities.

Massage therapy can facilitate relaxation, blood flow, and restoration of health to muscle and soft tissues. Osteopathic medicine involves a hands-on manipulative approach with techniques to alleviate pain, restore function, and promote health. The paradigm is one of symptoms arising from the bones, muscles, and connective tissues as they are integrated with our body's organ systems. Disturbance of this balance may affect function and health.

Alternative medical systems. These are therapies based on unique systems of theory, principle, and practice. For example, the ancient Indian tradition of *Ayurveda* ("ah-yur-vay-dah") has been practiced for more than five thousand years! And some people think of CAM as modern and novel. It includes diet and herbal remedies, emphasizing use of body, mind, and spirit in disease prevention and health promotion.

- *Homeopathic medicine* is based on the principle that administration of minute, highly diluted concentrations of substances, that ordinarily in much higher concentrations would cause similar symptoms, allows the body to respond in a curative fashion.

- *Naturopathic medicine* involves varied approaches including dietary, acupuncture, and massage, that facilitate the natural healing forces within the body.

My experience, like that of most clinicians, is that many people are receiving or have tried many of these types of therapies. It is important, in my view, for physicians to be open-minded and intellectually curious about CAM or integrative modalities. At a minimum there is a need to be informed, as many individuals, for example, take herbal "supplements," without knowledge of their potential risks, benefits, and interference with other prescribed medications. Physicians and allied health professionals have a wide range of interest and understanding of these modalities. This is a perfect example of how physicians and patients can effectively partner by openly communicating interests and concerns, as both may find themselves in uncharted waters. What follows is some practical advice to keep in mind as you contemplate embarking on CAM therapy:

- **Discuss all medical care and treatment with your primary provider.** If you are fearful of his or her response, then the nature of your therapeutic relationship needs to be examined. Withholding information could create potential danger if an unaddressed risk is allowed to continue. You might also deprive yourself of an opportunity to educate or enlighten your primary provider if you have researched an intervention. Which brings me to the next very, very important point.
- **Be as well informed as possible.** This cannot be overemphasized. This is of course true with regard to making any decision relating to your health. A tremendous amount of information is available for the health-care consumer (See chapter 15 on health-care literacy). Explore the extent to which scientific evidence adequately addresses both effectiveness and safety.
- **Check to see if insurance will cover your therapy.** Most therapies are not covered and will result in out-of-pocket expenses; however, some health insurance plans may cover a limited number of chiropractic or acupuncture visits.

If you are interested in a referral to a CAM practitioner such as a homeopath, myotherapist, naturalist, or Reiki therapist, ask your primary care provider if he or she can recommend someone. In my view, it is ideal to find a conventionally trained practitioner such as an M.D. with special training and experience in CAM. His or her approach will be inherently balanced and integrative. If you need more information about CAM therapy, look for professional organizations that publish standards of practice and explain the therapy. Many states may require licensure for certification to practice. Many professional organizations can be found by searching the Internet—for example, the Directory of Information Resources Online, or DIRLINE, at www.dirline.nim.nih.gov. Licensing, accreditation, and regulatory laws for CAM practices are becoming more common to ensure that practitioners are competent and provide quality services.

Please remember this very important point: *Natural is not the same as safe!* The U.S. Food and Drug Administration (FDA) does not require testing of dietary supplements prior to marketing. There are many products whose preparation may not be pure, whose claims may be unfounded and deceptive, and whose risks may be uncertain. With few exceptions, these substances have not been studied with the same scientific methodology that would be necessary, at a minimum, for knowledge of risks and benefits. They are not subject to post-marketing surveillance, and manufacturers are not required to report adverse outcomes.

Some have been studied. Below is a list that will grow significantly over time. Three excellent medical reviews have been published in the last year (see References). I offer the "Cliff Note" summary of best available medical evidence as of this writing:

- **Ginkgo:** The limited studies available are of questionable quality. Those of better quality show minimal to questionably mild benefits to memory, for example in early dementia; may be effective for tinnitus or ringing in the ears; possible benefit for leg pain from circulation problems. A proprietary multi-ingredient ginkgo preparation, ArginMax (Daily Wellness Co.), is an over-the-counter supplement containing ginkgo, L-arginine, ginseng, and Vitamins A, C, and E. Improvement in sexual function is reported in people taking prescription antidepressants including SSRI medications such as Prozac, Celexa, Paxil, and Zoloft, where sexual problems are common side effects.
  Cautions: Ginkgo has been associated, in uncommon case reports, with an increased tendency to bleed, particularly when used with aspirin, warfarin (a blood thinner), and anti-inflammatory medications.
- **St. John's Wort:** Studies suggest superiority over placebo as an effective treatment for mild to moderate depression and similar to low-dose "older" antidepressant medications. There is no data

comparing it to currently used antidepressants such as Prozac, Zoloft, Celexa, Paxil, and others.

Cautions: Potential risks include interference with the metabolism of several commonly used prescription medications including anticoagulants or blood thinners like coumadin or warfarin, oral contraceptives, and transplant medications like cyclosporin. It is very important to let your provider know if you are taking St. John's Wort with other medications. It is also very important *not to self-treat* symptoms of depression as it can be a dangerous problem, and more effective treatment may be available.

- **Ginseng:** Only one study of adequate quality (through October 2000) failed to show any benefit. Ginseng has been associated with reports of vaginal bleeding, particularly in women taking aspirin or aspirin-like products.

- **Echinacea:** Evidence is inconclusive in the treatment of colds and upper respiratory infections. Commercial products vary widely in their composition.

- **Saw Palmetto:** May have short-term effectiveness in reducing the symptoms of "benign" prostatic enlargement, also known as BPH. BPH is a very common disorder in older men, causing frequent urination and "nocturia" or getting up at night to urinate.

- **Kava:** There appears to be short-term effectiveness in treating anxiety.
  Caution: There have been reports of potentially serious liver damage.

- **Glucosamine-Chondroitin Sulfate:** Proven effectiveness in the treatment of degenerative arthritis, also known as "DJD." Glucosamine-chondroitin has been shown to be comparable to some anti-inflammatory medications, particularly for knee pain.

- **Sam-E (s-adenosylmethionine):** May be beneficial in the treatment of chronic musculoskeletal and joint pain, for example that seen in fibromyalgia. It may also have some effect on mood and energy level.

- **Garlic:** While better studies are necessary, garlic may have small, short-lived benefits for high cholesterol.
  Caution: *Rare* case reports of bleeding have been published, particularly in individuals taking the blood thinner warfarin.

- **For Symptoms of Menopause:** There are several good studies in the medical literature that have examined the efficacy of CAM for menopausal symptoms. Soy may have a modest effect on hot flashes. Black cohosh appears effective though there are no long-term data addressing its safety, as it behaves in a fashion similar to estrogen. Foods that contain phytoestrogens such as soy, some types of beans, clover, alfalfa, flaxseed, fruits, whole grains, rye, millet, and legumes have also demonstrated some benefit for treating hot flashes. Primrose oil, vitamin E, red clover, and acupuncture have not been proven effective.

Prepare some questions prior to seeing a CAM practitioner or having a particular CAM therapy, just as you would with any practitioner or treatment. For example:

- What is the therapist's background and training?
- Do they have a license or certification from a professional organization that has established standards of care?
- How much will the treatment cost?
- What are the risks and benefits?
- How many treatments will I need and how long might it take before I notice a change?
- Has there been much experience applying this particular CAM therapy to people with symptoms and conditions similar to mine? If so, how have the results been?
- Will this interfere with anything else I am currently doing or taking?
- How often will my progress or plan of treatment be assessed?
- Will I need to buy any special supplies or equipment?
- Will you collaborate with my primary care provider?

What if my physician does not believe in CAM?
In my experience, this is the exception and not the rule. There are some physicians who may be quick to dismiss any therapy that falls outside their area of expertise and professional training. I believe more physicians are open to this, in part because more than one out of three people, including physicians, will consider CAM for a particular problem. In my experience, any resistance from physicians tends to relate more to issues regarding safety, lack of vigorous study, and the realization that many people are exploited by virtue of their vulnerability with a health problem that conventional medicine has failed to remedy. An understandable desire to try something else is human nature.

Many people understand their health and wellness as a balance of mind, body, and spirit and seek to find modalities that nurture this. Many people want to avoid the potential toxicity of more potent pharmaceuticals or want to avoid more invasive approaches. There may be CAM therapies that are more aligned with your cultural tradition and identity. Whatever the reason, this is not something that should compromise the physician-patient relationship or result in "secretive" use of a particular botanical. Any difference of opinion between you and your physician with regard to this area should be viewed as an opportunity for mutual sharing, understanding, and growth. Your physician may ultimately be able to assist other patients with newfound insights and interests, or you may avoid potential risks through an explicit exchange of information. There is a difference between not recommending a particular therapy because of incomplete understanding or concern for safety and just being "anti-alternative." Physicians must attempt to balance the individual's right to nonstandard treatment with the ethical obligation to provide safe and effective care.

Useful Web Sites for Reliable Information on CAM

- www.nccam.nih.gov. Center for Complementary and Alternative Medicine, a subdivision of the National Institutes of Health. It is an excellent source for general questions, education, and research.
- www.ods.od.nih.gov. This is the NIH Office of Dietary Supplements. Here you can find public information as it relates to dietary supplements, their potential role in disease prevention, treatment, and health maintenance. Scientific research is compiled and displayed for reliable and objective information.
- www.drweil.com. A comprehensive Web site with excellent information from the pioneer and expert of integrative medicine. Dr. Weil is a leading educator, researcher, and advocate of integrative therapies, traditional in his training and background, innovative and holistic in his perspective on health and healing.
- www.nim.nih.gov/nccam/camonpubmed.html. CAM on PubMed is a database that contains scientifically based journals on CAM. You can search a particular topic, supplement, etc., and find a host of pertinent articles and research articles on CAM. This would be a good Web site to mention to your primary provider if he or she is in need of more information.
- www.cancure.org/naturopaths.htm. A non-profit organization providing information on alternative/integrative therapies, including referrals, since 1976. The term naturopath is used to describe a practitioner who uses natural methods to support the healing

process. This can include any number of a wide range of therapies, but typically most naturopaths work with diet/nutrition, nutritional supplementation, detoxification, herbology, and homeopathy. In addition, some have special training in bodywork, massage, acupressure, acupuncture, spinal manipulation, and mind-body therapies such as biofeedback, imagery, and visualization.

- www.ahha.org. The American Holistic Health Association (AHHA) is the leading national resource connecting people with vital solutions for reaching a higher level of wellness. The goal is to enjoy an enhanced quality of life with vitality, enthusiasm, confidence and self-worth. Creating wellness is an ongoing process. Wherever you are on this path, AHHA (pronounced ah-ha) assists you to become more informed about the many options available in the health-care arena today. You can explore those that feel appropriate for you and your situation.

- www.mca.gov.uk/ourwork/licensingmeds/herbalmeds/herbalsafety .htm. Licensing of medicines: policy on herbal medicines. Herbal safety news. London: Medicines Control Agency, 2002.

DO NOT MISS TAKE HOME POINTS

1. Be as informed as you can about the proven benefits and risks associated with an herbal, natural, or dietary supplement or treatment.
2. Tell your physician about any natural supplements or treatments you are taking.
3. Remember that "natural" does not mean "safe."
4. The potential to heal from within is remarkable. It is essential to be both critical and open-minded to integrative avenues to healing.

CHAPTER 15

HEALTH-CARE LITERACY
You Don't Know What You Don't Know

"The beginning of knowledge is the discovery of something we do not understand."

—Frank Herbert

THE OBJECTIVES of this chapter are:

- To review the importance of literacy as it relates to health care.
- To provide examples that link greater literacy skills with improved health outcomes.
- To share insights that will allow you to be better informed as a health-care consumer.

Not too long ago most people when ill went to their doctor for answers, guidance, and advice. Very few questions were asked and the spoken word was "gospel." It was not necessary to understand all there was to know about a particular problem. Insights were less complex and the options for diagnosis and treatment limited and few. "My doctor said this is what is going on and this is what I need to do." That "what I don't know can't hurt" mentality was acceptable, common, and made more comforting by the unquestioning trust in the physician. Asking too many questions of the doctor was tantamount to challenging the physician's veracity. "I don't want to upset my doctor by acting like I don't trust him," was a common sentiment. Many people still feel awkward about asking questions or challenging uncertain assumptions or inconsistent information.

I sometimes observe a generational pattern that reflects this cultural shift. "Seniors" experienced a culture where silent trust and acceptance was more the rule than the exception. Physicians did perhaps have more time and were the primary, if not the sole source, of information about health and disease. Baby boomers have been raised in an information revolution, questioning, challenging, and expecting to know more. For my twelve-year-old daughter, navigating computers and the Internet is as natural and comfortable as riding a bicycle.

Much has certainly changed. While the covenant of trust between a patient and a physician is paramount and necessary, it should not serve as a substitute for being as well-informed as possible. Never in the history of our existence has so much information become so readily available. And the majority of information out there, with respect to health, wellness, and disease, comes not directly from physicians, but from television, newspapers, books, journals, and the Internet. Science, technology, and diagnostic and treatment options are now more complex than ever before. There is appreciation for the fact that "what patients don't know can and may hurt them."

Physicians frequently assume, inaccurately, that patients understand what they are attempting to communicate to them. Evidence would suggest that patients may remember only 50 percent or less of the information given them immediately after being discharged from the hospital or after an outpatient visit. Poor health-care literacy is increasingly common among racial and ethnic minorities, the elderly, and in individuals with chronic medical conditions. According to the National Adult Literacy Survey, approximately one-fourth of adults in the United States lack sufficient ability to read, write, and speak in English. These are staggering statistics that have a profound impact on quality and cost of care. To make matters worse, we use a language in health care that makes literacy even more of an obstacle. A study at the Cleveland Clinic tested over 2,500 patients at two public hospitals. Thirty-five percent of English-speaking patients and 62 percent of Spanish-speaking patients had inadequate health literacy. A study published in 1998 and another study in 1999 demonstrated this:

1. Sixty-eight percent of patients studied did not know how to interpret a blood sugar value.
2. Twenty-seven percent could not identify their next appointment.
3. Forty-eight percent did not understand the instruction "take medicine every six hours."

4. Twenty-seven percent did not understand "take medication on an empty stomach."

The impact of health illiteracy on health outcomes may be profound. Problems with literacy may hinder one's ability to read pill bottle labels, appointment slips, education brochures, informed-consent forms, and other materials. Poor control of diabetes, blood sugar, with worsening damage to the eyes has been linked to poor health literacy. Compromised asthma care, for example, poor technique using an inhaler or "puffer," has also been linked to health illiteracy. In individuals with HIV-AIDS, compliance with medications, need for hospitalization, and diminished quality of life are strongly linked to issues of reading and comprehension.

What Can You Do to Improve Your Health Literacy?

I firmly believe that most medical problems are capable of being understood in a clear, satisfactory way. This means having enough information and understanding to allow you to make an informed decision that is consistent with your wishes, preferences, and values. This means being informed in a way that allows you and your family to be as comfortable as possible. This means feeling certain that no questions of importance to you are left unanswered, at least to the extent that they can be. We know that for many people, admitting difficulty with reading and comprehension is difficult. These are matters of pride, shame, and sometimes humiliation. The extent to which you can muster the courage to share these concerns will go a long way to bridge this gap in understanding. Here is some food for thought:

- Your physician may very well assume you understand when in fact you do not. Do not hesitate to ask for things to be re-explained. You may feel uncomfortable, awkward, or fearful. You may feel there is not enough time. You have no choice but to be an advocate for your health and wellness. This requires an adequate understanding.
- Ask for written materials or resources that can allow you to spend more time on your own, or with assistance from friends and family in reviewing the issues.

- If your physician is using medical jargon that you don't understand (this often occurs without physicians realizing it), ask him or her to clarify. For example, "Dr. Smith, when you say excessive bleeding, what do you mean," or "Dr. Smith, I am sorry my understanding is not clear. I know what you have to say is important. What do you mean by antihypertensive?" "What specifically do you mean when you say take this pill twice daily?"

- If your physician is communicating information too quickly, ask him or her to slow down. This is another common, unrecognized pattern that is an obstacle to literacy. For example, "Dr. Smith, I caught part of what you said, but did not understand everything. I appreciate your willingness to be more patient with me by explaining things a little more slowly."

- Try to make an effort to repeat what you are hearing and what your understanding is. This is a good method of testing your comprehension and allowing your physician to clarify any misunderstanding. For example, "Dr. Smith, if I hear you correctly, this may be pneumonia and the reason for the chest x-ray is to look for it."

- Many people may need help gathering the right information and putting it into perspective. Do not hesitate to ask caring family or friends to be present with you to ask questions and to assist you with your understanding. This is particularly important with regard to acute illness, as even the most skilled of individuals, when ill, may not be able to comfortably retain or understand all of the necessary information. This is particularly important for encounters such as an emergency department visit, hospital admission or discharge, an important decision concerning surgery, critical illness, or reviewing results of an important test.

- Write down questions in advance, if able. Bring a notebook to write down important information. Information that may be too difficult to put into perspective, particularly when you are overwhelmed or under stress, will often become clearer when the dust has a chance to settle.

- Consider a trusting and caring source of support and insight. This might be an R.N. in your church, synagogue, or mosque. Perhaps you have a neighbor with a medical background who can be of assistance. Whenever approached by a friend, neighbor, or faith community member for an opinion, I feel pleased to be in a position to offer some assistance. Never have I viewed this as an inconvenience.

- Do not hesitate to consider a second opinion, if you feel this will help you obtain a clearer and more comfortable assessment of the risks and benefits of whatever you may be confronting.
- Ask your provider about any available educational resources in your local community. In my experience, many resources are available that may not be readily recognized or taken full advantage of. For example, our community hospital has a terrific community education resource room. Here there are people who can assist with the use of printed materials and the Internet for finding health-care information.

In 2003, a large coalition of health-focused groups formed the Partnership for Clear Health Communication. Their Web site, www.askme3.org, provides simple advice for patients and families about managing their own care. Askme 3 is a tool that uses three simple questions that can assist in making sure you are getting enough information. They include:

- What is my main problem?
- What do I need to do?
- Why is it important for me to do this?

The Internet

There is more information available than ever on the Internet. We are in the midst of an information revolution. That is the good news. The downside is that a lot of the information out there may not be accurate or applicable to your specific circumstances. *The challenge is to know how to distinguish useful information from useless digital print.* A study by Baker, Wagner, and others (2003) examined the extent to which people use the Internet and e-mail for health-care information. This involved a survey done in December 2001, including almost five thousand responders. Approximately 40 percent reported using the Internet to look for advice or information about health or health care in 2001. Six percent reported using e-mail to contact a physician or other health-care professional. This is a number that is likely to rise dramatically in the future. About one third of those using the Internet for health research stated that it affected a decision. The number of physician visits was not significantly changed by use of the Internet. The majority of these individuals (80 percent) do not share their findings with their doctors, according to a recent report from the Center for Studying Health System

Change. In this study, the researchers surveyed 60,000 people in 33,000 families on how they research their health concerns. Fewer than one in six Americans turn to the Internet for this information. This study found that "educated" people and individuals with postgraduate degrees were seven times more likely to use the Internet compared to those who did not finish high school. Older people tended to rely more heavily on their physicians to provide them with medical information.

A recent report by the Pew Internet and American Life Project suggests that "80 percent of adult Internet users, or about 93 million Americans, have searched for at least one of sixteen major health topics online."

There are some misperceptions about physicians' views on patients who use the Internet to obtain information. First, physicians desire their patients to be as informed as possible. Second, the overwhelming majority of physicians (80 percent) are interested in what their patients find on the Internet. Third, many physicians are now beginning to recommend quality medical Web sites to their patients to obtain more information. Informed medical decision-making processes are in everyone's best interest. Physicians would, in fact, love for their patients to have access to quality information. Knowledge is power and was meant to be shared.

How to Evaluate Medical Resources on the Web

The National Institutes of Health has some excellent information on what to look for in a quality medical website (www.nih.gov). Here I have summarized some key questions to consider:

What is the purpose of this site? There are many reasons to provide information to the general public. An altruistic interest in the greater good may indeed be the predominant reason. Web sites from the federal government, for example a Web site or URL address with ".gov" on the end of it, are likely to provide more objective, unbiased information. Web sites from professional medical societies and organizations (.org) like the American Diabetes Association, the American Cancer Society, or the American Heart Association are excellent sources of "peer-reviewed" (reviewed and critiqued by many physicians and researchers) and published, high-quality medical information. If the site sells advertising, or is sponsored by a drug company, it may, of course, still be a superb site, though sources of funding can affect how the content is presented. Making money from the sale of advertising or receiving funding from private sources is perfectly legal and fair, though there are potential conflicts of interest inherent in the delicate balance of providing objective, quality information on one hand and the profit motive on the other. If possible, try to determine who runs the site from its title or the links provided, and who pays for or sponsors the site.

Where does the information come from? The best information in my experience is information created by the person or organization responsible for the site. Many health-related Web sites post information collected from other Web sites. The original source should be labeled.

How accurate are the sources of information? This is not always easy to determine, even for physicians. The best information comes from medical studies that are derived from excellent research, published in well-respected medical journals. Good information should have references to the studies and journals that the information came from. There might be a big difference between advice based on opinions and anecdotes and information that is "evidence-based" and research generated from accepted methodologies and thoughtful analysis.

How is the information selected? Do people with excellent medical, professional, and scientific qualifications review the material before it is posted? Again, research from reputable medical journals is most credible.

How current is the information? It is challenging for the most committed of physicians to stay on top of the medical literature. This is a rapidly changing landscape, to say the least. Much of the knowledge I acquired as a student, resident, and fellow has changed dramatically over the last twenty years! It is not uncommon for information to change significantly by the month in today's medical culture. Information, to be truly useful, must be up-to-date. The most recent update or review date should be clearly posted. Web sites updated on a regular basis are much more likely to be accurate.

Does the information I am obtaining relate to my individual circumstances? This is very important because the quality of information obtained is best if the studies upon which the information is based included people like you. For example, you might read information supporting the benefits of prostate surgery in the treatment of prostate cancer. Based on your age, stage of the cancer, other medical problems or conditions, quality of life, and personal preferences and values, this information, useful though it may be, might not be pertinent to you.

Does the Web site ask you for personal information? Health-care Web sites may ask for information for various reasons. It may be to create information more suitable to your needs, for example, based on age or gender, or to collect data used for marketing purposes. In either event, credible health sites asking for this kind of information should also inform you why they are asking and how the information will be used.

How does the site manage interactions with visitors? There should always be a way for you to contact the site owner if you run across problems or have questions or feedback. If the site hosts chat rooms or other online discussion areas, it should tell visitors what the terms of using this service area are. Is it moderated? If so, by whom and why? It is always a good idea to spend time reading the discussion before joining in, so that you feel comfortable with the environment before becoming a participant.

Looks do not equate with quality. In a recent study commissioned by Consumer Web Watch and led by Stanford University's Persuasive Technology Lab, nearly 42 percent of consumers tended to view online health information based on the site's visual design. The nicer it looked, the more credible the information was felt to be. Style should not be assumed to reflect substance.

In another study done by Sliced Bread Design LLC, Stanford University's Persuasive Technology Lab, Consumer Web Watch, consumers, and health-care experts were asked to assess the credibility of ten health sites. Here is how they were ranked:

Consumers	Experts
1. MayoClinic.com	1. National Institutes of Health
2. Intelihealth	2. MayoClinic.com
3. National Institutes of Health	3. WebMD
4. MDChoice	4. InteliHealth
5. Dr.Koop	5. MDChoice
6. WebMD	6. Dr.Koop
7. HealthWorld	7. HealthWorld and DrWeil tied
8. Dr. Weil	
9. Health Bulletin	9. Oxygen Health and Fitness
10. Oxygen Health and Fitness	10. Health Bulletin

There are far too many sites out there to include here, and the number is growing by the day. In addition to the excellent sites listed above, here are some additional sites I have personally used and have found to meet the quality criteria I just reviewed with you. Search engines will allow you to type in a particular topic and explore the various sources of information on that topic. While some of these sites have more sophisticated information, the content may be appropriate for your needs, interest, and background. These are also sites that can be mentioned to your provider as they are of reputable quality.

- **Healthfinder,** www.healthfinder.gov
  Resource from the U.S. Department of Health and Human Services provides prevention and self-care advice, government health news, and online journals.
- **FDA-MedWatch,** www.fda.gov/medwatch
  Find out what's going on with new medical products with the FDA's reporting program.
- **US National Library of Medicine,** www.nlm.nih.gov
  Index of resources for services, databases, publications, research activities, for the world's largest biomedical library. Services include Medline, NLM's bibliographic database covering the fields of medicine, nursing, dentistry, veterinary medicine, the health-care system, and pre-clinical science.
- **Clinical Trials,** www.clinicaltrials.gov
  This site provides patients, family members, health-care professionals, and the public access to information on clinical trials for a wide range of diseases and conditions. The National Institutes of Health (NIH), through its national Library of Medicine, has developed this site with the U.S. Food and Drug Administration. The site currently contains more than 6,200 clinical studies sponsored by the NIH, other federal agencies, and the pharmaceutical industry in over 69,000 locations worldwide.
- **MedHelp International,** www.medhelp.org
  A not-for-profit organization that provides a consumer health information library, medical specialty forums, patient-to-patient networking and daily medical and health news.
- **JAMA Information Centers,** www.ama-assn.org/special/infohome.htm
  The Journal of the America Medical Association maintains an archive of easy-to-use, peer-reviewed collections of resources on specific conditions.

- **American Medical Association,** www.ama-assn.org

  At the AMA's home page, click "Patients." Here you will have access to a wealth of information that will help you lead a healthy life and become an active participant in your health care, from nutritional and fitness articles to content about specific diseases and conditions.

- **American Cancer Society,** www.cancer.org

  This site provides an extensive network of services and organizations fighting cancer by providing education and support. There are many excellent resources for survivors, families, friends, and professionals.

- **American Heart Association,** www.americanheart.org

  This is a national directory of resources related to heart health and disease, including stroke. Resources include medical information and resources.

- **American Diabetes Association,** www.diabetes.org

  This is an important site for anyone with a history of diabetes. The ADA is a non-profit organization that provides up-to-date information on diabetes research, education, and advocacy. You can also receive important tips for healthier living with diabetes.

- **Arthritis Foundation,** www.arthritis.org

  Provides excellent news, research resources, and contacts for people with arthritis of all causes.

- **Agency for Health-Care Research and Quality,** www.ahcpr.gov/consumer

  This is an excellent site for quality news and information on consumer health. Well-established guidelines for current "best practices" are available.

- **WebMD Health,** www.webmd.com

  WebMD provides valuable health information, tools for managing your health, and support to those who seek information. Their content is timely and credible.

There is so much advertisement out there. How do I recognize bogus claims? There is a huge market for health products, many of which fall into the category of "natural remedies." As more people are willing to pay out of pocket for products they see advertised on TV and in newspapers and magazines, there is a high probability of getting ripped off. As there are many health problems for which there are no easy treatments, such as obesity or "muscle building" solutions, there are a growing number of unsuspecting people willing to try anything, particularly if it is a matter of just taking a pill. Billions of dollars are spent each year on fraudulent health products.

The Federal Drug Administration (FDA) shares federal oversight of health fraud products with the Federal Trade Commission (FTC). Safety, labeling, and package insert claims are under this oversight. FTC regulates advertisement of products. Paula Kurtzweil, a member of the FDA's public affairs staff, has reviewed some "Tip-Offs to Rip-Offs" that should raise flags around fraudulent claims and advertisements. For example:

1. Watch out for any product that claims to be a "miracle" drug. There is no such thing. If it sounds too good to be true, that is simply because it is not true. If you find yourself tempted to the extent that you are about to call that 1–800 number, click the purchase box in the Internet Web site, or respond favorably to the voice on the other end of the telephone, **STOP,** and ask yourself, "Can I afford to throw this money out the window?" At the very least, use some of the resources I have provided for a reality check and to obtain more information. Ask someone who is savvy how he or she would respond under similar circumstances.

2. Be suspicious of claims that the product treats a wide variety of unrelated diseases. Many fraudulent products recognize the desperation that people face when confronting a difficult to treat problem like obesity, AIDS, or perhaps Alzheimer's or dementia.

3. Be suspicious of personal testimonies. Many health problems ordinarily get better on their own, and have nothing to do with the particular therapy being advertised. There is no evidence weaker than hearsay.

4. Watch out for the "Quick Fix." Many minor problems can get better quickly (within a matter of days) by simply applying some common sense. Many of the "Quick Fixes" you hear about, again, are targeted at the more chronic, frustrating, hard-to-treat problems, where the demand for the quick fix is greatest, such as baldness, obesity, and arthritis. There are no rapid remedies for these problems.

5. Be leery of the "all natural" products. As I mentioned before, *natural* sure sounds nice, safe, and reassuring. Many natural substances can have significant toxic potential or may interfere in some way with important prescription medications you may be taking. These are not substances that are subjected to the rig-

orous FDA research process. Review any product you are considering with your primary care provider.

6. Watch out for the "new, revolutionary breakthroughs"! There is no place on earth where the research is more advanced, sophisticated, and committed to breakthroughs than the United States. Any revolutionary cure or breakthrough in health care *will not* come to you by way of an infomercial or Internet/newspaper advertisement. Again, if it sounds too good to be true . . . *forget about it*!

"Satisfaction guaranteed or your money back." When it comes to marketing fraudulent products with deceptive practices, I have two observations:

- Your satisfaction will fall far short of your expectations.
- Getting your money back will be easier said than done.

There is an interesting Web site called Quackwatch, Inc. (www.quack watch.org), founded by Dr. Stephen Barret in 1996. Quackwatch, Inc., "a member of Consumer Federation of America, is a non profit corporation whose purpose is to address health-related frauds, myths, fads, and fallacies."

Their activities include:

- Answering inquiries
- Investigating questionable claims
- Reporting illegal marketing
- Distributing reliable publications
- Improving the quality of health information on the Internet

Quackwatch is funded by donations and profits from the sale of publications. Their primary service is consumer advocacy and safety. If you have any questions or concerns about fraud, you might find this site very useful. You can also check the FDA Web site www.fda.gov/opacom/ 7alerts.html. The FDA can tell you whether the agency has taken action against the product or its marketer.

When it comes to your health, be as educated as you can. Ask questions. Choose to be empowered. Choose to know more.

DO NOT MISS TAKE HOME POINTS

1. If your doctor has given you instructions that you do not understand, do not hesitate to ask questions.
2. Having someone with you to participate in the sharing of important information is always a good idea, particularly if you feel that your ability to understand is limited.
3. Ask your doctor about practice or community resources that can assist in your understanding of disease education and management. Diabetes, for example, clearly responds better in individuals who participate in self-management programs.
4. If a medical advertisement looks too good to be true, it probably isn't true. Hold on to your money.
5. The Internet is an incredible source of information and communication. If you do not have a computer, you can find access to one in your local library or hospital health and information center. Do not be reluctant to ask for assistance—learning to use the Internet is not that difficult.

CHAPTER 16

MANAGING CONFLICT

Anger and Opportunity

"Speak when you are angry and you will make the best speech you'll ever regret."

—Ambrose Bierce

THE OBJECTIVES of this chapter are:

- To appreciate the root causes of conflict that can occur in a health-care encounter.
- To review common patterns of behavior underlying conflict with self, family members, or with your treatment team.
- To examine actual case-based scenarios, demonstrating the potential to transform conflict into greater understanding of self and others.
- To examine strategies that provide satisfying opportunities for growth, healing, and reconciliation.

You may be wondering what dealing with conflict has to do with navigating your health and our health-care system. Unfortunately, a lot! People confronting illness, from minor to very serious problems, encounter a system that is large, convoluted, highly sophisticated, sometimes impersonal, and very complex. It is much easier said than done to stay calm, cool, and focused when we or someone we love is sick. The human response to illness or loss encompasses fear, uncertainty, despair, profound change, and isolation. Those providing care, from front desk support staff to seasoned physicians and everyone along the spectrum, are immersed in high volume, high pressure, unpredictable, and complex clinical settings. Usually, when these sometimes harsh and indifferent realities meet, the result is positive. Unfortunately, the circumstances within which we meet and interact do not always lend themselves to smooth sailing. High stakes, high pressure, high emotions, high demand, and differences in perspective are conditions ripe for conflict. This is made even more likely when accompanied by communication breakdowns, all too common in the health-care encounter. Conflict is uncomfortable, consuming, and upsetting. It does not promote health. And conflict happens. The challenge for all involved in the health-care encounter is to transform conflict into a more positive outcome, particularly an outcome that serves your values without compromising the relationship. Most relationships are worth preserving. Our emotions have an agenda that can undermine our effectiveness when dealing with others such as our families, friends, and health-care professionals. When you think about it, the last thing anyone needs when dealing with illness or loss is to have their therapeutic energy shaken and consumed by conflict and interpersonal strife. The extent that one's "center," that point of equilibrium and harmony, is thrown off balance in illness, is made even worse when conflict enters the mix. In the health-care setting, conflict commonly falls into one or more of the following categories:

Inner Conflict

An example here is an individual who is torn about what the best decision or decisions may be for his or her health, such as proceeding with a major operation or deciding to be placed on dialysis. Another example is having an older relative such as a parent or grandparent who has deteriorated physically and is increasingly more confused and forgetful. You may have many growing concerns regarding his or her safety, independence, and quality of life. You may find yourself conflicted over the decision to keep the person at home, desperately clinging to a dwindling independence, or to seek placement in a skilled nursing facility or nursing home. You may have a loved one who is critically ill, and you despair over angry and bitter exchanges that occurred before this sudden and unexpected change in health status.

In the chapter examining spirituality and health I touch on the story of a woman deeply conflicted about her desire to end her life by stopping dialysis. She struggled to reconcile the conflict between her faith-based commitment to praise all life as a sacred gift under any circumstances and the painful reality of a life no longer "worth living."

Provider-Provider Conflict

Here you might observe two or more health-care professionals express-ing differences of opinion about a critical decision, such as to transfer a patient to another facility for treatment or about the best interventions to choose. The issues here relate more to conflicting opinions than they do conflicting personalities or attitudes, though these can occur as well. Occasionally health-care professionals confront complex medical cir-cumstances for which there is no clear and proven direction to take. As a patient you may hear varying opinions as to the best next steps. There may be varying degrees of medical evidence, leaving diagnosis and treat-ment strategies as well as prognosis open to significant variance. Inter-pretations of risks and benefits of a surgical procedure, for example, may conflict as you hear differences of opinion from members of your primary care group or involved consultants. This may leave you unset-tled or perhaps even untrusting as you try to figure out what exactly is going on and what best to do. Reconciling such differences, from a pa-tient's perspective, requires knowing what questions to ask, educating yourself, developing understanding from those you trust, and applying your values and preferences to the best options available to you.

Family Conflict

This is a very common source of conflict in people I have cared for. Often there are differences of opinion as to what would be best for a loved one, for example, to have surgery or not, to be placed in a nursing home or not, how "invasive" to be with attempts to diagnose, treat, or both. There may be conflicting views on whether a person should be resuscitated in the event of a cardiac arrest, whether a DNR order should be given. While conflict is the last thing a family needs when dealing with illness, it can serve as a basis for discussing issues that may be deeply rooted.

A lovely man I once cared for made the deliberate and well-informed decision not to have surgery for a large tumor. The surgery would not have cured his cancer. In the context of his other medical problems and in the context of his deep and certain preferences, he had had enough. There were two children. One lived with his father as a care provider. The other child was living at a great distance from his father and kept in regular touch with frequent phone calls and visits. The siblings struggled with their conflicting views of their father's decision to forego surgery. They were unable to support each other in what would turn out to be their father's last several weeks of life. I have found that it is common for siblings who are geographically distant to view circumstances, as they relate to their loved one's care, in significantly different ways. The sibling living nearby, perhaps responsible for daily care, has a perspective and understanding that daily observation, dialogue, and being in the trenches makes poignantly sharp and clear. A sibling geographically removed, loving and concerned as any sibling could be, may have a less clear understanding and "real-time" perspective, not having observed the decline in quality of life. Distance may have the unintentional effect of creating feelings of shame or guilt, making it difficult to separate the need to reconcile inner conflict with one's self from reconciling conflict with another. Two loving siblings, confronting the same harsh reality, with perhaps different values, preferences, and understanding, express these differences by a failure to agree on important decisions. The challenge here is to attempt to reconcile these differences through open, explicit, straightforward, and heartfelt communication, active listening, and hopefully, greater understanding.

Another example is feeling conflicted about a spouse who has a heart attack. On one hand you feel love and concern, and you pray for the best outcome possible. On the other hand you are increasingly angry about the poor lifestyle habits, choices, failure to follow through on advice about check-ups, testing, and treatment. You may harbor bitterness, caring for a loved one more than he or she seems to care.

Conflict Between a Patient/Family and the Health-Care System/Professionals

Many conflicts I observe among patients, families, and health-care personnel have in common a breakdown in the awareness and sensitivity of the fundamental needs of people. Issues here most often revolve around experiences lacking in empathy, clear communication, respect for values and preferences. They may be perceptions of inattentiveness, for example, long waits, outrageous bills, and the like. *These scenarios demonstrate significant gaps between patient/family expectations of what will or is likely to happen, how it should happen, and how it actually happens.* If you examine feedback from patients and families who are upset with a health-care professional, particularly a physician, there are certain consistencies in maladaptive interpersonal behaviors that emerge, for example:

- Lack of respect for values, preferences, and needs. This is a critical piece to the ethic of professionalism in health care. Your behavior or values, for example around smoking, drinking, or a sedentary lifestyle will conflict with the values of your physician-provider. While there is equal and intrinsic value in all people in need of care, conflicts sometimes play out when a physician expresses his or her value differences in a disrespectful and uncaring way. For example, "Mr. Long, it's obvious to me that the reason you are short of breath is because you smoke. If you can't stop you'll have to find another doctor to care for you. I cannot make you better." Or perhaps you have heard this, "If you cannot monitor your blood sugar, I cannot help you." I have found this to be an ineffective way of influencing a patient toward the desired behavior. While any hand reaching out deserves a hand reaching out in return, it may require patience and your contribution to the eventual success. For example, "Dr. Smith, I can sense your anger and dismay toward my smoking and other bad lifestyle habits. I need your help to understand what I need to do and how I can go about doing it. I have not been able to succeed on my own." Physicians love to see things go well! This is our *raison d'etre*. Greater awareness of your physician's expressed frustration as a genuine desire to see you get better and not a scolding (though it may be and feel like the latter) may allow you to take the first step forward. It is in your best interest to have a professional moving forward with you.

- Low therapeutic content, automated style, non-empathetic, and "disconnected." Here the health-care professional behaves as if he or she sees a problem more than they do a person with a problem. Perhaps this sounds familiar.

- Failure to read between the lines. Most communication is nonverbal. Physicians sometimes, unknowingly, miss signs or signals that may represent your important needs and concerns. As a consequence, many doors begging to be opened are left untouched. "Active listening" attempts to recognize the importance of these subtle, unspoken messages. Let me give you an example. A person is just starting chronic hemodialysis because her kidneys no longer function sufficiently to maintain health and wellness. The treatment requires placing two rather large needles into a shunt, which is a connection between an artery and a vein. It is of course natural for the patient to want to move her arm, sometimes requiring the nurse or technician to make repeated attempts. Failure to recognize fear and panic on the face of the individual as she sits in the dialysis chair means overlooking a profound form of nonverbal communication. There is a big difference between:

1. Failure to read the message: "Please don't move your arm, Mrs. Pettus! We won't be able to do your treatment and you'll feel sicker."
2. Aware and empathetic: "Hi, Mrs. Pettus. I know you have just started dialysis and this all must seem overwhelming to you. You must be frightened. You are in good hands here, and we will do all we can to help you feel better. I know these needles hurt a little bit. Close your eyes, breathe deeply, and relax, and I'll help you through it."

Scenario one cultivates more fear, anxiety, and technical challenge. Scenario two cultivates relationship, trust, and technical success, not to mention mutual satisfaction.

- Mission-oriented, high-control style. I refer to this as the Dragnet approach, that is, ". . . just the facts, ma'am." Many clinicians, in their need to "cut to the chase," ask targeted yes or no questions. Though often necessary, this style of inquiry leaves patients less able to elaborate on important details or to clarify information that may not be completely accurate. In outpatient clinic settings, studies have shown that physicians, after asking an individual what brought her to the office, will interrupt the person, on average, after eighteen seconds! The complete story or the story behind the story is never fully shared. For example:

The story: "I have been coughing for four weeks."
The story behind the story: "My father died of lung cancer and
   I am concerned that I might have cancer."

The paradox here is that many health-care professionals feel that it may takes too much time to allow individuals to speak freely without interruption. Feeling pressured for time and sometimes impatient, physicians and nurses may have a tendency to "cut to the chase." However, studies suggest that when physicians allow a more patient-centered interview, allowing the patient to talk until important issues are adequately communicated, more important information is shared and minimal extra time is required! Patient satisfaction, not surprisingly, is also improved with this approach.

- Failure to address potential barriers to effective communication:

- ❖ Environmental, for example lack of privacy or a noisy television nearby
- ❖ Physical, for example greater need to address comfort concerns
- ❖ Emotional, for example, there are better times to engage in certain sensitive and delicate conversations that I refer to as "ripeness"
- ❖ Sociocultural—we serve an ethnically and culturally diverse population that can create unique challenges with respect to communication and understanding

- • Studies, not surprising to you I am sure, consistently point to these issues deemed most important to patients in their health-care encounters:

- ❖ Respect for values, preferences, and expressed needs
- ❖ Communication
- ❖ Education
- ❖ Coordination and integration of care; keeping flow of information and care organized and clear
- ❖ Physical comfort
- ❖ Emotional support and alleviation of fears and anxiety
- ❖ Involvement of family and friends
- ❖ Continuity, having someone familiar with the key issues following your progress across the continuum of care. An example here is the frustration of keeping track with what is going on as an individual starts in the emergency department, is admitted to the CCU, is then transferred to a "step-down" heart monitoring floor, transferred to the rehabilitation unit, and eventually discharged home.

Most conflicts between patients, families, and health-care professionals could be effectively minimized by greater attention to these fundamental needs. You can see a familiar theme here. Understandably, you may see this as the responsibility of the health-care system and its personnel. Indeed, attention to these issues should occur as a matter of routine. Common sense however, is not common practice. Having these needs effectively met may require your tactful and explicit communication and willingness to partner with the system and the individuals who serve it. This will not come easily, particularly if you are feeling angry or hurt. The challenge for the patient and family is to partner in a way that is empathetic to those involved. This will run counter to your instincts to "dig in." In my experience, many health-care professionals are not aware of a particular style that may be affecting others in a negative way. Health-care professionals take a great deal of pride in what they do. Their mission and purpose are worthy ones. However, there is a lack of meaningful feedback in our system. This has the effect of masking awareness that a particular style or behavior is seriously impacting another.

There is still a prevailing cultural perception that physicians "walk on water." Quite frankly, I'm afraid to walk on ice. Many people, particularly seniors, feel that whatever physicians say and do should be accepted without question. One would never contemplate giving candid feedback. While this is still a common sentiment, baby boomers are more outspoken in expressing their needs and concerns. Still, many physicians have been unable to take advantage of the self-improvement potential of candid feedback, as the legacy of a health-care culture long past was "never to question the doctor." This is still an intimidating thing for many people to contemplate.

This will not come easily for most people. The physician-patient relationship is one that is not balanced with respect to power. Necessary though this may be as you desire to tap into the power of a physician's skill and expertise, the issues I am referring to here are not analytical or technical. These are "people skills" and should be the basis for interactions between people, regardless of title, position, or analytical expertise.

What we need to hear to become better providers of care is more likely to be kept silent than to be openly shared.

Ego, yours or the health-care provider's, should not be an obstacle to the flow of information between two people. This is true, by the way, in every aspect of our lives.

I am certain that many health-care professionals would be surprised and dismayed to know the impact their actions had on another. The impact of our behavior has a way of overshadowing even the best of intentions, from the finest of people, when it comes to conflict. Sure, there are arrogant, defensive, and egocentric health-care professionals out there, as there are in any profession. They are, however, a very small minority and I do not, for a minute, believe they are beyond greater awareness of their behavior, greater awareness of their impact on others, or beyond change.

There is no excuse for rudeness. You don't need that! Speak up. When it comes to physicians and hospitals, there are choices. I realize it is not easy to freely share feedback with a physician or nurse, particularly around awkward and sensitive issues. It should be in the best interest of everyone involved to make it work as effectively as possible. Despite the altruistic and compassionate foundation upon which our services should always stand, there are day-to-day realities that strain our human interactions. For example, when I observe these exchanges, these are the subtitles that emerge beneath the spoken words:

The patient/family are feeling:	The health-care professional is feeling:
Discomfort	*Physically fatigued*
Fear/confusion	*Mission oriented*
Uncertainty	*Unremitting responsibility and pressure*
Loss of control	*Need for more control*
In need of more time	*Short on time*
Overwhelmed	*Overwhelmed*
Hyper-aware	*Illness as a matter of routine*
Angry	*Frustrated*

When one examines emotionally charged health-care encounters, it is not difficult to understand how well-intentioned people lose sight and control of their behavior. It is not hard to understand how our mutual effectiveness can be undermined quickly. When you peel away the many layers of education, experience, and skill, you reveal the core.

People Treating People

It is in this domain that the quality of the encounter defines itself, that the harsh reality of a stressful environment allows conflict to set in, that understanding and reconciliation are made possible. This is where the rubber meets the road. It is natural for anyone who performs tasks day in and day out to take for granted how significant and indelible these events are in the lives of those they are treating. A few years ago I received a letter from a woman whose husband I met while doing my fellowship training. He was in his seventies and was very sick from advanced kidney failure. He was one of many people I had seen that day. His history and symptoms were similar to countless numbers of people I had seen and treated in the past. This could have easily been just another kidney failure patient. For Mr. and Mrs. G., this was the most frightening and unforgettable moment in their lives. In her letter to me, Mrs. G. elaborated in remarkable detail what happened that night, in The Massachusetts

General Hospital Emergency Department, more than sixteen years earlier! She recalled where I sat, how I addressed her husband, what we spoke about, and in a heightened, indelible way, recounted the details of the long night that followed. It is very easy for any health-care provider to lose sight of the overwhelming importance their "routine" interactions have on people who are experiencing a "once in a lifetime" medical encounter.

Here is an example of how conflict can be transformed by way of pursuing mutual understanding. While in our emergency department admitting a patient, I overheard a man who was talking to one of our nurses. He was visibly angry and upset. His wife, who was experiencing abdominal pain, was becoming increasingly uncomfortable. She had been told she would be going for a CAT scan almost an hour earlier. "What is going on here?" No one had been in to see her in over a half hour. "This is terrible care," he said, frustrated and impatient. The nurse he was addressing his concerns to was not directly involved in his wife's care. Her response was "Okay, let me look into it. We're doing the best we can." She was certainly being honest and truthful. She also failed to appreciate the lens through which he was looking at their circumstances. Five minutes later, no one had returned and the woman's husband was reaching a boiling point. I intercepted him as he again approached the nurse he had just conversed with. I introduced myself to him as a staff physician. "I overheard your concerns as I was seeing a patient in the adjacent room. The walls can be too thin at times. I understand your wife is very uncomfortable and you have had a long wait. I also appreciate that your expectation of what was to happen is miles apart from what your current reality is. Your wife's comfort is what is most important at the moment. I will help find someone caring for your wife who can address this right away."

Now I also knew there were four trauma victims from a motor vehicle accident who had arrived about an hour ago. I went on to share openly and honestly with Mr. Smith the trauma management occurring around the corner, beyond his view. "The E.D. physician who was evaluating your wife was unexpectedly diverted to address their needs. I know he would feel badly about your long wait and uncertainty. Some of these accident victims needed a CAT scan. This is the reason for your wife's delay. That, however, is no excuse for her being in a state of prolonged discomfort." He and his wife were visibly calmer, appreciative of an explanation, and actually contrite regarding their anger. Their feelings seemed to take a 180-degree turn.

What was required to totally transform this perception?

- Awareness of the emotions escalating
- Empathy, reflecting an understanding of how things looked through others' eyes
- Communicating an apology (a powerful resource) that specifically addressed their anticipated needs and concerns
- Broadening their perspective by offering an alternative lens through which to observe their environment
- Assurance that their needs and interests were heard, valued, and would soon be addressed

In the end . . . partners instead of adversaries. How long did it take? Sixty seconds.

This explanation also had the effect of putting in perspective their circumstances and that of the E.D. staff. This led to an almost immediate transformation. I subsequently found a covering nurse to give more pain medication. A near-infuriating and stressful encounter, ripe for escalating conflict, was transformed in a very short time to an experience characterized by empathy, mutual understanding, active listening, and fulfillment of the mutual interests at hand.

As Fisher and Ury so elegantly outline in *Getting to Yes*, every *position*—for example, the wait has been unacceptable—has many underlying *interests* and concerns—for example, I'm uncomfortable; I'm afraid; I'm uncertain. If you react or disagree with someone's position without an effort to more empathetically address and understand the interests beneath the position, you miss an enormous opportunity to realize the potential for mutual gain and reconciliation. This works both ways. For example, Mr. Smith might instead comment, "People are running around the department like crazy! Is there something going on that has made it more difficult to address the concerns my wife and I have? You are clearly very busy and distracted. Perhaps my wife's nurse and doctor have been unable, for good reason, to help us. Is there something you or perhaps another physician can do to address our needs? I am becoming increasingly concerned." Framed in this context, the concerns are more likely to draw in and engage a staff person than they are to elicit a defensive posture. *This defines the power of influence.*

> *Effective management of conflict transforms anger into empathy and understanding.*

Conflicts for both providers and patients are common in this complex environment, emotionally charged and with enormously high stakes. They make more difficult the opportunity to optimize the therapeutic partnership, trust, and alliance necessary for good experiences and meaningful outcomes.

There are many outstanding works by people who research, write, and lecture about conflict resolution and emotional management, for example, Fisher and Ury's *Getting to Yes*; Daniel Goleman's *Emotional Intelligence*; and Charles Dwyer's work on influence, to name a few. I have learned a lot from them and many others who reflect, write, and speak on these matters. My experience, both as a physician and as someone whose parents have encountered what can be a challenging system, has reminded me time and time again of the importance of basic human respect and the Golden Rule as it guides our relationships. As I always tell the medical students and residents we teach:

Humility Rules! Know when to leave your brain at the door.

If you find yourself confronting conflict, here are some observations and advice on moving effectively beyond it:

"The gem cannot be polished without friction, nor man perfected without trials."

—Chinese Proverb

Conflict is inevitable. There is no getting around this. Avoiding conflict may feel better and easier in the short term. Conflict can also escalate, internally and externally, in a way that will forever alter the quality of a relationship so necessary to nurture and maintain, for example with a physician or loved one. As an example, choosing to deal with a different M.D., R.N., or hospital is not always an option, nor does it necessarily make sense to risk compromising the stability of a patient where care is already fully engaged by those familiar with the circumstances. While your circumstances may force you to consider this, it should be a last resort.

You may be at odds with another family member who bitterly disagrees with a particular course of action, for example, diagnostic procedure or treatment. Times like this require your relationship to be shared and strong, not adversarial. *We are all hardwired to respond to conflict in a "fight or flight" mode.* Millions of years ago, in a hunter-gatherer society, this response served us well. One had to react quickly in an uncertain and harsh world to ensure survival. Though still necessary under some circumstances, these "reflex" responses do not always serve us as well in supporting a loved one by partnering with a medical team. Health-care encounters are characterized by the complex interactions and interdependence of many individuals. Dealing with others effectively is essential to the quality of the encounter.

When the conflict escalates, it is essential to:

- Detach yourself, physically and emotionally, from the moment. You may feel trapped, threatened, unsafe, and quickly overtaken by your feelings. If, for example, the choice you are about to make is certain to lead to an outcome that is miles apart from where you would really like to be, for example, crashing egos with strong words and anger as opposed to supporting each other under difficult circumstances, *retreat.* I refer to this as retreating to the bleachers. In the heat of the moment, the perspective looks very different from the bleachers than it does on the playing field. I apologize for reducing a difficult health-care encounter to a sports metaphor. Effective managers of conflict can adapt to changing circumstances with an awareness and control that enables effective emotional management. When the heat is turned up, it is almost impossible to link our choices with their consequences.
- Retreat to a private place such as a bathroom, solarium, hospital chapel, or meditation room.
- Close your eyes for a moment and take a few slow, deep breaths. This actually works quickly to calm.
- Suspend judgment. This is much easier said than done. You will be challenged to move in a direction opposite from what your emotions are telling you to do.
- Assume you have a perceptual blind spot. Understanding more points of view will often create enlightened perspective, more options, and will serve to sharpen your edge.
- Slow down, stop, and identify the emotions you are feeling. What are they telling you? Are they more or less likely to take you where you would like to be?
- Consider your options for responding and the consequences of each of these options. You may choose to express your anger toward a dear friend who chose not to have a recommended treatment and is

now confronting a serious health problem. Your anger, real and justified though it may be, could have the effect of condemning and distancing the person who, more than anything, needs your support and compassion.

Example scenario: You are angry and upset about the restrictive visiting hour policy in the ICU/CCU. Many hospitals, by the way, are examining the options of more flexible visiting policies.

Choice 1: Raise your voice in an angry tone to the charge nurse in the ICU/CCU about the restrictive visiting hour policy and how ridiculous and unfair it is. Other staff and family members of other patients hear you. (This particular choice is based on a true story.)

Consequence: Visiting hours do not change. The charge nurse feels defensive and becomes more distanced from you and your family. Word quickly spreads among the treatment team about the "angry" family disrupting other loved ones in the waiting areas.

Choice 2: Express your genuine sense of fear, lack of control, and anxiety as you wait to see your loved one on the other side of the closed ICU/CCU doors. Describe the slow and painful passage of time; each minute is like an hour and so hard to bear. "I know you are all very busy with many sick patients to care for and there must be a good reason for the visiting policy. I hope you understand the need I have to spend just a moment with my mother."

Consequence: Visiting hours do not change. Charge nurses are more sympathetic. A greater desire to support and nurture the needs of the family is elicited. A greater likelihood of flexibility around the policy is made possible through a shared and meaningful understanding. The time and connectedness between the loved one and the nursing team will be 180 degrees different, contingent on the choice made. I guarantee this. Which choice will better serve you and your loved one?

Example scenario: You are upset because a complication occurred during your husband's hospitalization. You have heard different explanations and are confused as to what is going on. You are frustrated and upset because you have been unable to talk with your treating physician. It has been impossible to reach the physician.

Choice 1: You see your husband's physician in the hospital hallway. You are angry and make clear your dissatisfaction with your husband's care. You threaten to "fire" the physician and say that you are considering transferring his care elsewhere.

Consequence: Justified though your feelings and comments may have been, the physician is put on the defensive. He or she reacts by withdrawing further, apprehensive that future encounters will be bitter and unpleasant. He or she feels the care has been of a good and reasonable standard and that this is "another potentially litigious family." They tell their colleagues to "be careful and stay clear of the patient's angry wife."

Choice 2: You ask the nurses caring for your husband to page the covering physician. You might also leave a message with the physician's office stating who you are and that you need a short period of time to address some very important concerns as they relate to your husband. "Dr. Logan, thank you for a moment of your time. I know you are busy and have many patients and families that need your attention. I feel frustrated and upset because my husband has had some complications that I do not fully understand and I have had trouble getting in touch with you (much more effective to focus on your feelings than to place blame). I'm sure you would understand if you were in my shoes. Here are my concerns. If there is a better way to reach you and to meet to review future concerns, please let me know. I want to be as informed as possible so that we can all be on the same page as we try to do what is best for my husband. Thanks for your time."

Consequence: Dr. Logan is more likely to respond in a favorable and less defensive way. You are more likely to share and receive timely, useful information. Your legitimate concerns will be framed in a way that makes clear your needs and expectations. You also demonstrate a willingness to hear and understand obstacles that may have interfered with more effective sharing of information by your physician. You appreciate that the complications were not a reflection of negligent care. Hopefully, this will prompt a more sensitive response in future encounters. A defensive, avoidance response is less likely to occur.

This is an epiphany that runs counter to everything our emotions and every cell in our body are telling us to do.

View conflict as an opportunity for greater understanding of yourself and those you are at odds with.

Short of being able to avoid a conflict scenario, which is often not possible or desirable, it is always best to choose the path of greater understanding and reconciliation. This is particularly true when you are in conflict with people you have to have repeated encounters with. If it is a situation that cannot be avoided, it is best to deal with it explicitly. The task will be difficult and perhaps frustrating. You have an opportunity to come out on the other end much better than where you started.

Some tips:
1. Look for a quiet/private place to engage the discussion.
2. Balance listening with the need to be heard.
3. Communicate clearly and explicitly.
4. If you have a number of issues and concerns that time may not allow you to address fully, select one or two to prioritize as agreed upon with your provider. You can then discuss a plan to address the other less urgent issues over time.
5. Focus on your feelings and how current circumstances have affected you, trying not to place blame or point fingers.
6. Take an active interest in understanding others involved and helping others to understand you.
7. Asking questions = Greater understanding

    a. "Help me to understand how you see things!"
    b. View empathy as a two-way street. Anger is a roadblock to empathy.

8. Be open to other possible explanations.
9. Try to identify and focus on shared interests and concerns—for example, "How can we relate more effectively in the future?" "What options are there for dealing with this?" "If you were in my shoes, how would you see this?" "What do you think I am feeling right now?"
10. A smile, easier said than done when confronting illness, confers a sense of warmth and will infect those around you. As someone once said, a smile is the shortest distance between two people. I know of many health-care professionals who would welcome a smile as they move through their hectic day.
11. If the relationship with the individual you are conflicted with is too important to undermine, channel your energies to preservation. You will be surprised to find that this is possible without having to compromise your principles.

12. If you feel there are gender or ethnic barriers, ask to speak to someone who may better relate to your needs and concerns.

13. This challenging process will hopefully lead to a greater understanding that will allow civility and mutual respect. Relationships emerge on the other side of the process more trusting, enduring, and effective.

There are resources available to channel these concerns to, depending on the nature, magnitude, and complexity of the process. These resources might include:

> *Sometimes, despite our best mutual efforts, we are unable to reconcile conflict.*

1. A hospital-patient relations director (ombudsperson)
2. A social services professional
3. An ethics committee—useful in confronting more challenging and difficult decisions about providing or withdrawing life-sustaining care.

I would like to conclude with a story that reflects a different kind of conflict. Mrs. Finn was a ninety-one-year-old woman visiting our area from New York City. She was the picture of marvelous health, sharp, independent, and very active. While visiting in our area she fell and broke her hip, requiring surgery. Soon after surgery she began to develop a series of complications. Within a couple of weeks I became increasingly concerned that the growing number of obstacles might be too numerous to overcome, at least to the point of regaining the independence so vital to *her* values and perspective of quality life. She was confronting more procedures and interventions and in a wise, aware, and poignant way began to confront her mortality. I could see she was torn about having more procedures. On one hand she was clearly clinging to life and the hope that she and her loving family had for her. She did not want to "disappoint her family" and at the same time did not "want to become a burden to them." She was at a crossroads in her life and was confronting some very difficult choices. Many people will find themselves at this crossroads. I have encountered it many times. Mrs. Finn and I had a growing relationship that allowed an open and frank discussion of her growing number of issues. She looked me in the eyes one morning and asked, "Dr. Pettus, am I dying?" I replied, "What do you think, Mrs. Finn?" She answered, "I believe I am."

I have observed many people under these circumstances and believe the process of death is recognizable to many people and their loved ones, as well as to many health-care providers. I replied while holding her hand, "While I can never be certain, Mrs. Finn, it is possible that you are dying, and I am here to support your needs and wishes in any way possible." "I am ready to die," she said. "I have had a long and wonderful life." After discussing options for her care in addition to emphasizing comfort, she was clear that enough was enough. Life for Mrs. Finn was a ninety-one-year independent and joyous journey. Anything short of full independence and autonomy from this moment forward would not be acceptable to her. She was concerned about how her family would respond to a decision to withhold further aggressive treatment, as many people are. When she understood and revealed what her heart and soul were telling her to do, she was clearer and very much at peace. Allowed enough space and support to contemplate, derive greater understanding, and weigh the options, Mrs. Finn was able to choose her path, to exercise the last vestige of control in her lifetime.

Her family was incredibly loving and supportive, though not in total agreement as to the "best" course. Some struggled with her decision and felt it was not yet time to "give up." Others accepted and supported her decision. Conflict of this nature is not uncommon. It unfairly adds to the pain and grief of the circumstances already at hand. This can be a terrible place to be. I felt my role was to inform the family as clearly as possible of the circumstances, our options for further diagnosis and treatment, and the likely consequences of those options. I also recognized the importance of our meeting together as a group with their mom and the importance of their being alone together.

Mrs. Finn's courage was an inspiration to me, and I know to her family. Through a process of sharing, an effort to mutually understand, and a commitment of total love and respect, Mrs. Finn and her family made that difficult journey to her death soon thereafter. While total reconciliation of the decisions made may not have been possible, the family remained bound by their shared love and support, and hopefully were able to move on with a sense of both great loss and inner peace.

DO NOT MISS TAKE HOME POINTS
(SEE FIGURE ON PAGE 231)

The schematic in the illustration is intended for both health-care professionals and for patients and families. The ingredients underlying conflict are plentiful in the average health-care encounter. While health-care

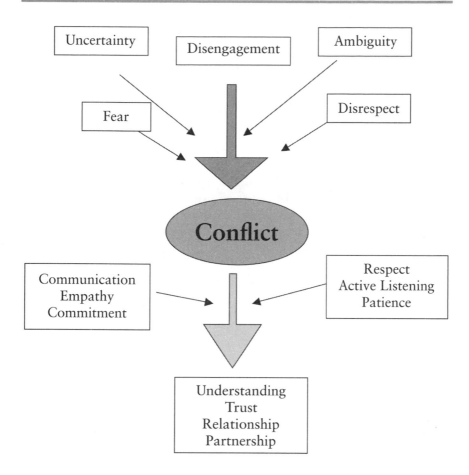

professionals should be held accountable for quality encounters, they too, are people whose skills may need to be developed more effectively. While you cannot change others, you can be empowered to help others and yourself by maintaining a greater awareness of the ingredients for greater understanding, trust, partnerships, and more effective relationships. Mutual emphasis on more effective communication, listening, empathy, and respect will help open these challenging doors.

1. Accept the reality and inevitability of conflict.
2. View conflict as an opportunity for greater understanding and growth.
3. Allow enough time to organize your thoughts and to manage your emotions.

4. Examine the consequences of the path you are on.
5. Candid feedback is crucial to the challenging process of self-awareness and self-improvement.
6. We can always be made more aware.
7. Self-improvement is a process that spans a lifetime.
8. Ask others you trust to share their thoughts and to be with you as you navigate through conflict.
9. Understanding others will make it more likely that you will be understood.
10. Communicate you concerns calmly and clearly.
11. Asking questions = Understanding
12. Understanding builds trust.
13. Trust is the foundation of an effective relationship.

CHAPTER 17

HEALTH-CARE COVERAGE

What Do You Got?

"Financial ruin from medical bills is almost exclusively an American disease."

—Roul Turley

THE OBJECTIVES of this chapter are:

- To review the different categories of health insurance that are generally available, with emphasis on Medicare.
- To provide an overview of COBRA (Consolidated Omnibus Budget Reconciliation Act), and the FMLA (Family and Medical Leave Act).
- To provide a general overview of long-term care insurance.

Health-care insurance will not make most people's top five list of interesting and stimulating topics. It is, however, one of the interests that should make the top five of one's list of priorities in life. Health care is very expensive. Health-care expenditures account for approximately 15 percent of our nation's gross national product (GNP)! This is the dollar value of all goods and services sold in the United States. The GNP of most countries is less than we spend on health care in the United States. More money is spent on health care per capita in the United States than any place else on earth. Costs continue to rise significantly as our society ages, as the demand for services and sophisticated technology continues to rise, and as the cost of prescription medications marches upward.

Health-care services are usually paid for by insurance companies and by the government, that is, by Medicare and Medicaid. Government programs are paid for by your tax contributions. Health-care insurance, for most people, is obtained by employer-based coverage offered to its workers. What this means is that people who do not have jobs or who work part time do not usually have health-care coverage that is both available and affordable. As the cost of insurance continues to rise dramatically, it is increasingly more difficult for employers to afford. As a consequence, the added financial strain of providing comprehensive health-care coverage is being realized by businesses everywhere. It is becoming harder for many employers to remain competitive because of these growing costs. There has been a dramatic increase in bankruptcy claims over the last ten years. Recent reviews of bankruptcy (personal and business) litigation reveal medical costs as a frequent contributor. To leverage this harsh reality, employers are passing more of the expense on to their workers. Spending on health care by employers in 2003 rose 10 to 14 percent, compared with a 15 percent rise in 2002. This is according to a survey of 3,000 small and large employers by Mercer Human Resource Consulting. More costs were passed along to employees. The average worker in a small firm paid $389 per month and at a large firm $224 per month for family health-care coverage. This means higher premiums, more deductibles and co-pays, and having insurance plans with less comprehensive coverage.

Recent statistics show that the number of people without health insurance rose for the second consecutive year. The U.S. Census Bureau reports that 15.2 percent of the population, or 43.6 million Americans, are uninsured. There has been a drop in the percentage of people covered by employment-based health insurance. Most of these people have jobs and many have children. Studies, not surprisingly, are clear on the relationship between health-care coverage and access to timely and comprehensive care, scope of services received, and health outcomes.

It is apparent that in some instances, people of lower socioeconomic class and ethnic minorities are at greater risk for poor outcomes because they do not have the same access to quality care. It is clear that many people who are uninsured will delay evaluation and treatment, sometimes resulting in serious complications and poorer outcomes. These are important and legitimate public health concerns. When it comes to health-care coverage and quality care, we are not created equal. I believe this is a *crisis* in America. I also believe that most Americans seriously under-

Basic health care should be a right, not a privilege.

appreciate the magnitude of this crisis. While health-care costs continue to escalate dramatically, more people are at risk for losing their coverage. Employers are finding it more difficult to afford coverage for their workers. Currently, most states in the United States are confronting enormous budget deficits—over $66 dollars in 2003! State and federally funded programs like Medicaid, which represent a large percentage of state expenditures, second only to education in many states, are inevitably going to cut back on coverage and services. It should be a social imperative to more openly discuss and debate how to apply our precious and plentiful resources to best meet the fundamental health needs of our citizens. But I digress.

This is a chapter about the different types of health-care coverage and what you should know. It is sort of an "Insurance 101" overview. Now, I must be honest. I am anything but expert on the topic of health-care insurance. The landscape is an increasingly confusing one. Much of the information in this chapter was gleaned from some subject review, experience, and some excellent government-sponsored Web sites such as the Center for Medicare and Medicaid Services (CMS). There is a wealth of good information on the government's Web site, www.medicare.gov for those who are comfortable with the Internet. This is a particularly good site if your parents or grandparents have only Medicare and require hospital or outpatient services. What is covered and to what extent can be very confusing. There are many contingencies. The "shock factor" when people receive their medical bills is accentuated by a failure to understand when, what, and how much health insurance covers. While there are many different types of health insurance, I will focus on the main types of coverage and their potential advantages and disadvantages. Added emphasis will be placed on our Medicare system. These are a few of the basic categories of health insurance coverage.

HMO—HEALTH MAINTENANCE ORGANIZATION

HMOs became popular in the1980s. They were developed to better organize, manage, and more cost effectively deliver care to people who enrolled. These plans offered purchasers of health-care insurance (employers) less expensive alternatives for providing coverage to their workers. In this model, you have access to a panel of participating physicians, allied health professionals, and participating hospitals. Care is "managed" within that network with an assigned primary care provider serving as the "hub" of the network, or "gatekeeper." If you need to see a specialist or require hospitalization, you are referred to participants hired, or who contract services with the HMO you belong to. Advantages include a "defined" network to navigate, often lower costs, and a model emphasizing primary care review/referral when more complex problems arise. A disadvantage is that you have less choice about which doctors you see and which hospitals you go to. The emphasis on primary care referral, for tests, consultations, and second opinions can sometimes feel more restraining and "hassled." More HMOs are offering options for members. For younger, healthy individuals and families, HMOs can be a very reasonable option.

PPOs — Preferred Provider Organizations

These are networks that are somewhat more flexible. Providers of care contract their services with the PPO for a predetermined fee. Unlike HMOs, PPOs allow evaluation and treatment outside the network. An increased out-of-pocket expense will be incurred compared to the cost of seeing a provider in the network. The main advantage here, however, is the potential to receive care with greater control over choice. PPOs generally will cover some of these costs. There is usually no deductible, but there is a co-payment for physician visits and prescriptions. These are increasingly popular models for health-care coverage and service.

Indemnity Plans

Indemnity plans have the greatest advantage of choice of physicians and health-care facilities. There is usually a deductible before the plan kicks in. The remainder of care is usually covered at 80 percent after the deductible. The price for free choice is generally greater with these plans as far as premiums go.

Coverage When You or Your Family are Out of Town

Most health plans will cover life-threatening emergencies regardless of your location, even outside an HMO/PPO network. For less emergent problems you may need to get prior authorization from your insurer before medical care is covered. It is important to review your policy before planned travel in order to minimize unexpected headaches and expenses.

Employer-Based vs. Individual Policy

Employer-based policies include options for coverage such as HMO, PPO, and indemnity plans, and they are usually less expensive because of cost-lowering leveraging with insurers to provide coverage for larger numbers of people. Individual policies provide similar options for coverage but are more expensive. "Individual" means that the policy is not purchased by an employer, but by the insured individual. While you can sometimes tailor the plan to meet your needs, individual plans are medically underwritten. The insurer can decline to insure you or add undesired contingencies because of preexisting or established health problems.

Medicare

Medicare is the largest health insurance program in the United States. The U.S. Social Security Administration offers it. It covers people age sixty-five and older, as well as people younger than sixty-five with permanent disabilities. There are approximately forty million Americans over sixty-five on Medicare. Eligibility for Social Security benefits (or railroad retirement benefits) means eligibility for Medicare. You are eligible for Part A if you are age sixty-five or older and you or your spouse worked and paid Medicare taxes for at least ten years. People can also be eligible if they worked for at least ten years in a government job at a federal, state, or local level.

MEDICARE PART A

This is the portion of Medicare that covers hospital fees, skilled nursing facilities, and hospice and home health care, assuming that the facilities and/or organizations are Medicare certified. Part A comes automatically with Medicare, and there is no premium for this coverage. In addition to semiprivate rooms, meals, general nursing, and other hospital services and supplies, SNF care is generally covered after a three-day related hospital stay. Private duty nursing, telephone, TV, and a private room (unless your doctor specifies this is "medically necessary") are not covered under Part A. Check the Medicare Web site www.medicare.gov and click the *Medicare & Your Mental Health Benefits* link for more information on inpatient mental health benefits. You can also click *Medicare & Home Health Care* for more information on these benefits. Part-time skilled nursing, physical therapy, occupational therapy, speech, home health aides, social services, and durable medical equipment (DME) such as wheelchairs, hospital beds, oxygen, and walkers are covered. This coverage at home may be contingent on an individual being "homebound" or unable to safely commute to ambulatory facilities to receive similar therapy.

MEDICARE PART B

This provides coverage for many non-hospital-related services and requires monthly premiums (approximately $54/month as of this writing). Premiums can be deducted automatically from your social security check.
    Examples of services covered include:

- Outpatient hospital services
- Emergency room visits
- Physician services (not routine physical exams)
- Laboratory and x-ray services
- Mammography and colonoscopy
- Ambulance transportation (with appropriate medical need and documentation)
- Medical equipment and supplies (it is important to make sure the pharmacy or supplier is participating with Medicare)
- Eyeglasses—one pair of standard frames after cataract surgery with an intraocular lens implant
- Kidney dialysis treatments
- Chiropractic services (limited—best to check with provider)

Medicare Part B covers 80 percent of an "approved charge" for covered services. You are responsible for the remaining 20 percent. Medicare is administered in some parts of the country as managed care plans, like HMOs.
    As there are many important health services not covered by Medicare, such as hospital/physician co-pays and deductibles, dental care, eye examinations, and others, people should strongly consider supplemental coverage if they can afford it.
    There are currently other ways for Medicare recipients to supplement coverage as a way to reduce out-of-pocket expenditures. Examples of supplemental coverage include:

- **Medigap Policies:** This is private insurance offering different combinations of benefits that Medicare does not cover. There are several standard policies from which to choose.
- **Medicare Select:** This is another type of insurance policy, supplemental in nature, sold by HMOs and insurance companies. Like the HMO insurance policies, the premiums can be less expensive and require that specific participating physicians and hospitals be chosen in order to receive full benefits.

The best time to apply for Medicare benefits is the six-month period around your sixty-fifth birthday, or three months before to three months after. There is also an open enrollment period in January of each year. The ideal time to enroll in a Medigap policy is during the six-month period after enrolling in Medicare part B. The federal government protects your right during this time period to choose a Medigap policy sold by any insurance company in your state, no matter what health problems you may have.

There is a national Medicare Hotline that operates seven days a week, twenty-four hours a day. This number, **1–800–633–4277**, can be used for any question regarding Medicare policy, coverage, grievances, etc. There are English and Spanish speaking assistants available. An ATT language line is available for other languages. Additionally, the Social Security Administration offers support at a toll free number, 1–800–772–1213, or online at www.ssa.gov. The government also has printed information, available from your local Social Security office: *Your Medicare Handbook: A guide to Health Insurance for People with Medicare.*

Medicare and Prescription Drug Coverage

The original Medicare Plan does not cover prescription drugs, except in unusual circumstances. At the time of this writing, Congress has passed a prescription coverage plan for Medicare recipients that will likely be modified with time. Congress has voted to allocate $400 billion in drug assistance over the next decade. This is estimated to represent approximately 25 percent of the amount seniors are expected to pay for prescription medications. This is clearly a legislative priority and a necessity. It is estimated that the average senior will have $3,160 in prescription drug costs per year in 2006. Starting in April 2004, all Medicare beneficiaries would be eligible to purchase a discount card for buying prescription drugs. Some Medicare recipients would see an immediate 10 to 15 percent cut in their prescription drug costs when filling prescriptions at their retail pharmacies. The card costs thirty dollars. The full entitlement plan would take effect in 2006. Participation is voluntary, though a penalty surcharge may be imposed if a senior defers the decision to participate. Once the new benefit takes effect in 2006, the law will prohibit sale of Medigap policies that seniors can currently purchase to supplement coverage and reduce out-of-pocket drug expenses. This new policy may be difficult to understand. Private insurers and HMOs will be encouraged to offer competitive plans that may create confusion as to what is covered and for how much. At the time of this writing, coverage would break down as follows:

- Medicare recipients pay the first $250 as a deductible.
- They then share 25 percent of the costs between $250 and $2,250.
- They are responsible for all costs between $2,250 and $5,100.
- For catastrophic costs (greater than $5,100) they share 5 percent of costs.

Individuals with incomes below $13,055 and couples with incomes below $17,619 and with assets no greater than $6,000 per individual and $9,000 per couple would pay no deductible and no monthly premium for their new drug benefit. Retirees with incomes above $80,000 for a single person and $100,000 for a couple would be required to pay more for their Part B benefits. Average premium costs will be $420 per year.

Many people without insurance are without jobs or struggling to make ends meet. The sad truth is that many medications are prohibitively expensive and as a consequence, are not taken, even with an understanding of the potential health risks. The best intentions cannot ensure compliance under these circumstances. Many pharmaceutical companies have financial assistance programs. Ask your physician and your pharmacist for some suggestions. It is important to know what your insurer will cover. Some health plans cover specific generic or trade brands that may be similar to what you were prescribed, if not covered, by your plan.

A new Web site, www.medicare.gov titled *Your Medicare Coverage* contains all of the current information regarding Medicare's coverage of prescription drugs. Coverage for prescription drugs is an enormous issue for many Americans. Many people over the age of sixty-five have only Medicare. It is increasingly common for people to be taking several different types of prescription medication that can cost hundreds of dollars per month! These are often life-sustaining medications that are involuntarily discontinued (or never filled in the first place) because of excessive cost.

If you are prescribed a medication or are already on a medication that you cannot afford, let your prescribing clinician know. It is hard for some people to admit to this as discussing financial hardship can be awkward and possibly embarrassing or shameful. There may be alternatives your physician can assist with such as free samples, prescription drug assistance programs, or less expensive alternatives. This is another very important public health concern that our legislators need to act upon. Check your Medigap or Medicare Plus Choice Supplemental Plan for policies regarding prescription drug coverage. Many have coverage with co-pays and certain dollar limits.

The Prescription Drug Assistance Programs Database on www .medicare.gov provides additional information on programs that offer discounts or free medications to individuals in need, including state prescription drug assistance programs, programs sponsored by pharmaceutical companies, and disease-specific programs.

MEDICARE—EXAMPLES OF SERVICES NOT ROUTINELY COVERED

* Acupuncture
* Dental care and dentures
* Cosmetic surgery
* Custodial care (help with "ADL" or activities of daily living, e.g., bathing, dressing, using the bathroom, eating)
* Hearing exams and hearing aids
* Orthopedic shoes
* Routine foot care
* Routine eye care
* Routine or annual physical exams

With respect to routine health maintenance and disease prevention screening tests including vaccinations, a list of covered services can be found at www.medicare.gov. Click the link *Medicare Preventive Services to Keep You Healthy.*

Tax Sheltered Health Savings Accounts

The Medicare prescription coverage bill passed by Congress in December 2003 makes available the option of developing Health Savings Accounts. Starting in 2004, taxpayers can shelter up to $4,500 annually (maximum $2,250 individual/$4,500 family). The catch is that in order to be eligible for these accounts, an individual or a family must meet a minimum high-range deductible on their insurance coverage. A high deductible would be $1,000 for an individual and $2,000 for a family. These accounts would grow (assuming a growing market, as they are like IRAs) tax deferred, until you need the money for health-care expenses. The new law has two requirements for opening an HSA:

- A taxpayer must be under the age of sixty-five.
- Your health insurance plan must meet the criteria for high deductible.

Contributions, investment growth, and withdrawals for health expenses are all tax-free. These funds can be used for:

- Physicians and dentists
- Hospitals
- Medications
- Eyeglasses
- X-Rays and blood tests
- Psychotherapy
- Chiropractic care
- Nursing home costs
- Physical, occupational, and speech therapy

While HSAs are not for everyone, they are attractive to individuals and families with few health-care spending needs, as well as those who spend more than $4,000 per year. Self-employed individuals and those who have individual health insurance coverage could save substantially. Purchasing insurance with high deductibles is cheaper. HSAs could grow until needed to offset health-care expenditures when they occur.

I should mention that many employers also offer Flex Accounts to employees. These are worker-funded accounts that can be used to pay out-of-pocket health expenses, like an HAS. Contributions are pre-tax from payroll withholding. However, these are "use it or lose it" policies. Money that is not used at the end of the year is lost.

How Do I Respond to a Claim That Is Denied?

How frustrating it is to require a health-care service and to seek care that you feel is appropriate, only to eventually learn that your insurer denied your claim and more out-of-pocket expenses are necessary. This is an inevitable experience for most of us, given the complexity of health-care coverage, the many contingencies around which coverage occurs, and the many changes with respect to coverage itself, as insurers struggle to contain escalating costs through greater scrutiny of claims. There are some steps worth considering in response to this frustrating experience.

Know your policy. Sometimes a denied claim is a reflection of simply not knowing what is covered and not covered by your policy. Before proceeding with any service whose coverage may not be guaranteed, such as a routine physical or chiropractic intervention, read your policy carefully, or check with your provider beforehand.

Inadequate documentation submitted. Sometimes a claim is denied because the insurer does not have enough documentation to deem the service "appropriate." The onus is on the patient and provider to fulfill the burden of proof. This may require a letter from you and your provider detailing the medical rationale for the service, such as a referral to a specialist or a repeat visit for the same diagnosis within a short time period. A hassle though this "burden of proof" can be, in my experience insurers will respond appropriately when documentation is complete.

Ask for an appeal of the claims determination process. A formal review may reveal a processing error. For example, medical treatments are submitted to insurers using a five-digit CPT (Current Procedural Terminology) code. These codes are catalogued in an enormous, changing, modified phonebook-like document that may be confusing to those attaching codes to the diagnosis or treatment. Physicians have to take courses just to keep up on the most appropriate codes relevant to their practices. If a clerk, for example, enters an inaccurate code, the claim will be denied. Make sure the insurer's code for your rejected claim matches the one on your doctor's bill. If not, there may be an error. If so, ask your provider's billing department to see if an "alternative CPT code might be appropriate to consider."

What Happens If My Employment Changes or I Lose My Job?

There are two federal regulations that should be understood in determining how best to continue your coverage after a change in employment. The first is **COBRA** (the Consolidated Omnibus Budget Reconciliation Act). COBRA mandates that an employer (with at least twenty employees) notify you before your current health-care benefits run out. You are able to continue your insurance under the company's health plan whether you are terminated, resign, or have your hours reduced. Your dependents can continue on this group coverage. You are responsible for paying for the coverage, however, and can pay up to 2 percent more for administrative costs than your employer was charged. Compared to an "individual" plan, this may still be less expensive. Compare COBRA pricing with "individual" policy pricing. COBRA coverage can continue for up to eighteen months (twenty-nine months if you are disabled). COBRA coverage can best be viewed as a "bridge" until you can obtain coverage under a new employer or Medicare, if eligible. If you want to continue the same coverage after eighteen months, federal law states that the insurer must offer you a conversion policy. Expect premiums, however, to go up substantially.

HIPAA (Health Insurance Portability and Accountability Act) is 1996 legislation that limits a health plan's ability to exclude coverage for a pre-existing medical condition. If your former employer had at least two employees and if under that employer's sponsored health plan you had continuous coverage for at least twelve months, your new plan cannot exclude coverage because of a pre-existing condition. Your former employer will need to provide a certificate of coverage, entitling you to the waiver. You will need to move to the new health plan within sixty-three days of termination of your previous coverage. HIPAA legislation addresses group employer-based coverage. There are fewer provisions made for people with pre-existing conditions who want to enroll in individual plans.

The most important thing to keep in mind is the *priority* of maintaining coverage of some kind. Whether under COBRA or an individual, non-employer-based plan, your maintaining "creditable" coverage is essential if you have a pre-existing condition and are to be protected under HIPAA. Hopefully this can serve as a bridge until you find new employment with coverage, or assume coverage under your spouse's plan.

Other strategies to assist with getting coverage with a pre-existing condition:

- During open enrollment periods, insurance must allow anyone to purchase a policy. There may be limitations placed on coverage, but at least you'll have some coverage.
- If you have been disabled for two years or longer, or are sixty-five or older and eligible, apply for Medicare coverage.
- If you meet low-income criteria (usually less than two times poverty level income), you may be eligible for Medicaid.
- Obtain dependent coverage through your spouse's insurance plan.

Not having health-care coverage is like walking on very thin ice. Countless times I have treated individuals who requested that tests not be ordered because of an inability to pay. Medications, many of them life-sustaining, are not taken because of an inability to pay. Follow-up appointments are missed because of an inability to pay. Health problems smolder and languish, often to a serious extent prior to treatment, because of an inability to pay.

There is surely no easy solution to what many health-care professionals and administrators view as a health-care system crisis.

Far more lives, both young and old, are at risk from this crisis than from any other threat. I do not wish to diminish the unique and potentially devastating threats that our society currently faces. These are issues that you, leaders in our communities, legislators, businesses, and legal and health-care systems must vigorously debate. These problems will not go away. They will continue to grow over time as costs rise and inequities in care widen.

Access to health care and affordable health-care coverage are among the major societal issues of our time.

What advice can I give you?

If you have health insurance, get a summary of what is covered and what is not. This can usually be obtained from the human resources department where you work if your insurance is employer based. Calling the insurance company directly for a summary of provided services, deductibles, co-pay, etc., is another option. Most government-sponsored and private programs have information available on the Internet with FAQ (frequently asked questions) sections. This can be an overwhelming task given the volume and complexity of information out there. Keep a personal file of all information regarding coverage and claims. Don't hesitate to ask for help from a family member or trusted friend, particularly if you are feeling confused or overwhelmed. Personnel working with billing in hospitals and physicians' offices are also often available to assist with any questions you might have.

If Medicare is your only insurance, you may be at risk for what can be extraordinary supplemental costs. Complementing this coverage is a good idea for those who can afford it. If Social Security is your primary source of income, as it is for about 35 percent of Medicare-covered individuals, you may be eligible for your state's Medicaid program. This can cover medications and skilled nursing facilities (nursing homes).

Veterans are usually able to obtain free or discounted medications from their local VA clinics. If you are a veteran, look into this option.

If you are income eligible (in many states, with an income of less than two times the poverty limit), your state's Medicaid coverage is an option. Information can be obtained from a local Department of Medical Assistance. Hospitals also have staff who can assist with questions about obtaining insurance, Medicaid eligibility/applications and in some areas, eligibility for free care.

As most insurance is linked to employment, inquire about health-care benefits when applying for any job. Anything is usually better than nothing. If you are unable to find or afford insurance, do not delay seeking care when ill. EMTALA, Emergency Medical Treatment and Active Labor Act laws, protect individuals from being turned away for insurance reasons. In my experience, most hospitals and physician practices are fair and willing to explore all options for payment.

If you are registered to vote, check to see who supports broadening access to health care and who seems passionately committed to working toward universal coverage and affordable prescription drugs. If a candidate cannot speak to these issues intelligently, informatively, and with purpose and conviction, move on to the next one.

Family Leave

The Family and Medical Leave Act (FMLA) was adopted in 1993. It requires any employer with at least fifty employees to ensure the job security of any worker who needs to take time off for the following reasons:

- Birth or adoption of a child
- "Serious" health condition of a family member
- One's own serious health condition

You are eligible for up to twelve weeks of unpaid leave in a given year if you have been employed for approximately twenty-five or more hours per week during the past twelve months. Your employer-based health-care coverage should not change during this leave. You may need to provide documentation by your treating physician to confirm the nature of the "serious health problem." Before considering FMLA leave, review any necessary information with the human resources department where you work.

Long-Term Care Insurance

Since the start of the twentieth century, our life expectancy has almost doubled. When I finished my training twenty years ago, it was uncommon to be treating a person in the hospital over the age of 90. It is now common to be treating people in their late eighties, nineties, and with greater frequency, at years one hundred years of age!

Most people, as they age, will confront a debilitating illness, such as a stroke, heart disease, or a chronic progressive illness such as Alzheimer's that limits their ability to care for themselves safely and independently. Long-term-care insurance (LTI) was conceived as a consequence of this reality. LTI provides coverage for care received at home as well as in a skilled nursing facility. Examples of covered services include:

- Home health aides assisting with bathing, dressing, etc.
- Homemakers who assist with chores such as cleaning, shopping, or meal preparation
- Long-term skilled nursing care
- Rehabilitative therapy

Most traditional insurance plans cover these services minimally or not at all. Medicare pays for home health care with time limitations and only under certain conditions. Medicaid covers skilled nursing in nursing homes. There are stringent financial criteria with respect to income. To become eligible, people often have to "spend down" their assets to less than $2,000. My father was forced to do this for transportation! Transportation is a real problem for many people who are unable to drive. My father required dialysis treatments that required transportation three times per week. As he was legally blind, he was unable to drive. The nearest dialysis center was twenty-five miles away. He had Medicare, and for many years paid expensive premiums for Blue Cross/Blue Shield, an excellent insurance plan. Transportation, however, was not covered. Taxi fare would have cost fifty dollars per round trip, three days a week, fifty-two weeks a year. You can do the math. On a fixed income with a meager pension and social security, this was simply not possible. As a consequence, he had to "spend down" to become eligible for Medicaid, as this was the only means of covering his transportation. It was a nightmare.

The cost of long-term care is expensive, as average annual nursing home costs are now in excess of $55,000 per year! Skilled nursing at home can cost approximately twenty-five dollars per hour and home health aides ten to twenty dollars per hour. This can add up quickly, depending on the nature of the underlying medical problems, the overall need for home support, and available additional resources, such as spouse and family to assist with care.

Premiums for long-term care are variable, depending on the range of benefits needed, age, and other factors. One consideration is the benefit period, such as three years to lifetime; the daily benefit, for example. $150 per day in a nursing home, plus $100 per day for home care; "inflation protection"—if nursing home costs rise, your benefits will rise as well. Expect your premiums to increase, as you get older. As of this writing, LTI premiums average approximately $2,200 per year.

In general, long-term-care insurance is a good idea if you can afford it. It can be a comforting safety net, particularly as chronic progressive health problems are increasingly common and not adequately addressed by most types of health-care insurance.

Disability

Though this is a topic that is not directly related to health-care coverage, it does relate to the impact one's health care can have on the ability to sustain work and to make a living. This usually has implications for health-care coverage. Briefly, the Social Security Administration (SSA) makes disability determinations. They will make a determination based on a thorough and systematic review of all details relating to your health problems and their effects on your ability to work. There are basic criteria and steps upon which this determination is made.

First, your condition has to render you unable to work earning more than five dollars per hour. Your medical condition will need to be on a list of "disabling impairments" that is maintained by the SSA. Examples include heart failure, stroke with neurological impairment, and lung or pulmonary insufficiency. Your condition will need to be sufficiently severe to make it impossible to do your usual work-related activities or a modification of these activities. For example, you may usually work as a custodian, and because of progressive lung problems are unable to maintain a reasonable activity level. If it is possible to respond effectively to vocational rehabilitation or if a sedentary job, such as light office work, filing, or computer work is an option, your claim for disability could be affected.

You will need extensive documentation, including blood work, x-rays, or other testing pertinent to your problem. You will also need supportive documentation from all physicians and providers on your care team, including consultants, if appropriate. The process of gathering information can be tedious and may be frustrating, particularly if many physicians are involved in your care. The effort will be worth it as the detail and extent of the documentation will allow reviewers to make a more accurate determination. It is important to keep in mind that your treating physician does not ultimately make the decision. He or she provides supporting documentation with recommendations. An independent team will review this information, along with specifics regarding your medical problem, previous employment, and prognosis.

You must be unable to work and your disability has to be expected to last at least a year. You can file a claim by going to the nearest Social Security office, or by calling and arranging for an interview (1–800–772–1213). You will be given a detailed list of information you will need to supply. If you are deemed unable to work, you can also apply for Medicare coverage, even if under the age of sixty-five.

DO NOT MISS TAKE HOME POINTS

1. Have a general sense of what your health-care insurance covers. At a minimum, keep that information available to avoid unpleasant surprises from your health-care services.
2. If you do not have health insurance, talk to personnel at your local hospital to look into Medicaid or free care support.

CHAPTER 18

TESTS

Getting to Know All About You,
What You Need to Know

"The art of medicine consists in amusing the patient while nature cures the disease."

—Voltaire

THE OBJECTIVES of this chapter are:

- To review the most common types of tests ordered by physicians.
- To provide an overview of the common reasons (indications) for ordering these tests.
- To point out inherent limitations that exist in the interpretation of tests.
- To provide a brief overview of the process involved with many common tests, including potential risks.

For a health-care provider, arriving at an accurate diagnosis is a lot like solving a mystery. I often remind medical students and residents I teach of the Sherlock Holmes nature of their work. Clinicians gather as many clues as possible from the questions they ask, the observations they make, and from the information you provide. Additional clues are obtained from the physical examination—looking into the ears, listening to the lungs, or examining the abdomen. Most often, the combination of a careful history and physical exam will provide enough information for a recognizable pattern to emerge. It is this pattern that points to a specific diagnosis or possible diagnoses, what we commonly refer to in the profession as a differential diagnosis.

As I have mentioned, people bring interesting and complex stories to their health-care providers. The clues provided may not point to a clear or certain diagnosis. The features may be so "non-specific" as to be caused by a whole host of possibilities, that vary from routine and non-urgent to potentially life threatening. For example, a person who is "weak and dizzy" may have a self-limited (will get better on its own in a matter of days) viral illness on one end of the spectrum, to a possible stroke on the other end, with many possible explanations that fall somewhere in between. Subsequent treatment and outlook will also vary greatly, of course, depending on the diagnosis.

Tests are generally considered to obtain more "clues" as a way of making a more certain, specific, and accurate diagnosis. Tests are also used as a means to follow the activity or progress, that is, response to therapy, of a particular problem. Examples are **Hemoglobin A1c** as a measurement of diabetic sugar or glucose control, **lipid profiles** as a measurement of cholesterol and triglyceride control, or **creatinine** level for the kidney function. It is beyond the scope of this chapter to describe all possible tests now available in health care and what specifically they are used for. I would, however, like to provide you with some basic information about some commonly ordered tests, reasons for ordering them, risks involved (if any), logistics of the testing procedure, and questions to ask that may assist in your understanding of the "what the test means and why the test is being ordered." An excellent book and Web site for a comprehensive review of medical tests is *The Harvard Medical School Family Health Guide,* www.health.harvard.edu/fhg/diagnostics.shtml.

First of all, it is important to keep in mind that very few tests in health care are perfect. I do marvel at the advances and sophistication of available technology and at the same time recognize that many commonly used tests may or may not bring you closer to a definitive diagnosis. At times a test result may lead to more confusion or uncertainty, or generate the need for more tests. We hope for clear answers and often get them. Before reviewing the general categories of commonly ordered tests and procedures, there are some important questions that the ordering clinician should be thinking of and that you should be aware of when tests are ordered. For example:

1. How vital is this test? Will it add important information to what we already know?

2. Is it likely that the results of this test will change the treatment options available to me, or are we likely to do anything different as a consequence of the results?

3. How accurate is this test? Is it likely to give us the information we need?

4. What are the risks of the test? If one hundred people like me undergo the test, how many might have a complication like this?

5. Is there anything special I need to do in preparation for the test, such as fasting or making a change in medication?

6. How much will this test cost, if you are able to tell me, and will my insurance cover the costs?

7. If the test comes back negative, or normal, how certain can we be that this diagnosis is ruled out or excluded?

8. If the test comes back positive, or abnormal, how certain can we be that I have this diagnosis?

9. How long will it take to get the results back?

10. How can I expect to receive the results of the tests?

11. Will other physicians involved in my care be getting the results of this/these tests?

As there are an enormous number of possible tests available, I want to focus on some of the typical or most common test categories.

Blood Work

The overwhelming majority of tests performed in health care require sampling of the blood. Adults have approximately five liters (quarts) of blood circulating in their systems. There are many, many clues to diagnosing disease, monitoring response to treatment, disease prevention, and health maintenance that can be obtained by sampling blood. A needle is used to sample blood from a vein, usually in the arm. Sometimes multiple samples can be obtained from the same needle stick if several tests are ordered. A sampling of commonly ordered blood work includes:

- **White blood cells or WBC**—is ordered to check for a possible sign of infection. When the number of WBC is high, it suggests the possibility of an infection though it does not tell the doctor where the infection is coming from.

- **H&H**—hemoglobin and hematocrit to check for anemia, which is a low red blood cell count.
- **CBC**—complete blood count checks all of these and in addition checks platelet counts. Platelets are another type of blood cell that helps the body make blood clots.
- **Chemistry panel**—sugar or glucose, sodium and potassium levels, kidney function (BUN and Creatinine). This is very important when screening for diabetes, a kidney problem, or changes in electrolytes, e.g., a low potassium level from a diuretic like HCTZ (hydrochlorothiazide).
- **Liver function tests**—a panel of tests that check for inflammation or damage to the liver from a hepatitis virus or medication, for example.
- **PT (prothrombin time) or INR (international ratio)**—a commonly ordered and very important test to see how well your blood clots. This is usually used to monitor adequacy of blood thinning in people taking coumadin or warfarin, commonly used blood thinners to prevent blood clots from forming in people with an irregular heart beat such as atrial fibrillation, for example.
- **Lipid Profile**—a panel of tests for blood cholesterol types and for triglyceride fat levels. It is often obtained after an overnight fasting state as this is when lipid levels are at their lowest.
- **Albumin or pre albumin**—a test to assess nutritional status or how your body's nutritional protein stores are doing: "How full is the cupboard?"
- **Cardiac enzymes**—important tests to measure leaking of specific proteins from the heart due to damage caused by a heart attack (MI or myocardial infarction). We refer to these tests as **CPK and Troponin** levels.
- **Hemoglobin A1C (HbA1c)**—a test to examine glucose or sugar control in the months prior to sampling, unlike a simple blood sugar test that checks your sugar level at that point in time.
- **PSA**—Prostatic Specific Antigen is a blood test used to screen for prostate cancer in men. (See chapter 20, Parting Wisdom for more details on this). If this test shows a high value, your physician will recommend consultation with a urologist and a biopsy of the prostate will likely be advised.
- **C-Reactive Protein (CRP)**—This is a test you will be hearing more about. Though its ideal use is still uncertain, it appears to be a very good "marker" for inflammation in the body. A high level suggests more inflammation than a low level. More specifically, the greatest

interest is in the connection between CRP levels and coronary artery disease (CAD) or risk of having a heart attack. While the jury is still out on this, people at risk for CAD, for example with high blood pressure, diabetes, high cholesterol, smoking, etc., with an elevated CRP level in their blood, may be at an even higher risk for having cardiovascular disease. Some medications such as the statins (an effective class of medications used to treat high cholesterol, e.g. Lipitor), in addition to lowering cholesterol, lower CRP levels. The benefits of lowering CRP levels, at this time, are uncertain.

- **Fasting Blood Sugar (FBS)**—Blood sugar results will also come with "chemistry profile testing." The best screening test for diabetes is the FBS. You are asked to fast, that is, have nothing to eat after 9 P.M. the evening before. The following morning your blood sample is obtained (see chapter 20 for a more detailed discussion of these very important test results).

- **Thyroid Function Tests (TFTs)**—an important, commonly ordered, and very accurate test to diagnose thyroid disease. The thyroid gland is in our neck (right below our "Adam's apple"). It is "dumbbell-shaped" and usually not obvious in appearance. Most people with thyroid problems have an under-functioning gland, with the minority having an over-functioning gland. **TFTs** are an excellent screen for both. If the test is abnormal, you can anticipate having more blood work and possibly a "thyroid scan" obtained. Medications can very effectively treat these common conditions.

Imaging: A Picture Is Worth a Thousand Words

Imaging refers to the testing technology that creates pictures or images. Advances in imaging technology are coming more rapidly and are very sophisticated. Most practicing physicians who have been around for awhile would have never thought possible the detail now routinely available with current technology. The thriving marriage of science and technology makes possible detailed examination of virtually any part of the human body. The pace of these advances has been rapid and as is true for many aspects of our burgeoning sophistication, we are always trying to determine who will most benefit from this testing technology and under what circumstances. The social dividend is marvelous from a diagnostic standpoint, and our profession greatly benefits from the insights these technological breakthroughs offer. The costs are also substantial, therefore our understanding of how to apply these tests, an appreciation of their limitations, and a shared responsibility with respect to utilization, are essential. Many headaches, for example, do not require a CAT scan or MRI of the brain.

As is true with blood work, there are far too many specific types of imaging to review in detail here (www.health.harvard.edu/fhg/diagnostics.shtml). My goal is to provide an overview of the common categories of imaging tests available, common reasons why they are ordered and risks, if any, you need to know about.

PLAIN FILMS

Plain films or "traditional" x-rays were once the only category of imaging tests available to assist a physician with diagnosis. Common types of plain films used include:

- **CXR or chest x-ray:** These are used to examine the lungs for signs of pneumonia, fluid congestion (or CHF, congestive heart failure), abnormal masses that might indicate cancer, enlarged lymph nodes, and others.
- **Bone and joints:** These x-rays are ordered to examine a specific area of the skeletal system, usually for a fracture (break), dislocation, or signs of arthritic damage.
- **KUB:** Though historically used to look at the kidneys, the ureters (the tube that connects the kidneys to the bladder), and the bladder, it does none of the above very well. It is like a chest x-ray of the abdomen, used much less often, as there are much better ways to image the abdomen (e.g., a CAT scan). It can be a useful screen for blockage, or perforation, of the small intestine or colon (large intestine).

CAT SCANS (COMPUTERIZED AXIAL TOMOGRAPHY)

CAT technology catapulted diagnostic imaging by providing much more detail than plain films. Like plain films, they are painless procedures, though some require an IV or drinking of chalk-like liquid (see below). While you are lying flat, a large donut-like structure will encircle you. X-ray images are taken and images are created by computer regeneration. The images look like slices, much like a loaf of bread is sliced. Radiologists are able to examine these slices as they go through whatever is being imaged. CAT scans are usually used to examine the brain, chest, abdomen, spine, and sometimes the joints, though MRI is often used here. CAT scans sometimes require an intravenous infusion of "contrast," a dye-like material that circulates through the blood, creating more detail and information as the images are obtained, for example of the brain or lungs. There are a few things you should be aware of if IV contrast is used:

1. *If you have ever had contrast before and experienced an allergic reaction such as hives, itching, tightness in your throat, trouble breathing, etc.,* **tell your doctor, as you should avoid further contrast exposure.**

2. IV contrast can cause impairment of kidney function. Its approximate risk is ten to fifteen percent in people who already have kidney damage, for example from high blood pressure or diabetes. The more advanced the underlying kidney problem, the greater the risk, sometimes as high as 50 to 70 percent. **It is important, therefore, that you have your kidney function checked prior to receiving IV contrast. This can be achieved by checking blood tests known as BUN and Creatinine.** If use of intravenous contrast is absolutely necessary (as it sometimes can be—see cardiac catheterization or arteriogram), your physician can take steps to minimize, though not eliminate, this risk. These steps should include giving a lot of fluids (IV or by mouth), limiting the amount of contrast material used, and perhaps holding some of your usual medication before and for one to two days after the test. A medication called Mucomyst (acetylcysteine), taken before and after exposure to IV contrast may also reduce the risk of toxicity to the kidneys.

3. Contrast can sometimes give you a "flushed," warm sensation, not to be confused with an allergy.

If you and your treating physician have concerns about your kidney function, consider an alternative imaging test if appropriate, for example an MRI or ultrasound.

CAT scans of the abdomen often require drinking contrast by mouth. This is not dangerous to your kidneys. This is a chalk-like substance that fills the stomach and the small and large intestines, allowing radiologists to examine more accurately both bowel and non-bowel structures in the abdomen.

CAT scans are often used to look for a stroke or bleeding in the brain; blood clots (pulmonary embolus) in the lungs; diagnosing infections such as appendicitis or diverticulitis in the abdomen; abscesses—infections enclosed as a pocket of pus and bacteria; kidney stones; and tumors. CAT scans can look from head to toe in evaluating people with cancer or to evaluate for serious injuries after trauma such as a motor vehicle accident.

Ultrasound

The beauty, safety, and simplicity of sound waves have been an invaluable tool in diagnostic imaging. Unlike plain film and CT or CAT scans, there is no radiation exposure with ultrasound. Ultrasound is safe, painless, and inexpensive. The technician performing the test will place a thick, clear, jelly-like substance on the skin over the area to be examined. A microphone-like object is placed through the jelly and pressed against the skin. A nearby screen allows the technician to position the probe in a way that will provide the best image. Ultrasound focuses sound waves that are reflected back and create an image of where the ultrasound is directed. Common indications for ultrasound include:

- Use in pregnancy to assess fetal growth, position, and development
- Examining the gallbladder for gallstones
- Examining the abdomen for an aneurysm, or for presence of fluid in the abdominal cavity, called ascites
- Examining the ovaries for cysts
- Examining the female reproductive system for an ectopic pregnancy (fetus that is in the fallopian tube instead of the uterus) or for abscess
- Examining the kidneys for blockage or obstruction, and for kidney stones
- For use with guidance of a biopsy procedure, for example a biopsy of the prostate gland

Another type of sound wave test called DUPLEX scanning is often used to check the legs for blood clots (deep venous thrombosis or DVT) and checking the arterial system for circulation problems that can lead to a stroke.

Mammography

Mammography is a specific type of imaging that uses low doses of x-rays to produce detailed images of the breasts. Mammography plays a critical role in the early detection of breast cancers, most often revealing changes in the breast before a patient or physician can feel them. It is important for the ordering physician to be aware of any new findings in your breasts before the mammogram. It is best to schedule mammography one week following your period to minimize any breast tenderness. You should inform your physician or x-ray technologist if there is any possibility that you are pregnant. Before the exam you will be asked to remove all jewelry and clothing above the waist and will be given a gown that opens in the front.

A mammography unit has a box with a device that holds and compresses the breast and positions it so images can be taken at different angles. The examination process should take about half an hour. The radiation dose a woman receives from a routine mammogram is about the same as the average person receives from background radiation in three months. The risks are negligibly small relative to the benefits.

The American Cancer Society recommends:

- Avoid use of deodorant, talcum powder, or lotion under your arms on the day of the exam as these can appear on the x-ray film as calcium spots.
- Describe any breast symptoms to the technologist performing the exam.
- If you have had prior mammograms done at another facility, try to have them sent to the imaging center where you are having your current exam for comparison.
- Ask when the results will be available. Do not assume the exam was normal if you do not hear anything.

It is important to appreciate that approximately 5 to 10 percent of mammogram results are abnormal and require more testing—more mammograms, ultrasound, needle sampling, or biopsy. Usually, repeat testing is reassuringly normal. It is also important, as has been emphasized in all of the aforementioned testing, that mammograms are not perfect. A "normal" test might miss a cancer if a woman has large, "dense" breasts, prior surgery, or implants.

2-D CARDIAC (HEART) ECHO

The two-dimensional cardiac echo is a commonly ordered test to examine how well the heart is pumping and how well the heart valves are working. The cardiologist gets a nice visualization of the heart and heart valves that can be particularly useful in settings of heart murmurs, congestive heart failure, and in the assessment of damage to the heart after a heart attack. The ECHO can also be used as part of a stress test to see if the heart is contracting or pumping uniformly and vigorously in response to a "stimulant" called Dobutamine.

A second type of heart ECHO is referred to as a TEE or trans-esophageal echo. This procedure also uses sound waves, though instead of positioning the probe over the breastbone and chest, it is placed into the esophagus, by swallowing. The main advantage here is the ability to visualize the heart valves in more detail. This is usually recommended when looking for a blood clot or infection that is "sticking" to the heart valves and poses a risk of breaking off, traveling to the brain, and causing a stroke.

MRI (MAGNETIC RESONANCE IMAGING)

MRIs have been another revolutionary breakthrough in the use of imaging for diagnosis. MRIs work by the application of a super-powerful magnet that, when applied to a particular part of the body, aligns the molecules of the tissues in a way that creates exquisite detail in imaging. There is no radiation involved with an MRI. Because a powerful magnetic field is created, any metallic device inside you, such as a pacemaker, may preclude use of MRI. You will be asked to complete a detailed questionnaire beforehand to screen for any such "hardware." Some MRI machines involve being inside a very confining space that can easily lead to a claustrophobic feeling. Not everyone can tolerate this, particularly having to lie perfectly still for fifteen to twenty minutes, which can feel like an eternity when there is little space between you and the machine. Some newer MRIs are "open" and thus much more comfortable. If you are anticipating an MRI and have a tendency to feel claustrophobic, check to see if the machine is an "open" one. If not, let your physician know. There may be an alternative test to get the required information, for example a CAT scan. It is better to deal with this in advance than to become claustrophobic at the time of the test, after waiting some time to get it done in the first place and then feeling badly about the circumstances. This could result in an even longer wait for an alternative test to be scheduled and a diagnosis made.

It is fair to say that the full potential of MRI has yet to be realized. Frequent uses include:

- Brain—to diagnosis strokes, tumors, infections
- Abdomen—to diagnose tumors, abscesses
- Joints, e.g., shoulders, hips, knees—to diagnose structural damage to cartilage or ligaments
- Spine—to diagnose disc disease and pinched nerves, usually in the neck or lower back

A special type of magnetic resonance imaging can look specifically at blood vessels. This is called an MRA, or magnetic resonance arteriogram. This is used most commonly in the neck and brain to look for blocked arteries that may be causing or could lead to a stroke. It is sometimes used in the legs to diagnose blocked or narrowed arteries in people with circulation problems.

ARTERIOGRAM

An arteriogram is an x-ray that involves placing an IV into an artery in the groin. This is done using a local anesthetic. Any discomfort is similar to that of having a blood sample drawn. Contrast or "dye" is injected into the blood vessels, creating a roadmap-like picture of the arteries. It is used to most accurately diagnose blockage or narrowing in an artery. Typically, this is used to look at the legs in people with circulation problems, or in the renal (kidney) arteries to diagnose a narrowed/blocked area. A radiologist who specializes in "interventions" does this testing. We cleverly refer to this individual as an *interventional radiologist*. Depending on the circumstances, the interventional radiologist may place a balloon in a narrowed blood vessel and inflate it to open up the narrowed area. This is called angioplasty.

A similar procedure is routinely performed in the heart and is referred to as *cardiac catheterization*. When a balloon or percutaneous transluminal coronary angioplasty (PTCA) is used in the heart, a stent or straw-like metallic mesh is placed into the area to help keep the artery open after the balloon has pushed open the narrowed area.

After an arteriogram or cardiac catheterization, you can anticipate being restricted to bed rest for approximately four to six hours with a sandbag on your groin area. This is a precaution to minimize any bleeding after the procedure. It is unusual for bleeding to require anything other than rest and direct pressure to the site where the study was performed.

STRESS TESTING ON THE HEART

Another common category of testing is stress testing to look for heart disease. Stress testing is ordered for a few common reasons:

- Evaluation of chest discomfort or shortness of breath to determine if the cause is a narrowed or blocked artery in your heart.

- Follow-up evaluation after a balloon angioplasty or heart bypass operation in an individual having symptoms of chest discomfort or shortness of breath, again, to determine whether the coronary arteries that were previously opened have closed again.
- Evaluation for heart risk prior to major surgery, especially if you are having symptoms as previously described or if you have multiple risk factors for a heart complication, such as high blood pressure, diabetes, smoking, high cholesterol, prior history of heart disease, and a positive family history.

There are a few different ways a stress test can be performed.

1. **Exercise treadmill test**—Here you will walk on a treadmill until fatigue, shortness of breath, or chest discomfort limits your capacity to continue. A continuous cardiogram tracing will be recorded by sticky electrodes or pads attached to your chest. The accuracy of the test is enhanced the longer you exercise and the higher your blood pressure and heart rate go, that is, as normally seen with exercise. You may need to withhold some of your medications twenty-four hours prior to the test. Discuss this with the ordering M.D. beforehand.
2. **Exercise test as above with injection of a "radio nuclide tracer"** called cardiolite, sestamibi, or thallium. Pictures are taken during and after exercise to see if parts of the heart may not be getting enough blood flow, suggestive of a narrowed or blocked coronary artery.
3. **Persantine-Cardiolite stress test.** This is a type of stress test for people unable to tolerate exercise on a treadmill due to arthritis, circulation problems in the legs, obesity, lung disease, or deconditioning. Here, Persantine (a pharmaceutical that opens up or dilates blood vessels) is used in a way that mimics exercise.
4. **Dobutamine ECHO.** This uses ECHO or sound waves to visualize the heart pumping. Dobutamine stimulates the heart as exercise would. Normally when the heart pumps, the heart muscle contracts in its entirety, as if you were opening and closing the fingers on your hand to make a tight fist. If part of the heart that was contracting or squeezing normally before the infusion of Dobutamine changes after infusion of Dobutamine, it suggests a narrowed coronary artery.

Significant symptoms such as chest discomfort, shortness of breath, light-headedness, or excessive fatigue, with or without an abnormal stress test, may lead to the recommendation of a cardiac catheterization (see below), if appropriate for your circumstances. The cardiac catheterization continues to be the "gold standard," or the best test to diagnose narrowed or blocked coronary arteries. As described in the section on arteriograms, the coronary catheterization is done using a local anesthetic. An IV or catheter is then placed into the artery in your groin. Using x-ray imaging, the IV catheter is threaded into the heart arteries and an injection of IV contrast is given. The arteries of the heart "light up," revealing areas that are narrowed or blocked. Balloon angioplasty and stenting are considered at that time, if appropriate.

There is a great deal of interest in the potential use of high resolution CAT scanning to examine the coronary arteries more accurately. While not yet adequately studied with comparison to the gold standard arteriogram, you may read about this in the lay press.

PET Scans (Positron Emission Tomography)

PET scanning is the newest addition to available imaging technology. Simply stated, PET scanning involves an injection of an isotope, a minute amount of radioactive substance that circulates into the body and is taken up by the cells in various locations. While the optimal utilization of PET scanning is still a work in progress, its most common use is in looking for evidence of cancer that has spread to other areas, for example to the lung. It is useful also in examining responses after chemotherapy or radiation therapy, in an individual who has already been diagnosed with cancer. It works on the principle that a tumor cell dividing more rapidly has a higher metabolism than a normal cell, and as a result, will take up more of the isotope and "light up" in the scan.

Endoscopy

Endoscopy is a test that allows visualization of the inside lining of the esophagus (connects the mouth to the stomach), the stomach, and the first part of the small intestine. It is also referred to as an EGD, very short for esophagogastroduodenoscopy. This procedure is performed using a fiber optic scope, approximately the diameter of your finger. This test is ordered most commonly to evaluate:

- Anemia, such as loss of blood from an ulcer; gastritis (inflammation of the stomach); or tumor
- To provide a diagnosis for individuals with symptoms of "dyspepsia." Causes might include reflux, also known as GERD; an ulcer; or tumor.
- To evaluate individuals with a possible blockage, for example, difficulty in swallowing, with food or drink getting stuck on the way down.

The procedure involves gargling with an anesthetic that numbs the back of the throat to prevent the "gag reflex." A light sedative is sometimes used for relaxation. The test itself usually takes less than thirty minutes. Visualization usually allows diagnosis or exclusion of any of the above concerns. EGD also allows potential treatment, such as cauterization of a bleeding ulcer, in appropriate individuals.

COLONOSCOPY

Technically, colonoscopy is similar to endoscopy, except that the gastroenterologist is looking into the colon. Again, the procedure usually does not take long and is tolerable with the use of sedation. The preparation for colonoscopy is generally worse than the colonoscopy itself, as the test requires drinking several quarts of a cathartic to clean out the colon beforehand. The prep is extremely important, as a "clean colon" allows for better visualization, diagnosis, and treatment.

As you may know, colonoscopy has emerged as a vital screening test for colon cancer and is recommended for everyone at age fifty (see chapter 20, Parting Wisdom), or age forty-five if there is a positive family history. Colonoscopy is also extremely useful in diagnosing pre-existing problems with the colon, such as bleeding from a polyp or tumor, or for diverticulosis, an outpouching of the colon, very common as we age.

BIOPSY

A biopsy is a sampling of tissue from somewhere in the body, that is done to determine the cause or nature of something seen on an imaging study such as an x-ray or CAT scan, or something felt on exam, for example a lump in the breast or an enlarged lymph node. Most of the time, a biopsy is done to distinguish a "benign growth," of absolutely no concern, from a possible tumor, cancer, or infection.

The other reason to do a biopsy is to make a diagnosis and determine the extent of damage in a particular organ. For example, blood testing may demonstrate abnormalities of liver or kidney function, or an abnormal urinalysis or routine test of the urine may demonstrate the presence of blood and/or protein, neither of which a person may know exists. While these routine tests point to a problem, they do not necessarily clarify the cause or extent of the problem. This is where the biopsy can potentially add useful information. This information may significantly affect how the problem is treated and may allow important prognostic information to emerge.

For example, the most common reason to biopsy the liver is in a person with a history of viral hepatitis B or C. Hepatitis C is now much more common. Because the treatment of hepatitis C, for example, is continued over a long period of time, six months to a year, and has the potential for nasty side effects, the biopsy helps you and the gastroenterologist determine how beneficial treatment might be.

In the kidneys, an abnormal urinalysis and/or blood work may not have an obvious cause. Here the biopsy can shed more light on the diagnosis, prognosis, and best way to treat.

Regardless of the circumstances, a biopsy ordinarily involves use of a local anesthetic to numb the surrounding skin and soft tissues beneath the skin. A needle, not unlike an IV in diameter, is inserted into the organ or area of concern and samples of tissue are obtained. Depending on the location of the area being biopsied, imaging—CAT scan or ultrasound—may be used to guide the placement of the biopsy needle. Once the tissue is sampled, it is placed in a special container and sent to the pathology laboratory for analysis. Depending on the circumstances, a final pathology report might take about one week; a preliminary diagnosis may be possible within hours, with more specific information in a few days.

DO NOT MISS TAKE HOME POINTS

1. You should have as much understanding as possible of any test being done.
2. If the test results are "normal," what does that mean?
3. If the results are "abnormal," what does that mean?
4. What are the risks, if any, of the tests?
5. Keep a record of all your test results, such as blood tests, electrocardiogram, and x-ray reports. These can be obtained from your physician's office. These records are vital and can assist those involved in your care.

CHAPTER 19

MEDICAL EDUCATION

Patient as Teacher

"To acquire knowledge, one must study; but to acquire wisdom, one must observe."

—Marilyn vos Savant

THE OBJECTIVES of this chapter are:

- To review the importance of medical education in the health-care setting.
- To emphasize the role of patient as informer and teacher.

During your encounters with the health-care system, you will probably meet an individual who is in some phase of his or her educational training. Medical students, residents, nurses, pastoral care students, LPNs, technical staff, and many other allied health trainees require the acquisition of principles, knowledge, skills, and clinical experience that can be obtained only "in the trenches." An understanding of our health-care system as a venue for patient care and for educational training is an important one. I have been very lucky to have as one of my primary responsibilities the teaching of nurses, medical students, and residents. Recognizing the essential role patients play in this educational process, I want to share a few brief insights regarding medical education.

If you have ever been admitted to a teaching hospital, you were probably seen by a host of people who were both participating in your care and in the process of training. For everyone from third-year medical students, experiencing clinics and hospital wards for the first time, to seasoned veterans, you, the patient, are the main focus of attention. When you are ill, particularly if physically and emotionally distressed, it may not be easy to interact with trainees in an enthusiastic, participatory way. Individuals in training are likely to ask more questions, take more time, and perhaps require more than one attempt to satisfactorily complete their tasks, for example, blood drawing, starting an IV, or doing an EKG. When ill, your patience for questions and on-the-job performance improvement may understandably be limited.

The training of physicians and other health-care professionals is an integral part of the health-care enterprise. This elaborate process will often be occurring behind the scenes, in conference rooms, teaching rounds, and other activities. Occasionally, though not nearly often enough, the teaching occurs at the bedside. The greatest potential for learning will occur at your bedside. The bedside is where it is happening from my perspective as a clinical educator. It is that coveted shared space between you the patient and all involved in your care that the greatest opportunity for learning exists. The bedside is where all are connected, where the observations are direct and genuine and where unspoken communication is at its poignant best.

The increasingly hectic lives of physicians and medical students, combined with the sophistication of applied science and technology, have shifted the ultimate "classroom" for teaching from the bedside to the conference room. I believe this is also true for hospital administrators, who spend an inordinate amount of time developing strategies for high-quality, efficient, and cost-effective care, with less time spent in direct contact with the environment where care is occurring and with the individuals whose lives their mission is to make better. We can improve our system both clinically and administratively only by being in touch with those we serve.

Your patience and willingness to share with those who are in training will develop more experienced and skilled practitioners. Many other people will eventually benefit from this experience. The wisdom of experience we want in those to whom we entrust our care ultimately came as a consequence of hundreds of people before us, sharing their stories and themselves, with the then medical student (third or fourth year), resident (three to five years after medical school), fellow (two to three years after residency training to specialize, for example in cardiology or vascular surgery), and junior attending (starting practice).

If your nurse or physician is a more experienced veteran, many patients before you contributed to the development of these refined skills. You probably do not realize how important your role is as teacher when you encounter a health-care professional. You may also be thinking, "C'mon, Pettus, when I'm sick, I want to focus on being the patient, not the teacher. I want to feel better, not teach." By feeling sick, seeking care, and by a natural desire to heal, you choose to share your story with others. Some will be seasoned professionals, some new to their practices, and many still in training.

It is in the sharing of your story that you both teach and allow others to best assist you.

The more information shared, the better. Think of health-care providers as specialized chefs in a large kitchen that prepares a wide range of simple to very sophisticated entrees. Think of your shared information, input, and thoughts as the ingredients. Chefs can create some marvelous entrees, more likely to suit your taste, by having an abundant source of ingredients. There, I have done the injustice of reducing the health-care encounter to the preparation of a meal.

Students, residents, and fellows, as a means of learning, may in fact have a little more time and interest in talking with you. As we participate in the learning process and to the extent that your circumstances allow, view these encounters as opportunities for someone to learn about you in a way that will also help others. I feel it is also very important to see yourself as a source of feedback, responding to skills (or lack thereof) in areas of active listening, communication, decision making, and interpersonal style. Across the spectrum of training and experience, we health-care professionals need your feedback, both positive and constructive. It is clear that many health-care professionals are unaware of or not appreciative of the impact of certain "practice styles," both positive and negative. Health-care personnel are sometimes uncertain about what they are doing well and what they need to improve. Awkward though providing candid feedback may feel, I believe most health-care professionals will be appreciative. Most genuinely wish to be more effective, to improve the satisfaction of the encounter with you and other patients and families to follow. The patient as teacher can go a long way in making these "improvable behavior patterns" more effective.

Health-care training in the United States is the envy of the world. Research and clinical scholars from all over the world wish to gain experience in the United States because of the incredible legacy of basic science research and applied sophisticated clinical knowledge. I look into the eyes of medical students I teach and I am filled with hope for the future. Ours is a profession that, now more than ever, needs leaders who are bright, compassionate, and interpersonally strong. We need young leaders who advocate with compassion and purpose. One of the greatest sources of inspiration and motivation will come from you, in your state of need. Though you may sometimes "feel like a number," your story is unique, interesting, and vital to the success of the health-care encounter. Though in a vulnerable state, reliant on the clinical skills and expertise of those to whom you entrust your care, you are just on the other side of the very fine line that separates those of us who treat from those of us in need of treatment.

So if you see someone at your bedside who looks young, interested, uncertain, or overwhelmed, extend your hand and heart if able, and welcome yourself as patient and teacher.

DO NOT MISS TAKE HOME POINTS

1. As a patient, you are a storyteller. Share your story. You will help yourself and those assisting you, many in various levels of training.
2. The experience and wisdom we desire in our doctors is made possible by your sharing with those less experienced, on the path of wisdom.

CHAPTER 20

PARTING WISDOM

The Best Advice I Can Give Anyone for a Long and Happy Life

"I don't want to achieve immortality through my work . . . I want to achieve it through not dying."

—Woody Allen

THE OBJECTIVES of this chapter are:

- To empower you with self-management insight and action steps that could profoundly change the way you live.
- To provide an antedote to inertia, the enemy of action and getting things done.
- To lay out a roadmap for health maintenance and disease prevention with "pearls" that will make your journey more informed and satisfying.
- To add years to your life.

The Savvy Patient was written to help you recognize the potential for more effective control of your health and your health-care encounters. Our choices in life are critical in creating positive life experiences and in serving our deepest values. Good choices can allow us to live longer. While good choices are necessary, they are not, unfortunately, enough to provide full control of the outcome. There is no such thing as full control. Instead, control what you can . . . your relationship to self and others. I have always enjoyed writing, and in large part, this book has been a therapeutic endeavor. It has lifted me from some of the stress of "life at the shop" . . . much cheaper than Prozac and with far fewer side effects.

If you had to pay for this book, it is my goal to make it worth every penny spent and then some. If you re-read or periodically re-examine, as reference only, one chapter in this book, this is the one.

The advice I am about to share could significantly change the quality and possibly the length of your life. Medical knowledge is always changing rapidly and at times unpredictably. I would have given anything twenty years ago to be able to apply the knowledge I am about to share with my parents and my extended family. The truth is that many of these insights were waiting to be born. Sharing these insights with you may help to reduce illness and disease-related complications and provide greater potential for good health and happiness.

In truth, you have more control over your health than you perhaps ever imagined. You have much more potential to impact your health and wellness than any physician, medication, or hospital ever will. That is not to say, of course, that modern medicine has not accomplished marvelous breakthroughs. Life expectancy has almost doubled since the turn of the twentieth century and disease prevention and treatment, once unimaginable, are now reality. Awareness and improvements in public health measures, cleaner water and sanitization, have had a lot to do with this.

Americans have understandably come to expect a lot from our health-care system. Not a day goes by without reading or hearing about a remarkable breakthrough in health care. Our health-care system is more commonly examined as a "provider/consumer" model these days. From a business standpoint (and at 15 percent of our Gross National Product, medicine is big business) this paradigm makes perfect sense. All service industries aim to please their customers. This is the first commandment of the marketplace. People deserve quality care, shorter waiting times, reductions in medical errors, best possible outcomes, and more than anything, access and compassion. And while people in need of health care can be thought of as customers, health promotion and disease prevention are not exactly like buying a television or going out to a restaurant. At the risk of sounding self-righteous and unfair, many people I encounter in my work expect much more from the system than they do from themselves. For some people there is a passive tendency to take their health for granted with the expectation that the system will be able to fix it when it's broken.

Compassionate caring should always be at the core of the health-care encounter. The point, and perhaps the most important message from this book, is the notion that you can be marvelously empowered by taking an active role in your health and wellness. While you are a consumer or "customer" of health care, your greatest health-care service is to yourself. Consumption of health care is not the same as consumption of fast food or technology. The stakes are much higher, the responsibility much greater, and the yield on the investment priceless. It is in this spirit of sharing what I can that I offer the following advice . . . the best medical advice I can give you. But before I do I want to touch briefly on the topic of "watchful waiting."

Watchful waiting overcoming the inertia to action. (He/she who hesitates misses a huge opportunity.)

As you focus your commitment to greater understanding of your health, you will begin to see many opportunities for change. Trying to close the gap from where we are in our lives to where we desire to be requires tremendous awareness, understanding, motivation, and action. If your efforts and those of your physician do not translate into positives change, it is time for action. *Action is the only way to get things done!* Lip service and mind games are not your friends. Action is where it is happening.

For example, I have, many times as a physician, recommended a watch-and-wait attitude in my approach to patients with "borderline" high blood pressure, diabetes, and high cholesterol. Watchful waiting is appropriate when lifestyle and behavior modification are working to bring you closer to your health goals and are likely to succeed. It may not be appropriate, however, when progress is slow or nonexistent, and the risk of "doing nothing" is substantial. Like many physicians I have deferred starting new medication due to reluctance on my patient's part to take medications. There may be cost issues or a history of side affects that create obstacles to action. For whatever reason, it is common, perhaps too common, for the physician-patient partnership to be reluctant to act in a more timely and aggressive manner, especially when available medical evidence strongly supports an intervention.

While many physicians point to patient preferences as reason not to take action, it is actually more common for physicians themselves to be reluctant to start or intensify treatment. There is a psychology to "minimizing" concern from a physician perspective. Patients and families are less likely to be upset if the problem is framed as "mild." Potential concerns, from a patient perspective, about taking new medications, can be avoided. Perhaps the time and "hassle" involved with starting a new intervention, for example, starting insulin in a diabetic whose sugar control is poor, can be delayed until another time. Positive though this approach may feel to everyone involved, it commonly results in under-treatment.

While you may not feel different, as symptoms go, the cumulative effect could be devastating—having a stroke, heart attack, or developing kidney damage.

In the old paternalistic model of delivering health care, it was appropriate to simply accept the decision of the treating physician, no questions asked. This is not a model that works well now, a recurrent theme in *The Savvy Patient*. So what am I suggesting? As you will see in the remainder of this chapter, there are many vital signs or numbers that you must know about. These are your goals for successful treatment and good health. If you are not at these goals, talk to your doctor about taking action. If you hear "It's okay, this is just a touch of diabetes or borderline high blood pressure, let's keep an eye on things," speak up! The expression "mild" may need to be interpreted as a call for action. It may feel awkward, but it's the right thing to do. Having been guilty of this many times myself, I know that physicians may be near the tipping point to treat, reluctant to move into action out of concern for how you might interpret the need for changes. As partners in your health, physicians should recommend timely and aggressive intervention with any treatment that can prolong your life and reduce complications. If lifestyle changes and behavioral modification begin to work more effectively, the decision to withdraw medication and other treatments is always an option. Here are some examples where watchful waiting of the status quo may not be in your best interest:

- Borderline high blood pressure
- Failure to intensify treatment when high blood pressure is already being treated and not in good control
- "Pre-diabetes" or borderline diabetes
- Failure to intensify treatment, such as starting insulin or adding oral medications, in an established diabetic whose control is poor
- Borderline high cholesterol and triglycerides
- "Mild" kidney disease. "Mild" in the eyes of many primary care physicians is not considered mild by nephrologists or kidney specialists.
- "Mild emphysema." Once signs of emphysema are seen on a chest x-ray, a lot of water has gone under the bridge.

Remember these three principles and do not hesitate to raise them in conversations with your physician:

1. Normal is always better than borderline!
2. A "mild" problem should receive maximum attention, including consultation by a specialist who can work with your primary care provider to see that all that can be done, is being done.
3. Small action steps can make very large differences.

Ask your doctor, when on the fence about whether to intervene or watch and wait, "What would you do if you were in my shoes or if I was your parent/grandparent?" While many mild medical problems may not require or have proven treatments, many do.

So here we go, you and me. The advice you are about to read may add years to your life. It will however, take a lot of work. This will not come easily. *Do not, I repeat, do not put your health on autopilot.* While there are no guarantees, your odds of improved quality and quantity of life could go up considerably. Now I have to include a disclaimer. I hate to do this because I am most sincere in the advice I am about to give. Best medical evidence is always rapidly evolving. Best medical advice is always changing and for some individuals, the best advice will vary. You may need to discuss some of these suggestions with your physician to ensure their safety and appropriateness as they apply to you.

Some of this advice is ancient wisdom, wisdom that has been powerfully reaffirmed in what I have done and seen over the last twenty years. It is wisdom that cannot be overstated. What I am attempting to do is to distill all that I know into the most important, most meaningful advice possible. It is hard for me to list this advice in order of importance, as all of it is important. If some suggestions do not seem relevant to you, move on to the next. Remember, discuss any questions you may have about this with your primary care provider. Here we go. This reads like David Letterman's top ten insights as they relate to your health.

Wash Your Hands!

If God spoke to me by saying, "Mark, you're down to your last three words: what do you want to say to your fellow humans that would make the most positive impact?" It would be a close call between *Love Thy Neighbor* and *Wash Your Hands*. A close third would be *Move, Move, Move*. All would actually have a profound impact on your health and wellness, and when all are combined? Watch out! You're off to the races. The sky is the limit!

Most respiratory and common gastrointestinal infections are spread from contamination of our hands. It is no coincidence that surgeons scrub their hands for several minutes before performing surgery. Now, it is not necessary to perform a "surgical scrub" several times a day. Good hand washing, however, before every meal, after every visit to the bathroom, and after repetitive contact with others, cannot be overemphasized. You do not have to be an obsessive-compulsive knucklehead about this. Washing your hands, however, whenever possible, will most definitely improve the quality of your life. A great breakthrough of late, in my opinion, has been the development of alcohol-based antiseptic hand cleansers. These are the cleansers that do not require water. They are an excellent way to clean, they are convenient, and they dry within seconds. I have had fewer colds, GI (gastrointestinal) infections, and respiratory infections by keeping this stuff handy and readily available. I keep it in my glove compartment, briefcase, and at the office. In addition, keep your hands out of your nose, your mouth, and your eyes. Okay, so now you may think I am a little off balance. I'm a doctor—trust me. What this advice will save you, in cold and cough remedies alone, will more than pay for this book.

Walk 150 Minutes a Week: Move, Move, Move

That would be thirty minutes a day, five days a week, or approximately forty-five minutes three days a week. If you exercise more than this, great. If not, make this your goal! Start with ten to fifteen minutes per session and increase every one or two weeks until you are at your target. Humans were meant for mobility. Is it a coincidence we have evolved into two-legged creatures? Can you imagine how long our prehistoric ancestors would have lasted if they had sat around all day? Instead of eating, they would have been the meal. *We owe it to all the people who walked this earth before us to keep moving!* Resist gravity and resist immobilization. Move, move, move. Motion is the lotion. Before I touch on some recent medical evidence linking exercise with reductions in risks of diabetes, heart disease, and stroke, I want you to consider the phenomenon of "pain leading to gain."

Anyone who exercises regularly will be quick to notice the phenomenon of pain leading to gain. The hypothesis goes something like this. As we start to engage in any activity, regardless of the shape we are in, we will experience some discomfort as we stretch and work muscles, bones, tendons, ligaments, and other "connective tissues." This will be a source of local mechanical signals to the brain that translate as discomfort, stiffness, and sometimes, significant pain. Mentally we may feel tired, lethargic, and sluggish. The mind and body will make its strong case to cease. And indeed, ceasing will diminish these undesirable feelings. Our stopping is positively reinforced in the short term. We conclude, "I can't do this. My body can't take this. I'm stuck here." The consequences are a disaster! We convince ourselves that we cannot elevate ourselves to a more active place. We become resigned to immobility, content to do only what our bodies suggest we can do.

The breakthrough comes when we transcend these powerful physical, emotional, and mental hurdles. Within ten minutes of starting activity, areas of the brain are "turned on" and a remarkable transformation occurs. I know because of what many people who have been there have shared with me and because of what I have personally experienced. When these areas in the brain are turned on, we tend to notice our discomfort less. Our brain actually modulates our perception of pain. Neurotransmitters are produced that create a satisfying feeling of euphoria, motivation, and strength. This in turn becomes a powerfully positive biological effect that sends the message KEEP GOING, DON'T STOP! When people refer to an addiction to exercise, they are literally describing a remarkable neurobiologic phenomenon that takes the message of "I must stop, I can't do this, it hurts too much," and transforms it into "I feel soooo good and I look forward to the next opportunity." This phenomenon is within you! It takes only ten minutes a day for a few weeks to recognize and strengthen.

I have seen other remarkable examples of this phenomenon in action. People who are able, for example, to reduce salt and sweets in their diets in a consistent and disciplined fashion, for as little as three weeks, will soon notice how incredibly salty and sweet things taste when these foods are reintroduced. Again, the body adapts biologically to these changes in a manner that reinforces the changed behavior. If a patient tells me they could not tolerate reducing salt in their diet because of taste, I know they did not give it much of an effort. Whether it is exercise, dieting, or any other behavioral or lifestyle change, if it will improve your health, *the more you do, the more you do.* We seem to be hardwired for this. All most of us need is to be aware of this power within and to develop the desire to tap into it. The key is to start small and build momentum.

Even if your health makes it difficult to walk, find a position that is comfortable and keep those arms and legs moving. Your ultimate goal should be at least 150 minutes a week. The evidence is clear; simple walking improves health and wellness through greater mobility of your joints, enhanced muscle tone, improved bone strength, and emotional wellness. If you are at risk for diabetes (and recent data suggests that approximately 6 to 8 percent of adults in the United States are diabetic and as many as 10 to 12 percent are at risk as "pre-diabetics"!), *evidence suggests that losing 7 percent of your weight (if overweight) and walking 150 minutes per week, reduces your risk of progressing to diabetes by almost 50 percent! No medication is this effective.* In other words, you could perhaps cut your risk of having diabetes in half by walking regularly and by losing a relatively small amount of weight. This is a pretty good yield on the investment! The other important message here is that *small steps lead to large gains.*

Walking is a good way to clear your head. Music can be a stimulating motivator while walking. You can walk anywhere, even standing in place while at home. I should add that walking at work or while shopping, for example, doesn't count. While it may help, exercise time should be special time reserved for you. Say to yourself, today and most days, "I have an appointment with me! It's an appointment I cannot break." Walk at the maximum pace that is comfortable for you.

The National Academy of Sciences has recently published guidelines on "New Exercise Recommendations for Health." Ideally, spend one hour each day in "moderately intense physical activity." This is twice the daily minimum established by the 1996 Surgeon General's report.

Examples of moderate intensity activity include:

- Stair walking for fifteen minutes
- Walking two miles in thirty minutes
- Pushing a stroller 1.5 miles in thirty minutes
- Bicycling five miles in thirty minutes
- Dancing fast for thirty minutes. I like this one. Music and movement are a potent combination!

Get your Butts Kicked!

Smoking is a brutal habit. I mean Brutal with a capital "B." It is wicked, wicked, wicked. Nicotine is a potent and strongly addictive drug. It is clearly very, very hard to quit, even with the knowledge that your life is surely being shortened by the habit. To say, "quit smoking" to someone whose very life revolves around the habit is well intentioned and usually ineffective advice. The key ingredient here is *motivation,* true for much of the advice I am giving you. There may be many sources of motivation within you such as education, illness in you or other family members, love for your children and spouse, loss of a loved one, love of life, or negative social stigma. The greatest reason of all is self. *Motivation ultimately has to come from within.* Motivation comes from having a value in life—to be smoke free—that takes on too much meaning to ignore. Motivation has to emerge from the awareness that the overwhelming consumption and hassle that accumulate from thinking about quitting can no longer be offset by the pleasure smoking gives you. In other words, the hassle of continuing to smoke, such as the negative impact on your health, and the emotional, physical, and financial consequences, become much worse than the challenge of quitting itself.

There is no easy or surefire way to kick this unforgiving habit. I've seen too many people after heart attacks, strokes, or breathlessness with minimal activity such as a trip to the bathroom, cling to the habit with a hopeless sense of having no control. That is what addiction is. It is a biologic and emotionally consuming response that replaces hope with loss of control. People do get over addictions. People can overcome the intense habitual craving and conquer the seemingly impossible. People can do it. People have done it. These are people just like you and me! This will not be easy. Do not expect it to be easy. You will spend every waking moment of every day consumed by it. That is beside the point! If you feel ready to make the choice to quit, here are some suggestions to increase your chances. I must also add that if you do not succeed initially, discouraging and hopeless though it may seem, keep the faith. I have seen many people successfully quit even after several failed attempts. Advice physicians are given when they want to try to help their patients quit smoking includes "**The 5 A's**," developed by the U.S. Public Health Service:

1. **ASK** every patient about tobacco use.
2. **ADVISE** all tobacco users to quit.
3. **ASSESS** each patient's willingness to make a quit attempt.
4. **ASSIST** the patient in quitting by providing medication and resources.
5. **ARRANGE** for the patient to return for follow-up.

The key is to want it to badly happen. Physician advice, support, and prescribed treatment can have a significant impact on your success. It is estimated that only 3 percent of people who quit cold turkey remain smoke free at one year. With the support outlined below and with your total commitment, these results can go up by a factor of ten, or 25 to 35 percent!

- Pick a date to celebrate the end of an old nemesis and the beginning of a new life. Consider this the birth date of your new life!
- Talk to your physician about a medication that may help with the emotional roller coaster of cravings and desire. This should be started approximately two weeks prior to quitting. It is not my purpose to promote specific brands of medication, though I can tell you that one exists. It is called Brupropion sustained-release. Your provider will know which one. This medication may also limit the increased appetite and weight gain that so often accompany smoking cessation.
- Also take, at the time you quit, nicotine replacement medication. There are different forms of this, most commonly patches, chewing gum, and lozenges, available without a prescription. Nicotine replacement is also available by prescription as a nasal spray or in inhaled form. This is key to reducing the symptoms of withdrawal that are strongest in the first few days after quitting. They will not eliminate cravings and withdrawal symptoms in their entirety, though they will help. Physical symptoms from withdrawal are at their worse in the first two to four days after stopping.
- Strap yourself in and hold on! The next forty-eight to seventy-two hours are critical! You will feel like you are going out of your mind! You will tell yourself you cannot do it! You will confront habitual patterns that will leave you wondering how you will ever make it through the day. You will confront the minutes, the hours, and eventually the days and weeks. *Remember, you do have a choice. This is your life. You have one body for living that life.* When the temptation is overwhelming, call a friend. Talk to your spouse. If he or she smokes, it is critical that he or she rise to the challenge with you. You are much more likely to be successful if your significant other can quit with you. You then increase the odds of being together longer. I am assuming that is an important goal for you. Carry a picture of your children, your spouse, or perhaps a younger picture of yourself. Repeat a meaningful prayer.

Some people try hypnosis. I am certified in hypnotherapy and have seen some success in this area. I find that there are many misperceptions about hypnosis. Hypnosis is a state of deep relaxation and focused awareness that can foster the mental and emotional energy to resist craving and to maintain control while fighting the urge to light up. Hypnosis is not some magical spell that you will emerge from never craving a cigarette again. All hypnosis is self-hypnosis. You will still crave and struggle with the challenges of abstention, and hypnosis can take the edge off. Remember, motivation is the key to success regardless of the strategies you try.

Go for a ride, or better yet, a forty-five-minute walk! Day by day, in every way, your desire to smoke will be replaced by the growing control you have over it. This can work. People have done this. People do succeed. These are people just like you.

The Weight is Over

This is another one of those "impossible dream" categories and again, I do not mean to suggest this is easy to do or a simple matter of understanding its importance. As difficult as it is to lose weight, it is even more challenging to maintain weight loss. We are just beginning to understand the complex biologic system in our brains that regulates hunger and energy expenditure, that is, how we burn calories and lose weight. In the words of John Bantle, M.D., who researches weight control, "When we ask patients to restrict energy intake (food consumption) and increase energy expenditure through exercise to lose weight, we are asking them to override a powerful biologic control system."

Obesity is an epidemic in our society. Recent data would suggest that approximately 30 percent of American adults are significantly overweight, that is, obese, based on weight and height. More than 60 percent of Americans are overweight! Many, many more young adults of middle school and high school age, and older adults are being diagnosed with early and more advanced signs of diabetes and high blood pressure. For example, the percentage of children and adolescents defined as overweight has doubled since the early 1970s! About 15 percent, or nine million young children between the ages of six and nineteen, have weights that are at or above the ninety-fifth percentile! In other words, they are almost off the charts. More than 10 percent of preschool children ages two to five are overweight, up from 7 percent in 1994. These are very, very, disturbing statistics! This is truly a cultural epidemic and arguably public enemy number one. Diabetes and hypertension, clearly related to weight, are two potent risk factors for heart disease, stroke, kidney failure requiring dialysis, loss of vision, and amputation. So common are these health problems that for health-care professionals they are a "dime a dozen." The impact on the health of our society, costs, and quality of life are immeasurable. We are a society consuming far more calories than we burn. *Ours is a societal "bank account" where the caloric deposits far exceed the caloric withdrawals.*

There is so much said, written, and advertised on weight reduction that it would be meaningless for me to tell you what you already know. None of the fads, the frauds, or the many quick fixes will get you where you want to be and keep you there. It's a matter of simply eating less and doing more. It is a matter of fundamental behavioral change. This is much easier said than done. As noted, our brain's hunger center is turned on as we eat what is necessary to maintain our current weight. This physiologic equilibrium challenges us to consume more than we need to maintain adequate nutrition. It does not help that ours is a society of convenience, fast food, and fast calories. Some foods turn our biochemistry "on," resulting in a "good" feeling, as anyone experiences who eats when feeling "down." This transient "high" is inevitably followed by the "low" of weight gain, diminished self-esteem, and so on. Unfortunately there is no quick fix for the problem of craving a quick fix. I have been there and done that, and so have you.

Taking inventory of your calories on an average day can be an eye opener. I find that people almost always think they eat less than they do. Imagine your caloric account as you would your budget. Where, over the course of the day, can you save 500 calories by depositing less into the caloric bank? Where over the course of the week can you withdraw more with exercise? *Make your goals doable.* You know yourself. Choose a realistic target—think long-term, over many months and years, not just in terms of a few weeks. The goal is a *lifetime* of effective behavioral modification. The strategies around which a quick plummet provides short-term results are less likely to sustain long-term results because they do not address fundamental behavioral change. There is nothing more challenging for you or your physician than successfully facilitating behavioral and lifestyle change. Drink a lot of water. Keep moving. Eat as many fruits, vegetables, and *whole* grains as you can tolerate.

A brief word on diets. Historically, strategies have focused on reducing calories from fat in our diets to less than 25 percent of total calories consumed, for example less than five hundred calories per day of fat, assuming two thousand calories per day total consumption. Most Americans eat much more than this. The Atkins diet, currently very popular, suggests the opposite. Restrict carbohydrates and be more liberal with protein and fat calories.

A recent comparison of these dietary approaches demonstrated greater success with the Atkins diet (7 percent versus 3.2 percent weight reduction) at six months. At one year, however, the difference between these dietary strategies was not significant. Regardless of the approach, people tended to "drift" from the diet. Long-term adherence to the Atkins diet and its "monotony" is difficult. The South Beach Diet, a variation on the Atkins plan, has not yet been extensively studied.

What about "meal replacement" strategies? One popular strategy is Slim-Fast®. The idea here is to replace one or two meals with liquid or a bar of some kind. One study on overweight diabetics demonstrated good results that were sustained for over two years. Meal replacement products resulted in fewer calories consumed. Safety and cost do not appear to be concerns for people using these products.

The rewards to successful decreases in weight and maintenance of weight loss are absolutely profound! In addition to how much better you will feel emotionally, you will positively reward your self-esteem, sense of control, and inner confidence. This is another example of the pain leading to gain phenomenon. You will realize dramatic potential health benefits. For example, if you can lose 7 to 10 percent of your current weight, assuming you are overweight—for example, ten to fifteen pounds if you weigh 150 lbs, you will dramatically reduce your risk of developing diabetes, high blood pressure, high blood lipids (cholesterol and triglycerides), heart disease, and premature death! Wow . . . think two to four pounds a month. Be patient! Slow and steady win the race. Small positive doable steps will be reinforcing and will lead to further steps that will eventually bring you to your goal. Losing weight and maintaining it should be viewed as a series of victories over the long haul, not a rapid sprint to the finish line.

You will be hearing and reading more about the BMI or body mass index. BMI is a measurement of weight as it relates to height. It is a practical marker to assess obesity and an indicator of optimal weight for health. Overweight adults age eighteen and older with a BMI of higher than 25 are at greater risk for diabetic and cardiovascular disease. A BMI of over 30 is reason for serious pause. A BMI of over 35 is trouble for sure. There is a recently described medical entity known as the *metabolic syndrome* or *lifestyle syndrome* that you will be hearing and reading a lot about in the media. Though still not completely understood, the metabolic or lifestyle syndrome is notable:

- High triglycerides (a particular type of blood fat)
- High blood pressure
- Obesity (BMI > 30)
- Being large around the waistline—women with waist size >35 inches and men > 40 inches

- Low blood levels of the "good cholesterol" or HDL
- Resistance of the body to insulin, or a pre-diabetic state

People with the metabolic syndrome are more likely to become diabetics and to have cardiovascular complications down the road. The good news is that this may, at least for some people, be preventable with weight loss and regular exercise. Sound familiar?

The Body Mass Index Chart on the following page will show you where your BMI currently is.

Questions frequently arise regarding weight-loss medications. For understandable reasons, both public health and market opportunity, there is tremendous interest and research in this area. Wouldn't a quick-fix in the form of a pill be fantastic? Earlier products were prohibited by the FDA because of concern about heart-valve disease. Sibutramine acts on the brain to reduce appetite and can effectively work with diet to enhance weight reduction. Increases in pulse rate and blood pressure have been reported. Orlistat intereferes with absorption of fat and can assist with modest reductions in weight. Common side effects include increased gas and bloating. It is fair to say that medications have not yet been the Holy Grail. They can be expensive and must be continued indefinitely.

The greatest interest and success to date has been with bariatric surgery. These operations involve "bypassing" the stomach, thus interfering with the absorption of calories. While the results of medical studies using bariatric surgery have been impressive (in some instances weight loss of well over 100 pounds), there are concerns about safety. Complications, including death, have been reported. Who best to select for these procedures and who best to perform this is currently an active area of discussion. Techniques are now employing laparoscopes that have the potential to reduce complications and costs.

Nutrition: We Are What We Eat!

Good nutrition is essential to health and wellness. The amount of information out there can be overwhelming. While there may always be some debate and uncertainty about the ideal constituents and proportions in our diets, the basics have held true and should be the basis for your daily meal planning. You may have a particular health problem that requires special dietary needs, like restricting refined sugars if a diabetic (not a bad idea for anyone), or moderating salt if you have high blood pressure.

Body Mass Index Chart

Weight in pounds / Height	100	105	110	115	120	125	130	135	140	145	150	155	160	165	170	175	180	185	190	195	200	205	210	215
5'0"	19	20	21	22	23	24	25	26	27	28	29	30	31	32	33	34	35	36	37	38	39	40	41	42
5'1"	18	19	20	21	22	23	24	25	26	27	28	29	30	31	32	33	34	35	36	36	37	38	39	40
5'2"	18	19	20	21	22	22	23	24	25	26	27	28	29	30	31	32	33	33	34	35	36	37	38	39
5'3"	17	18	19	20	21	22	23	24	24	25	26	27	28	29	30	31	32	32	33	34	35	36	37	38
5'4"	17	18	19	20	20	21	22	23	24	24	25	26	27	28	29	30	31	31	32	33	34	35	36	37
5'5"	16	17	18	19	20	20	21	22	23	24	25	25	26	27	28	29	30	30	31	32	33	34	35	35
5'6"	16	17	18	18	19	20	21	21	22	23	24	25	25	26	27	28	29	29	30	31	32	33	34	34
5'7"	15	16	17	18	18	19	20	21	22	22	23	24	25	26	26	27	28	29	29	30	31	32	33	33
5'8"	15	16	16	17	18	19	19	20	21	22	22	23	24	25	25	26	27	28	28	29	30	31	32	32
5'9"	14	15	16	17	17	18	19	20	20	21	22	22	23	24	25	25	26	27	28	28	29	30	31	31
5'10"	14	15	15	16	17	18	18	19	20	20	21	22	23	23	24	25	25	26	27	28	28	29	30	30
5'11"	14	14	15	16	16	17	18	18	19	20	21	21	22	23	23	24	25	25	26	27	28	28	29	30
6'0"	13	14	14	15	16	17	17	18	19	19	20	21	22	22	23	23	24	25	25	26	27	27	28	29
6'1"	13	13	14	15	15	16	17	17	18	19	19	20	21	21	22	23	23	24	25	25	26	27	27	28
6'2"	12	13	14	14	15	16	16	17	18	18	19	19	20	21	21	22	23	23	24	25	25	26	27	27

Moderating fats is important if your lipid levels are high. In truth, it is beneficial to moderate fats under any circumstances.

A great Web site for excellent nutritional information, complete with a rating guide, is from the Tufts Center on Nutrition Communication (Gerald J. and Dorothy R. Friedman School of Nutrition Science and Policy). Many excellent links to various informative sites are provided. Site reviews for women, men, family, seniors, general nutrition; weight management, and special dietary needs are included at www.navigator.tufts.edu/. Handouts, brochures, fact sheets, reprints, and hundreds of educational materials are available as you explore these excellent links. You can even find recipes. General principles of a nutritionally balanced diet include:

- Reduce fat to 30 percent or less of your total caloric intake. For instance, eat no more than 600 calories from fat in a 2000-calorie-per-day diet. Each gram of fat has approximately 9 calories.
- Increase fiber to twenty to thirty grams a day. Whole grains are an excellent source of fiber, vitamins, minerals, and protein. They are low in fat. Choose a hot or cold cereal that provides at least four grams of fiber per serving. Have whole-wheat varieties of pancakes or waffles. In recipes calling for flour, use at lest 50 percent whole wheat flour. For dinner, at least twice a week, serve whole-wheat noodles or brown rice. They are high in vitamins, minerals, and protein. They are low in fat. A whole grain still has its outer covering, which contains most of the fiber, vitamins and minerals. Whole grains can be found as whole wheat, bran, oatmeal, and multigrain. READ THE LABEL! If it does not say "whole grain" or "whole wheat," it is not the real deal. Try high fiber cracker varieties like whole rye or multigrain. Once or more per week, try a low-fat meatless meal or main dish that features whole grains such as spinach lasagna, red beans over brown rice, and vegetable stir fry.
- Include a variety of fruits and vegetables. Fruits and veggies are a great source of fiber, vitamins, and minerals. They are low in calories and fat. They may reduce cancer risk! Buy a variety to discover those that you like most. Buy frozen, dried, canned, or fresh fruits and vegetables, based on your needs. Keep a fruit bowl, raisins or fresh-cut vegetables nearby for snacking.
- Minimize consumption of salt-cured, salt-pickled, and smoked foods.
- There are as many diets out there as there are people interested in losing weight.

The above guidelines are time tested.

A recent review, published in *The Journal of The American Medical Association*, examined the "Optimal Diets for Prevention of Coronary Disease." They came away with three dietary strategies proven effective in preventing heart disease based upon an extensive review and analysis of the published medical evidence:

1. Substitute nonhydrogenated unsaturated fats for saturated and trans-fats. Examples of nonhydrogenated unsaturated fats include flax, corn, safflower, sesame, and sunflower. Nonhydrogenated fats are liquid at room temperature. Trans-fats are found in hydrogenated foods such as margarine, shortening, microwave popcorn, pastries, crackers, and other snack and fast foods.
2. Increase consumption of omega-3 fatty acids from fish, fish oil supplements, or plant sources such as corn, safflower, sunflower, and soybean. Omega-3 fatty acids are considered "essential fatty acids" because our bodies cannot make them. Good natural sources and recommended amounts would include three or more three-ounce servings of fish per week plus another source such as flax seeds or walnuts. Omega-3 fish oil capsule supplements are not generally recommended as natural sources e. g., fatty fish and plant sources also contain other beneficial nutrients not found in capsules.
3. Increase fruits, vegetables, nuts, whole grains, and reduce refined grain products. Some terrific information and "action suggestions" can be obtained at the Federal Consumer Information Center, www.pueblo.gsa.gov/. Click the link to food.

Don't Despair!

Depression is a common, debilitating, under-recognized, and very treatable disease. There are few medical problems I have ever encountered with as profound an impact on quality of life as depression. It is estimated that at any point in time, approximately 5 percent of our population are experiencing symptoms of depression! While we will all have a tendency to "feel down" on occasion, depression is defined by recurrent symptoms that last at least a few weeks at a time. This is different from feeling temporarily down due to a specific circumstance such as bereavement after losing a loved one. *It is very important to appreciate that depression is a biologic problem, not unlike high blood pressure or diabetes. If you are feeling blue, it is not your fault!* Feelings of despair cannot simply be turned off as you would a light with a light switch.

Because it is awkward to talk about mood and emotions and because people often feel they can just "snap out of it," depression frequently goes unrecognized and untreated. This is a terrible dilemma, given the impact depression has on quality of life and the extent to which many people are tormented who could otherwise be helped. Depression also accounts for an enormous social burden as defined by loss of life, loss of days at work, negative impact on other health problems such as heart disease, and frequent association with other problems such as anxiety and substance abuse. Because mood is not easily communicated or measured like blood pressure or blood sugar, we need much greater awareness of the magnitude of this problem. We know that many physicians fail to recognize and diagnose depression. We know that many people have symptoms and never seek care for them. We know that depression can be easily masked by other physical symptoms such as changes in sleep pattern, appetite, energy level, or effectiveness of relationships at home, work, and school. In 1997 (see references), a study was published that defined the following two questions as a screen for possible depression.

Have you ever, for at least a two-week continuous stretch:

- **Felt down, sad, or hopeless?**
- **Noticed little interest or pleasure in doing things?**

A "yes" answer to these questions is not proof that you are depressed, though it may serve as a warning to take seriously. You should discuss this with your physician, family, or a trusted friend. One difficulty in dealing with depression is that the very nature of the disease makes it difficult to seek help. As a result, those most in need of help are least able to reach out for it.

The overwhelming majority of individuals with depression will improve considerably with therapy and/or medications. The medication options for treating depression have never been more effective. Your life can be made so much better by treatment.

The take home message is this: *If your life is feeling very dark and filled with despair, a source of light, hope, and contentment may be much closer than you realize.*

If You Have Diabetes or You Are at Risk for Diabetes . . . Listen Up

The number of people with diabetes in America is rising at an alarming rate; it is triple what it was some thirty years ago! These are remarkable and disturbing statistics. This rise in diabetes correlates with the growing problem of obesity in America. The overwhelming majority of people who develop diabetes are overweight. We now recognize that this risk can appear in adolescence and early adulthood. This risk rises further as people age. As mentioned earlier, diabetes in some people may be reversible or preventable with activity, good nutritional habits, and loss of weight. Diabetes is associated with the following conditions, among others:

- The number one cause of kidney failure requiring dialysis and kidney transplantation in the United States
- Increased risk for heart disease. A person with diabetes has the same risk of a heart attack as someone who has already had a heart attack.
- Increased risk for stroke
- Number one cause of loss of vision in the United States
- A major risk factor for amputation of a toe, foot, or leg
- Much greater likelihood of dying at an earlier than average age

Though it is not my intent to scare the living daylights out of you, diabetes is the ultimate enemy. It can slowly and surely progress over many years toward some or all of the complications above. I have treated countless individuals with some or all of these complications. I watched diabetes bring my mother down. The good news, and there is always a positive side, is that much can be done to prevent these devastating outcomes, particularly if recognized and treated at an early stage.

As I mentioned, my mother had diabetes, probably unrecognized for many years. It is not uncommon to have diabetes and not know it. I have cared for scores of hundreds of people with diabetes just like my mother, just like your mother, grandmother, or sister. So much more is known now than ten or fifteen years ago. And though there is still no cure for diabetes, much more will be researched and understood in the years to come. Helping you or your loved one to help yourself is my purpose. For me, this is personal. The best I can do is to provide what I believe to be the current best medical evidence to empower you to take control.

Some ethnic groups are at a particularly high risk of diabetes and need to be aware of this risk. These include Native Americans, African Americans, Hispanic Americans, and Asian/South Pacific Islanders. It is absolutely essential to appreciate that many of the life altering and life threatening medical events that occur later in life are from problems that are mostly *silent*, until their "downstream" effects rear their ugly heads.

Diabetes, high blood pressure, high cholesterol, obesity, smoking, and a sedentary lifestyle will not leave you feeling lousy or create symptoms until the damage is well under way.

Your car may be running safely and smoothly right up until the lights of the oncoming train appear. Again, I do not mean to overstate this; however, fear can be a motivator. I have seen too much not to react in this manner. These are some very important things to think about if you have or are at risk for diabetes. These are critical life-improving and possibly live-saving goals. These recommendations, as of 2003, can best be summarized as follows:

- DO NOT wait for symptoms to trigger your need to be checked for diabetes.
- If you are overweight (from adolescence and older), talk to your doctor about being tested for diabetes. This should be done with one or more fasting blood tests or a blood test taken about two hours after a meal.
- In 2004, the American Diabetes Association updated guidelines for defining diabetes, and just as important, "pre-diabetes." *Know these numbers.*

Blood sugar	Normal	Pre-diabetic	Diabetic
Fasting sugar (first thing in the morning, before eating)	Under 100	100–125	126 or more
2 hours postprandial (after eating)	Under 140	140–199	200 or more

- If you fall into the pre-diabetic category, and it is estimated that approximately 10 to12 percent of Americans do, heed the warning. This should be seen as a bright, flashing light accompanied by a loud bell, warning you of an oncoming train!

- If you are in the pre-diabetes range, and overweight, commit your-self to attempting to lose 7–10 percent of your current weight and walking 150 minutes per week.

If you have diabetes, here's a checklist to help you with essential aspects of your care. There is no reason why you and your providers cannot be establishing the shared goal of getting "straight As" on the report card.

✓ **Talk to your primary care provider about a possible referral to a diabetes specialist or endocrinologist.** Your primary provider will probably be able to handle most aspects of your care. However, endocrinologists are specifically trained as experts in diabetes care and can address more challenging issues around education, medication treatment, and newer research and insight. You, your primary care team, and your endocrinologist should form the "triangle" of care in the management of your diabetes.

✓ **Hemoglobin A1c**—This is a blood test that checks average ranges of blood sugar over a two to three-month period. *Your goal is less than 6–6.5.* We have very good medical evidence that many diabetic complications involving eyes, kidneys, heart, and circulation are reduced when blood values are in this range. Your provider should check it regularly, two or three times a year. *Know your number and know where you want to be.* Partner with your providers to get there.

✓ **Blood Pressure**—Your pressure should average **no higher than 130/80**. This is critical in reducing your risk of cardiovascular disease, stroke, circulation, and kidney disease. It is also much easier said than done. Lower is better as long as you feel okay. Feeling dizzy or lightheaded, like you may "pass out" can be a sign of low blood pressure. You may notice this when changing from a lying to sitting to standing posture. As it can take a minute for your body to adjust to these changes, allow yourself a moment to sit before standing. When you do stand, stay near your bed or chair for another moment so you can sit or lie down if you feel lightheaded. This might prevent a serious injury from falling or passing out. When it comes to blood pressure control, be prepared . . . you may need as many as two to four different classes of blood pressure medications, depending on your readings. This takes time and patience for you and your care provider. Blood pressure control is extremely important, especially in people with diabetes. The risk of having a stroke, heart attack, kidney failure, and death are dramatically reduced. This goal, challenging though it may be, is very achievable, requiring perseverance, commitment, and clear communication with your provider. Ask your doctor if you might benefit from being on a blood pressure medication in the *ACE inhibitor or ARB* category, as these agents may have important vascular and kidney protective effects in addition to their blood pressure lowering effects.

✓ **Have your eyes checked annually.** This is so important! I have seen people suffer dramatic loss of vision over a short period of time. Your ophthalmologist will be able to identify potential risks for visual loss and do all possible to lessen this risk. How important is your vision to you? If an ophthalmologist has not seen you, ask for a referral.

✓ Talk to your doctor about being on a **baby aspirin (81 mg per day)** if you are not already. Aspirin can have important benefits in preventing heart attack or stroke. However, it can also increase the risk of a bleeding ulcer. The benefits, for most diabetics, will far outweigh the risks.

✓ **Know your lipids.** These are the different types of blood fats in your system. Though the recommendations continue to evolve, as of this writing, there are two important numbers for you to know about.

LDL cholesterol—lowest appears best
Triglycerides < 150

Ask your doctor if you might benefit from a medication in a class called *statins*. As risks for heart disease and stroke are much higher with diabetes, lipid control is particularly essential. A recently published clinical trial from Oxford University, referred to as the Heart Outcomes Trial, suggests that any diabetic, regardless of blood lipid level, may benefit (decreased risk of stroke, heart attack, and death) from being on a statin. Talk to your doctor about this important study.

✓ Protect your kidneys! As a nephrologist, this is an issue near and dear to my heart. Like many disease processes that affect the kidney, such as diabetes and high blood pressure, the two most common, *you will not have any symptoms! Do not wait for symptoms! At a minimum,* you should have an annual blood test for:

BUN (Blood Urea Nitrogen)
LYTES (Sodium, Potassium)
CREATININE (A muscle protein that allows estimates of kidney function)

And a urine sample for:

Microalbumin or a protein/creatinine ratio. These tests look for any sign of kidney damage, causing leakage of protein into the urine. The kidneys are like filters that continuously clean the blood of impurities that occur from things we eat and drink. Under normal circumstances these filters do not allow protein into the urine. Most people with protein in their urine are unaware of it. Large amounts of protein can make the water in the toilet bowl very foamy after urinating. Sometimes swelling around the eyes (especially in the morning right after awakening) or in the feet and ankles can be signs of protein in the urine.

Any, and I mean any, abnormality here should raise these questions for your doctor/provider:

- **Would I benefit from being on a medication, if I am not already, in a class called ACE inhibitors or ARBs?** Most of the time the answer is yes. If you are a diabetic over the age of fifty-five, or any age with evidence of protein or albumin in your urine, you should be strongly considered for one of these classes of agents. Be prepared to have some blood work checked more frequently as a matter of routine monitoring.
- **Should I be referred to a nephrologist?** In my humble, objective opinion, the answer here is a definite yes!

✓ **Protect Your Heart!** You do this with all the aforementioned interventions such as weight loss, better sugar control, ASA (aspirin), lower lipids on a statin, perhaps being on an ACE or ARB medication if over the age of fifty-five, and stopping smoking.

✓ **Maximize your Control!** Self-understanding, awareness, and self-management are critical in the management of any chronic medical problem, particularly diabetes. Of course, not everyone is capable. There may be, in addition to caring family and friends, community services available to assist in your self-management, such as physician office support staff, community services through local hospital programs, VNA (visiting nurse association), Elder Services, parish nursing–faith communities, and others. The goal is to help people realize the potential they have to help themselves. Taking on a disease like diabetes can be daunting, particularly as you first begin to deal with it physically and emotionally. Ask your doctor what resources may be available to assist in your self-care and education. Once you begin to gain greater understanding and develop trusting relationships with yourself and others, you will know the satisfaction of being in greater control of your life. You will begin to see the positive rewards of better blood work, better emotional and physical well being, greater confidence, more choices, and the power unleashed from the gratifying collaboration with others vested in your health and wellness. I know this is not easy. This is a challenge. This is a major commitment. There will be frustration and peaks and valleys along the way. I also know that it is possible. I have seen countless numbers of patients and families rise to the challenge. Ask yourself, "Is my life worth this effort? Is anyone more responsible than I am for effectively navigating this challenging journey? If professionals involved in my care are telling me it is important and I am capable of doing it, is their faith in me greater than my faith in myself?"

Self-management is not a one-time deal—it is ongoing. You should have a relationship, in addition to your doctor of course, with:

1. A diabetes educator
2. A nutritionist
3. Another individual you know and trust who is going through something similar and can serve as a mutual mentor or supporter

You should target your long-term goals around the following:

*   Finger stick sugar measurements, if necessary, are essential to monitor your sugar control and can assist in correlating any potential symptoms, such as dizziness, with a sugar that may be too low or too high. The roller coaster of sugar highs and lows can be a difficult one for diabetics and providers alike. The health benefits of tight control are increasingly clear—that is, a fasting level of <120; two hours after eating <140–160; and Hemoglobin A1C (HbA1c) <6 to 6.5. The potential tradeoff here is a greater risk of having a low blood sugar reaction. We refer to this as symptomatic hypoglycemia. This is a very scary thing for anyone who has ever experienced or observed such a reaction. A low blood sugar

reaction can occur with pills as well as with insulin injections. People often experience overwhelming fatigue, tremulousness or shakiness, excessive sweating, altered cognition, and palpitations. There are many strategies for treating diabetes, including different classes of oral medication and different types of insulin given as a shot under the skin. You may get by with oral medication alone, insulin alone, or a combination of the two.

Never forget the importance of diet, weight loss, and activity.

If you are prone to peaks and valleys, careful finger stick sugars and documentation to recognize important patterns will allow you and your provider to tailor your diabetic regimen. This can take time and great patience. It will, however, serve to greatly improve the quality of your life in the long run.

✓ **Take Your Shoes Off.** If you have diabetes, your shoes should be off with every physician or allied health professional visit. Chances are you will not be asked to do this. That is okay. Do it anyway. Your feet may forever be fine; however, many diabetics lose feeling in their feet. We call this neuropathy. Many diabetics may have impairment of vision that can make it difficult to appreciate an early (or perhaps advanced, as I have seen many times) problem. There may be an unnoticed fungal infection around the nails or webs of the toes. These skin and nail problems are now recognized to increase the risk of bacterial infection—much more common in diabetics. When is the last time you really looked at your feet and spread your toes to examine the dark and distant space between them? If your nurse or physician asks why your shoes and socks are off, tell them, "This is a preventive care reminder for me and for you. Dr. Pettus said so." Hopefully you'll get a smile and receive the quick check you need and deserve.

Blood Pressure—Get it checked!

Over 40 million Americans have high blood pressure. Most people recognize that high blood pressure (HBP) is a significant risk factor for heart disease and stroke. Did you know that HBP is a leading cause, like diabetes, of progressive kidney failure requiring dialysis or transplantation? Did you know that HBP could lead to heart failure, a problem of the heart not relaxing and contracting properly? Did you know that HBP could increase the risk of death from cardiovascular causes such as heart attacks, heart failure, and stroke?

HBP, like so many chronic health problems, is *deceptively silent* until the volcano erupts, or until the lights of the oncoming train appear. Headaches, by the way, are usually not related to HBP. The overwhelming majority of individuals with headaches, even if they have HBP, will have other causes for their symptoms. The take-home message here is don't wait for a headache to be concerned about your blood pressure.

Let me give you an example, albeit an extreme one, of how unrecognized and untreated HBP can affect a person. I first met L. P. several years ago. He was thirty-eight at the time and had never seen a health-care professional. He came to our local emergency department with a several-week history notable for increasing fatigue, increasing shortness of breath with minimal activity, particularly worse at night, diminished appetite and changes in vision, making it hard to read even the headline print of our local newspaper. I was called by our emergency department staff because his blood pressure was 240/150; he had fluid congestion in his lungs; his kidneys were functioning at less than 10 percent of normal; and examination of his eyes revealed leaking of blood and protein (we call these hemorrhages and exudates or "retinopathy"). It was shocking to enter the life of this young man under such circumstances. In retrospect, HBP ran in his family and he had probably developed HBP himself ten or fifteen years earlier. It accelerated to the extreme of causing irreversible damage to his eyes, his heart, and to his kidneys. He was probably within days to weeks of dying. With a number of BP medications and initiation of chronic hemodialysis, he stabilized and began to feel much better. The damage, however, was not reversible. He died, despite our best efforts, six years later at the age of forty-four. He was a lovely guy, sweet, sincere, engaging, and somewhat limited in his understanding. He never knew what hit him. None of this had to happen, and I believe none of this would have happened if his blood pressure had been checked long ago, followed, and adequately managed. For many reasons it did not happen. Though this is a less common scenario, I see people all the time with milder, progressive problems because of blood pressures that are not where they need to be. Here are some words of wisdom as they relate to HBP and, as you will see, some familiar themes as they relate to health maintenance and disease prevention.

- Have your blood pressure taken during adolescence, particularly if your parents have a history of HBP or if you are overweight.

- Have your blood pressure taken annually as a minimum screen. This will take five minutes out of 525,600 minutes/year. There is simply no excuse for not having your BP checked. This can be done at your physician's office, through various free community screening offerings, or by friends or family members who can measure your pressure. The USPSTF strongly recommends screening by age eighteen at the oldest.
- If your blood pressure is borderline, e.g., 130–140 systolic and/or 80–90 diastolic, have it repeated periodically, at least every month for the next three months to establish a consistent pattern. Remember, do not minimize the importance of your readings being referred to as "borderline."
- You may come across the expression "white coat hypertension." This refers to the phenomenon of readings in a medical office setting being higher than outside the medical office setting. Though sometimes dismissed as an insignificant concern, white coat hypertension may reflect true hypertension. While it may be milder in its severity, an increased risk of complications over time may indeed exist. My best advice? If you are labeled with white coat hypertension, have frequent readings taken and documented both outside and in medical office settings. I would strongly consider treatment if consistently higher than normal readings occur, regardless of what setting they are taken in.
- Recent published guidelines make note that some individuals with a top number (systolic) between 120 and 130 and a bottom (diastolic) between 80 and 85 may be at increased risk for developing high blood pressure in the future. There is some controversy about this among experts in the field. If your BP is in this range, particularly if your parents have HBP, if you are overweight, or if you have another risk factor for heart disease such as high cholesterol, have your pressure checked regularly, at least once a year, as a matter of routine.
- Under any circumstance, losing as little as 5 percent of your current weight, if overweight, with regular activity such as walking 150 minutes a week (sound familiar?) and for some people, moderating salt in your diet, could be the difference between needing medication and not needing medication.

Here is an HBP checklist to assist in your management.

   ✓ BP can be screened at any age, usually starting in adolescence. If normal, it should be repeated every one to two years, with more frequent testing as noted if borderline, for example 130/85.

✓ If your BP, on at least three separate readings, is >140/90 (or greater than 130/80 if you are a diabetic or have kidney disease), you may need to be on medication or have your medication adjusted.

✓ If you are a diabetic, your goal for BP control should be <130/80, or as low as you can tolerate.

✓ As noted above, and worthy of reemphasis, if you have a history of kidney disease your BP goal, like a diabetic's, should be <130/80.

✓ If you are a diabetic or have kidney disease, particularly if you have evidence of protein in your urine, ask your doctor if you are taking a medication of a class called ACEs or ARBs. If you are not, should this be considered? I think it should.

✓ Are you having an annual check of important blood work, such as kidney tests—BUN, Creatinine, urinalysis, and lipid profile? Do you know these results? You should.

✓ *If you have resistant, or hard to control HBP, have kidney disease, and are a diabetic or have heart disease, you may require at least three different classes of medication to control your pressure. This is a lot of medication to take, but it is often necessary.* Costs, inconvenience, and side effects can make it difficult to comply with such a complicated medication regimen. If you are unable to take what you need for any reason, talk to your prescribing provider and negotiate the best plan to get you where you need to be.

✓ Invest, if possible, in an automated cuff for home readings, or try to have someone take periodic readings outside of a physician's office. This is important, as there are sometimes discrepancies in readings between home and office, the latter of which may drive the decision for more medication. This could lead to over-medication if your home readings are lower. As noted previously, we call this white coat hypertension.

Home readings are very important and in my view, are essential aspects of the self-management mindset, just as a glucometer for home sugar monitoring is for the diabetic. If a patient calls me with a symptom such as headache, fatigue, or dizziness, and they have BP readings at home while they are symptomatic, we can, together, best determine whether the BP has anything to do with how they are feeling. I am more likely to cut back on a dose of medication if the fatigue and dizziness are correlated with a BP of 90/60, than I am if it is 180/100. The latter scenario, perhaps, may require more medication or a modification of the current regimen.

Some home cuffs may be less accurate or lose accuracy over time. When in doubt, bring it with you to your provider's office and ask the nurse to compare readings with your cuff and the office cuff.

✓ If you have HBP and are taking a BP medication that is a diuretic, for example HCTZ or Lasix (furosemide) or ACE/ARB, be cautious about long-term (several weeks to months) use of anti-inflammatory medications. Some anti-inflammatory medications, or "NSAIDS," as we call them, (ibuprofen and Naproxen are common examples) can interfere with the effectiveness of the BP lowering medication. If you have questions about potential interaction, talk to your doctor about them.

✓ If you're having side effects, talk to your doctor. They may or may not be related to your medication. If so, there are many options. Treating HBP should be viewed as having a suit tailored to give you the best individual fit. Almost always, this should be possible.

✓ Never just stop a BP medication without first discussing it with your provider. Remember, HBP is usually without symptoms. You may be tempted to say, "I feel just as well without it." Who needs the added expense or possible side effects? Who needs a stroke, an MI (myocardial infarction or heart attack), kidney failure, or heart failure?

Treating, controlling, and maintaining blood pressure with the fewest side effects, number of medications, and most acceptable costs, can require time and patience. A trusting and open relationship with your physician will enable this process to be successful and effective.

✓ If you are taking more than one medication for your blood pressure and are struggling with compliance due to the number of pills you take, ask your doctor if a "combination" medication might be reasonable for you.

Trim the Fats

Make sure you have regular checks of your **lipid profile.** This is a blood test. It includes your total cholesterol, broken down into the good "HDL," the bad "LDL," and the ugly "triglycerides." Recommendations for the safest "targets" are continuously evolving and your target will depend on your age, cardiovascular risk factors, and medical history. Discuss where your targets should be with your physician, and how best to get there. While the ideal age to start checking lipids is debated, in my view, if you are old enough to be legally drinking, you're old enough to have your lipids checked. The USPSTF (U.S. Preventive Service Task Force) recommends starting at age twenty in both men and women, particularly if there are risk factors for coronary artery disease (CAD), such as diabetes, smoking, family history of high cholesterol or heart disease, or hypertension. This should be repeated every three to five years if results are in a normal range. There are more effective medications than ever before for controlling abnormal blood lipid or fat levels. Remember the class of medications called *statins*. There are other classes of effective lipid-lowering medications as well.

An Ounce of Prevention is Worth a Pound of Cure

It is important to stay up to date on disease prevention and health maintenance issues. These are proven, safe, and very effective measures to stay healthy and to decrease the risk of developing more serious health problems. Some considerations here would include (based on the U.S. Preventive Service Task Force and The American College of Physicians—American Society of Internal Medicine 2002 recommendations):

Screening:

- Periodic height and weight screening. Ask to have your Body Mass Index (BMI) calculated. A number greater than thirty should elicit the warning sound of a distant train drawing nearer.
- Screening for coronary artery disease. The U.S. Preventive Services Task Force, in a 2004 update, recommends against routine screening with an electrocardiogram, stress testing (treadmill test), or electron-beam computerized tomography (EBCT) for coronary calcium in individuals at low risk for coronary artery disease (such as the absence of or limited risk factors).
- See lipid screening and blood pressure-screening guidelines explained earlier.
- Fecal occult blood screening: this is checking a stool sample for blood, which may provide an early clue to colon cancer. Your

doctor will provide you with three cards to take home. Three separate samples should be checked. Current recommendations are every year after the age of fifty.

- Colonoscopy: As of this writing, colonoscopy is the best test to screen for colon cancer. It is recommended at age fifty and if normal, perhaps every ten years (American College of Gastroenterology). You can discuss the ideal frequency for you with your gastroenterologist. If there is a family history of colon cancer of if you have inflammatory bowel disease such as Crohn's Disease or ulcerative colitis, you should start screening at an earlier age, around forty, and may need more frequent follow-up than someone with low-average risk.

- PAP Smear: This is an evolving story. The good news is that deaths from cervical cancer have gone down tremendously over the last sixty years. Cervical cancer was once a common and lethal cancer. Appropriate attention to screening can virtually eliminate this risk. The American Cancer Society has recently modified its recommendations. Any sexually active woman should have a PAP done within three years of onset of sexual activity or by age twenty-one. The interval of time between PAPs will vary between six months and three years, depending on the findings and your risks. High risk factors would include prior cervical or vaginal cancer, history of sexually transmitted diseases (STDs) like chlamydia, gonorrhea, or human papilloma virus (HPV). An abnormal PAP or high risk warrants more frequent follow-up. Any woman over the age of thirty who has had three normal annual PAPs in the preceding years, and who does not fall into a high-risk category, can safely wait three years between subsequent PAPs. The upper age limit at this time is seventy if a woman has had three or more normal PAPs within the preceding ten years. Some recommend sixty-five as an upper limit. This is based more on consensus than hard data.

- Self breast exam/mammography: All post-pubertal women should be taught breast self-exam (BSE). You are never too young and should become comfortable with your body and what is normal for you. Mammography continues to be debated with respect to the ideal age for starting. There are recent guidelines proposed by the American Cancer Society for breast cancer screening. For women at average risk, mammography should begin at age forty. Evidence is insufficient to recommend for or against teaching or performing routine breast self-examination (BSE). Annual mammography exams are appropriate. Women with a higher risk, such as a first-degree relative with a history of breast cancer, should start screening at an earlier age, around thirty or thirty-five. A review article published in 2003 examined the effectiveness of screening women after age sixty-five. There is a suggestion that biennial screening beyond the age of sixty-five can save lives. This continues to be a work in progress as age becomes relative in a society that is living longer

- Digital Rectal Exam and PSA screening for prostate cancer: I must say this is a controversial area. The controversy stems from the fact that that the PSA test is pretty good at picking up cancer, which is obviously a good thing. What has made this controversial is that it is unclear how best to treat many cases. An elevated PSA will lead to the recommendation of a biopsy of the prostate to determine if cancer is present and to what extent. Cancer that is localized (confined to the prostate gland), as is often the case, can progress at very different rates over time, sometimes very slowly. Surgery to remove the prostate, called radical subtotal prostatectomy, is a curative treatment, though it can sometimes lead to side effects such as impotence and urinary incontinence. The challenge is that there is no way to predict or distinguish who will progress very slowly and thus make less aggressive treatments more desirable, from those who will progress more quickly, where surgery is clearly the way to go. Current best evidence suggests that the risk of dying from prostate cancer can be reduced, if the cancer is localized to the prostate gland, by undergoing surgery. Many men however, may do just as well with less aggressive intervention. This controversy is reflected in differences of opinion by many specialty societies. The bottom line here, as with many medical decisions, is to learn as much as you can about the test and the implications if the test is positive or negative. Discuss this with your primary care provider. If your doctor is a male, ask him what he would do. This is not, in my view, a decision that is right or wrong. There are simply more questions than answers. Personally, if my risks were higher—for example, if my father or grandfather or men in my extended family had a history of prostate cancer, or if I were African American (a higher risk)—I would strongly consider surgery. Get the facts, weigh them from an advantage/disadvantage perspective, and test that analysis against your preferences, values, and wishes.

- Bone densitometry: This is an important test to screen for osteoporosis. It is recommended by the American Association of Clinical Endocrinology, for women in estrogen-deficient states (post menopausal or with surgical removal of the ovaries) or other high-risk states, such as taking corticosteroids like Prednisone on a chronic basis. You can discuss how often to request this with your treating physician. Osteoporosis is a significant health problem as women age beyond their post-menopausal years. Osteoporosis increases the risk for fracturing bones in the back (vertebrae) or hip. There are excellent strategies to minimize these risks that you can discuss with your doctor. Recently published recommendations by the U.S. Preventive Services Task Force suggest screening in all women sixty-five years and older. Currently, Medicare part B covers screening for women sixty-five and older once every two years. The cost-effectiveness of screening women in their fifties is controversial, as the average age of menopause is fifty-one. Some younger women will have evidence of osteoporosis.

- Vision and hearing: This should be done routinely at and beyond the age of sixty-five in most people. Frequency of retesting will depend on your circumstances.
- Rubella Screening: Any woman of childbearing age should have this checked. A history of vaccination or blood testing can confirm this.
- STD (sexually transmitted disease) screening: This is recommended for women with a history of STDs, and in women under twenty-five with two or more sex partners in the last year. Many women will be without symptoms and treatment is important to prevent potential fertility problems due to chronic infection. STD testing is usually done with a GYN exam/PAP.
- Influenza Vaccine: This is the "flu shot" to protect against strains of influenza viruses, most prevalent between November and March. In 2001, the Centers for Disease Control (CDC) guidelines recommended vaccination of all adults fifty and older. It is also recommended regardless of age for individuals at higher risk:

  ❖ Residents of chronic care facilities
  ❖ Individuals with diabetes
  ❖ Individuals with kidney disease
  ❖ Individuals with pulmonary diseases like asthma or emphysema
  ❖ Individuals with impairment of the immune system, such as cancer being treated with chemotherapy; HIV
  ❖ Health-care workers when at risk for exposure or transmission

- Pneumococcal Vaccine: This is a vaccine that can reduce the risk of acquiring a common form of *bacterial* pneumonia. This requires some clarification as I have encountered many patients whose understanding of this vaccine and the flu vaccine is inaccurate. The pneumococcal bacterium is one of the more common bacterial causes of pneumonia. It can be serious, even fatal, if it spreads from the lungs to the bloodstream, particularly if you have other health problems. As there are other types of bacterial pneumonia, *the pneumococcal vaccine will not prevent all types of pneumonia*. It decreases the occurrence of this particular kind. Similarly, the flu refers to influenza, just one of many types of *viruses* that can cause pneumonia or flu-like symptoms. Both pneumococcal and influenza infections can be serious and their risks substantially diminished by these vaccines. There is simply no excuse for not getting these vaccines. They can usually be obtained free or at minimal costs and are readily available in offices, community clinics, and hospital settings. Unlike the flu vaccine, which is given every year, the pneumococcal vaccine is usually given just once for people sixty-five or older. Younger individuals with chronic pulmonary (lung) and kidney diseases, diabetes, or impaired immune function (chemotherapy for cancer, blood cancers, removal of the spleen), should also receive this. Boosters can be given if the first dose was received under the age of sixty-five and more than five years prior.

- Tetanus vaccine is recommended every ten years.
- **Folic acid at 0.4 mg/day** is recommended for any woman who could become pregnant to prevent a specific "neural tube" congenital defect in the fetus. Folic acid is a B-vitamin and has many other potential health benefits that are being studied. It can be obtained in this higher dose, by prescription. While folic acid is available in non-prescription multivitamins, it is in a lower dose.

Awareness and Mindfulness Practice . . . Stress Overboard!

Nothing, and I mean nothing, will have a more immediate, lasting, and profound impact on the quality of your life than unloading as much stress as possible. Admittedly much easier said than done, I have become more aware of the need to pause, take inventory, and make it a priority to unload all that is unnecessary or simply not worth the consumption. I liken this to the analogy of floating in a hot air balloon, cruising at times, only to lose altitude and risk crashing as the weight of life diminishes our buoyancy. As the excess weight of stress is thrown overboard, the balloon lifts and moves forward in a more effective way.

Try this: take inventory of the top ten or twenty sources of stress in your life. Examine the sources. Do the benefits derived from these sources outweigh the drawbacks? Asked another way, is the loss of altitude worth it? If not, are there reasonable and acceptable options? If there are, make choices that bring you closer to the "buoyant altitude and attitude" you desire and move on. If the benefits are substantial, despite the stress, examine ways to transform all that is within your influence, to reduce as much stress as possible. For example, focus your energy on relationship building, an awareness of "non-self," and non-judgment. See forgiveness not as something deserved, but as an avenue to peace, your peace. Try to maintain a goal of negative stress balance—that is, unloading > acquiring. If your hot air balloon of life is losing altitude, throw as much stress as possible overboard. Open the hatch and let it fly! Soon thereafter your spirits will start to soar!

Over time, I have gradually learned more about the peace, potential health benefits, and necessity for allowing quiet reflection and stillness into one's life. As a young boy, I often retreated to a nearby lake where I would sit alone, collect my thoughts, sometimes fish, and become connected with the stillness around me. I would usually choose to do this when I needed to regroup. It was a comforting way to cope with my mother's depression and the pain and despair I felt as she and my father often struggled with daily life. These were some very dark moments for me. I would have appeared alone and isolated to an outsider observing me, sitting in the woods, solitary and quiet. In a paradoxical way, the more deeply I immersed myself, the less alone I felt. Over time, I actually felt a greater sense of connectedness to the life around me, to nature's steadfast and consoling presence. These "mindfulness retreats" became a consistent source of comfort, always waiting to receive me, like a friend, in an otherwise indifferent and harsh world around me. I felt anything but alone. There was a comforting force, a spirit that was very much alive and present. Something very meaningful was "lit" within me, connected in a natural way to the beauty of the trees, birds, fish, air, and tapestry of life around me.

I appreciate, more and more, the importance of knowing one's self. Life can be so hectic and distracting. It is too easy, at times, to lose touch with those things that mean the most to us. It is too easy to lose touch with one's self. Our awareness of our inherent connection to all life, to each other and all that surrounds us, is so easily deflected and diminished in today's crazy pace. Stillness has a way of enhancing that awareness.

Ancient disciplines of meditation and yoga in their various forms, religious worship, and prayer, are based on the awareness and faith that a divine energy and purpose are the essence of our being.

There are well-documented physiologic and biologic expressions of meditation and prayer, for example, that have health benefits. Improvements in mood disturbance, anxiety, depression, anger, and confusion have been well documented. In general, total stress was significantly reduced in these clinical studies. Improvements in pain are also noted. In some patients studied with breast or prostate cancer, additional positive changes were seen in the bodies' immune system. Parts of the brain that "light up" during meditation and prayer on brain scanning, correlate with feelings of "non-self." Non-self is expressed as a greater feeling of connectedness to life around us. Non-self is awareness of our being, in the context of much greater and broader purpose. I strongly believe that making time, even as little as five minutes per day, to be still, silent, quiet, reflective, and at peace will serve to relax, rejuvenate, and restore.

Mindfulness meditation involves deep breathing and heightened attention to physical and emotional sensations, with the goal of easing stress and pain. There is a growing body of medical evidence supporting the benefits of meditation in many types of chronic disease, including cancer. Jon Kabat-Zinn directs the stress reduction clinic at the University of Massachusetts Medical Center. He introduced this program in 1979 and now more than 240 programs exist in the United States. His technique is somewhat different than traditional forms of meditation. Most traditional forms of meditation focus on the release of all external thoughts while entering into a passive state of relaxation. In mindfulness meditation, focusing on the process of breathing is also key. In addition, however, the individual attends to all thoughts, feelings, images, and sensations as they arise. The goal here is to become more acutely aware of the details in one's awareness, including sensations of pain and stress. The goal is to develop another context to accept what one is feeling.

Discomfort is managed more effectively as one "relaxes into it" instead of struggling to avoid or diminish it. According to Dr. Kabat-Zinn, patients learn to pay closer attention to the present moment. In doing this they can separate the physical experience of pain from emotions such as anger, resentment, and fear.

The most common method for practicing mindfulness meditation is the "body scan." In this technique a person sits or lies comfortably, directing his or her awareness of the sensations of breathing throughout the entire body, from head to toe. Any discomfort noted during the deep breathing body scan is "let go."

There are many instructional books (I highly recommend Jon Kabat-Zinn's *Full Catastrophe Living: Using the Wisdom of Your Body and Mind to Face Stress, Pain, and Illness*. New York: Dell Publishing, 1990), videotapes, and classes on meditation and yoga. There are many places of worship, if you are so inclined, whose doors are open. There is an abundance of beautiful literature, places to walk and sit, music to listen to, all of which can effectively allow you to transcend the chaos of your life. When it comes to healing and wellness, listen to the silence.

Make a list of the greatest sources of joy and happiness in your life. Take inventory of your most deeply held values. Examine the many options and choices you have in your life. Life is about choices, each with a consequence. Are your actions and choices a reflection of your values? Are you living your life in a way that fully nurtures your greatest sources of joy? Are you committed to changing the deeply rooted behavior patterns that widen the gap between real and ideal? If so, a more fulfilling and satisfying life awaits you! It is not beyond your reach. It is already within your grasp.

DO NOT MISS TAKE HOME POINTS

1. Strongly consider what you need to know to partner more effectively with your physician to achieve maximum health. These questions to your physician can assist in this purpose: What are the most important issues affecting my health? What would we like the outcome to be? What do we need to do to get there?
2. Anything that can be done to prevent disease is better than treating the disease once it occurs, as summarized in this chapter.
3. If you have diabetes, high blood pressure, or high cholesterol, understand what your treatment goals are. There is no reason you and your doctor cannot achieve high marks on your health report card.
4. Inertia and rationalization are the enemies of action and results!
5. Believe in yourself.

EPILOGUE

"We're on a mission from God."

—Jake and Elwood Blues

OUR HEALTH-CARE system is under tremendous stress. I do not think it would be an overstatement to say that we are in a crisis. We continue to confront escalating costs, obstacles to access, and widening disparities in quality care. I believe that many consumers of health care are unaware of the myriad issues currently gripping our system. I also believe that many consumers of health care see the health-care system's problems as the health-care system's problems. This is a societal challenge, big time. These are challenges that are shared by those who serve health care with those being served. As I have emphasized, ours is an aging society. We will experience longevity as none before us ever have. We are also a society under tremendous physical, mental, emotional, and spiritual stress! The net effect is a burgeoning demand for health-care services. We consume a lot of health care. The costs of applying more sophisticated technology, research, and information technology to a greater number of people, are becoming untenable to those who purchase health care—you, your employer, and the government.

Escalating costs for health care put us all at an economic disadvantage. Businesses lose their competitive edge and individuals struggle to find affordable coverage. Our government spends more on health care while fewer individuals are covered and necessary services cut back. While this is an enormously complex problem for all of us, we can each make a big contribution toward improvement by being savvy consumers (see the figure on page 317). Any system, in the end, needs to ensure universal coverage of agreed-upon basic, fundamental services. Funding will have to come from public and private sources.

The payers of health care—insurance companies, health maintenance organizations, the government—are scrambling to control escalating costs in the setting of escalating demand. This has led to dramatic inflationary pressures on premiums for employers and employees. As a result, higher co-pays, deductibles, and premiums are being passed on to employees. There are now an unprecedented number of bankruptcy filings, many of which are rooted in financial crisis created by devastating health-care expenditures. Major cuts are being made in covered services such as medications, home care, mental health, substance abuse, and addiction services that are offered by health plans. Many of our most vulnerable citizens such as the elderly, those with disabilities, and the uninsured are without protection or seeing their protection threatened as federal and state budgets have been forced to cut back on necessary services.

Despite a whopping 15 percent of our GNP being spent on health care—a phenomenal sum of money—more than 41 million Americans, many of whom work and have children, are without any coverage. It is estimated that at some point in the year 2002, 75 million Americans were without health insurance! The cost of prescription medications is becoming prohibitive and is frequently not covered or is associated with higher co-pays. Many states are examining strategies to obtain prescription medications from Canada, as many medications there are considerably cheaper.

As a nation we have incredible resources in health care. Ours is an immensely gifted and committed workforce. Unfortunately, our health-care system works much better for some people than for others. There is a marked and very worrying disparity with respect to access to care, resource utilization, and health outcomes between the well-insured and the uninsured. Ethnic minorities and people in lower socioeconomic groups often do not receive the same standards of care that exist for others. Employment is no longer a guarantee of health-care coverage as the costs of premiums are shifting, out of necessity, from employers to employees. More people have to piece together several part-time jobs to make ends meet, none of which provide health-care benefits. In many instances, health-care outcomes are better in countries that spend far less than we do to cover more of their citizens. Despite our resources abound, citizens more than ever before in the United States are in need of basic, fundamental services. As citizens of this remark-

"We're tired and we're not going to take it anymore!" . . . take a deep, cleansing breath . . . and repeat . . .

able country, we are all vested in the systems that ensure our health and wellness. It is time for people everywhere to stand up and say . . .

"What Can I Do to Help?"

At the risk of overstating my point, our health-care system is confronting a crisis that has a major consumer contribution. Improving our health-care system will not be possible without a significant shift in social awareness, understanding, and thinking about resource availability and utilization. There is potential for profoundly positive change to occur. The truth is this: Health-care systems—hospitals, clinics, administrators, physicians, nurses, researchers, and allied health professionals and management teams, cannot, as a system in isolation, sufficiently tend to the growing and complex needs of our communities. It is simply more than our system can handle. I believe this point deserves reemphasis. The American health-care system cannot, by itself, meet the growing needs, concerns, and disparities that currently exist in our communities.

These are complex problems, easily oversimplified in an effort to understand and debate. There are many powerful stakeholders who currently benefit from the status quo and who powerfully influence legislative policy. Uninformed, uncommitted, and uninspiring leadership here will continue to fail miserably. We seriously need grassroots dialogue, most importantly at a local level, where the "smallest," most effective unit of social capital can begin to leverage available resources to promote healthier communities more effectively. State and federal policy makers need to become informed and educated, and to debate these issues with greater understanding and conviction. With that said, and I do feel better, here are some parting thoughts on ways that we can "be closer than we currently are to organizing and applying our resources toward measurable improvements in community health.

1. Dispel the myth that the health-care system is solely responsible for the health of our communities.

Existing health-care systems should be viewed as being at the hub of many other community resources that have the potential to extend the reach of health and wellness. There are many other sources of community outreach, such as schools, workplace, senior centers, faith communities, and human services that could more effectively partner with our health-care resources in the fulfillment of these needs. Currently, in most communities, these resources are not "linked" in purpose, planning, resource utilization, data management, and quality improvement efforts. We are at a defining moment in the evolution of our health-care system. While I am not a sociologist, the community is a special, time-tested, fluid, adaptable, and very powerful social construct. Communities are what connect people. When people are connected, energy and information begin to flow.

Community coalitions of leaders in health care, business, pastoral care, education, government, and human services (to name a few) are "ripe" for linkage and alignment of vision, purpose, and creative exploration of options and opportunities as they relate to the leveraging of available resources to meet the needs of our communities. A spontaneous combustion of ideas could emerge, allowing greater alignment of goals, interests, and mission. There would be a sobering recognition of duplication of time, energy, human and financial resources that would allow more efficient options to emerge. There would be a sobering affirmation of shared frustrations, obstacles, and limitations. There would also be an inspiration and motivation emerging that like-minded people, when linked together, can bring about—new, different, and very exciting. Relationships would be strengthened and purpose more shared and focused. This could only serve to strengthen the foundation upon which our community health stands.

2. Health care in America is mired down with waste.

At the risk of pontificating, many of the resources funneled through our gigantic enterprise are not well spent. For example, it is estimated that approximately twenty-five cents of every dollar spent in health care is an administrative price tag. There are far too many people involved with billing, insurance claims, referral processes, pre-approval processes, and so on. We need to examine ways to trim this incredible waste. The avalanche of information, documentation, and health-care management has served to mire down our system in excessive expense, duplication, and inefficiency. We need to move toward a system where information is reliable, consistent, secure, easily retrieved, manageable, and universal. One of the great innovations in health care is the integration of information technology. While other industries have realized the incredible potential of this technology, health care is just catching on. Electronic information, data storage and management, and communication will revolutionize the way medicine is practiced.

Physicians order a lot of unnecessary tests, and as technology has become more sophisticated and expensive, this adds up to a lot of money. There are many reasons for this—a defensive posture for fear of litigation, consumer demand and expectation, ready availability, market demand, and profit motive. Science and technology have galloped ahead faster than our ability to apply it in a more cost effective fashion. We need to develop practice efficiencies that will allow us all to make better use of our available resources. We need to reinvigorate trust as the currency with which our relationships are based and our decisions made.

3. Consumer responsibility

The theme woven throughout *The Savvy Patient* is that of our vital and shared responsibility for improving the effectiveness of our health-care encounters and indeed, our health-care system. As consumers, we have a profound role in both the contribution to health care's problems and in shaping the necessary changes to more effectively meet the needs of an aging, more complex society. So how can we as individuals more effectively meet these challenges?

- Be educated about our health-care system and how best to utilize its precious resources.
- Be informed about your health care, your medications, your insurance, and your available diagnostic and treatment options. An informed consumer clearly has an edge in navigating health-care encounters.
- Be responsible for your health, wellness, disease prevention, and treatment! Take steps, literally and figuratively, to become healthier.
- Consider, when appropriate, the option of consuming less, again literally and figuratively. I do not mean to sound facetious. Americans are master consumers, of all things, health care and otherwise. I, too, am a member of this large club. Consumption drives up prices, given the inflationary pressures of an open market. I am not at all opposed to open markets in health care. There is no incentive greater than competition to improve quality, service, and efficiency. It is over-consumption that drives much of the duplicative waste in health care. Many health-care dollars are spent on minor health problems such as cold and cough symptoms, sore throat, and back strain, and on unnecessary testing, for problems that would normally get better on their own.
- Enormous sums of money are spent treating problems that could dramatically and profoundly be altered by behavioral and lifestyle changes. These changes, for example, activity, caloric restraint, and better health choices are the key to both successful primary prevention of diseases in people at risk—activity and nutritional

changes decrease and may prevent diabetes in many people, and secondary prevention such as reducing the risk of another heart attack, stroke, or death by application of evidence-based medical information.

- If you have values, wishes, and preferences regarding advance directives, your desire for or against "heroic measures," or organ donation, make those who care for you aware of these wishes. Tell your physician. You are never "locked in" and always have the option and right to change your thoughts and wishes at any time. There are far too many unspoken conversations that need to be had between family members and between you and your physician.

- If you are lost and need help understanding how to get Medicaid or free care (if available), call your local hospital or community elder services or local division of human services. *Be patient. Be prepared for frustration. Persevere.* You may be surprised at what you are eligible for once you are directed to the appropriate community resources and understand the processes involved. If you are uninsured and need medical attention, call your local hospital and inquire if there is a community clinic that will see you and perhaps assist with pursuit of coverage, forms to be filled out, and free care.

- In the decision-making process, feel comfortable discussing explicitly the "risk-benefit and cost-effectiveness" of the test or treatment under consideration. A physician might order a test, for example a CAT scan of the brain for a headache or an MRI for your back pain, that will not likely change the overall diagnosis, prognosis, or treatment plan. Tests are sometimes expected by consumers, necessary for reassurance, or insisted upon by a demanding consumer. A lot of tests could be avoided with clear, trusting communication, understanding, appropriate attention to follow-up, and reasonable contingency plans.

- Ask for equivalent generic prescription alternatives, when available, and definitely compare nonprescription store brands with national brand names when it comes to price and ingredients.

- Avoid antibiotics whenever the suspicion is greatest for a viral infection, particularly in the first seven to ten days. If you and your physician agree, you will avoid many unnecessary antibiotics for problems that would get better anyway with time. You also diminish the risk of promoting "resistant strains" of bacteria that increasingly posing a serious threat to people at risk.

- *Feeling well does not mean all is well!* Many potentially serious health-care problems are silent—high blood pressure, diabetes, high cholesterol, and colon cancer, to name a few. *Be proactive! This is about you, your precious life! People care about you. People need you. Care about yourself!* Promote your health. Make health promotion and disease prevention a mission in your life. Prevention is so much more effective than treatment once the problem develops.

- Write, call, and tell your legislators that you want reform, open dialogue, and debate and that the status quo is no longer acceptable.

4. Reform of Our Malpractice System

Health-care providers spend enormous sums of money in an effort to lower the risk of getting sued. Unnecessary tests are ordered and more energy is placed on securing evidence to cover all possible outcomes than in securing trusting relationships that in the end are more lasting, effective, and therapeutic. Physicians are leaving communities because of rapidly escalating malpractice insurance premium costs. This is a significant problem in my home state of Massachusetts. Some clinicians are cutting back on their scope of practice to reduce the medical-legal risk. Not a day goes by when a physician does not consider the possibility of a lawsuit.

I could not agree more that people need vigorous assurance that licensed physicians and allied health professionals meet and maintain an acceptable standard of care. However, it is not necessary to spend scores of billions of dollars "just to be on the safe side." There should be better quality management processes for health-care professionals to more effectively reduce medical errors and improve patient safety.

We desperately need reform of our malpractice system. Litigation, necessary though it is at times, is not always the best option to resolve disputes. Nor has our current litigation system reduced medical errors. It has not served patients well either, as a very small percentage of malpractice claims actually end up in court providing justice to those who are victims of substandard care. Most medical errors do not occur because of clinical incompetence. They occur because of flawed systems that allow a sequence of remediable warnings to march forward, resulting in eventual harm. Improving health-care systems and processes are the best way to prevent errors from occurring in the first place. Other industries have known this for many years. There are also alternative dispute resolution options that are more effective and efficient than our current system of litigation.

Mediation, a process involving a neutral facilitator, allows all parties involved to openly exchange thoughts, concerns, and options for reconciliation. In mediation, the parties craft the outcome. These processes may reduce the costs of time, money, and diminished relationships. They may also allow opportunity for systems and behavioral change that would serve to decrease the likelihood of a similar event happening to someone else. Some people have advocated removing medical malpractice cases from the current court system altogether. Instead, having a separate, independent panel or tribunal of medical experts reviewing and deciding on the case could lead to more fair, balanced, and less expensive outcomes.

With tremendous work, perseverance, patience, and a long-term perspective, our health-care system can achieve its greatest potential ever. You are an important contributor. In conclusion, we need renewed emphasis on:

- Health-care professional skill development in communication, conflict management, empathy, and relationship building
- Development of health-care leadership
- Greater consumer education and awareness
- Greater consumer empowerment and understanding
- Greater consumer savvy in knowledge and practice
- Greater trust as the antidote to defensive medical practices
- Attitude shifts that view health care as an active partnership instead of a passive exchange of services and information
- Leveraging social capital to create healthier communities through creative partnerships and interdisciplinary collaboration

Oh yes, I almost forgot. Our health-care system could use a lot of prayer, if you are so inclined. There is however, reason for hope. After all, as Jake and Elwood Blues said, in their noble effort to resurrect The Blues Brothers . . . "we're on a mission from God."

Figure 1: The Economic Implications of Being a Savvy Health-Care Consumer

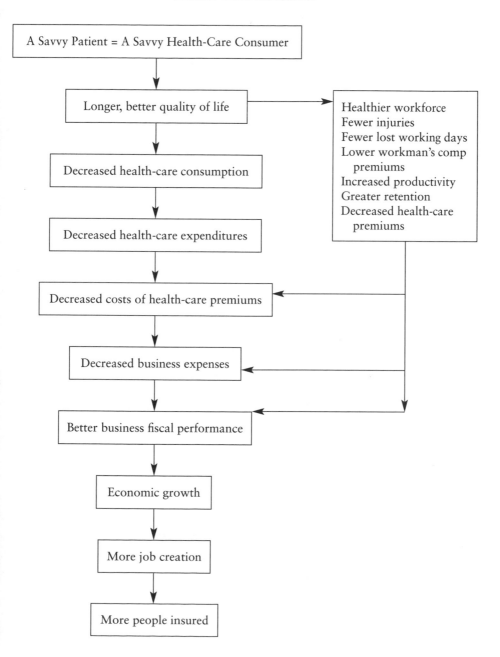

SUGGESTED READING

August, Yosaif, and Siegel, Bernie. *Help Me to Heal: A Practical Guidebook for Patients, Visitors, and Caregivers: Essential Tools, Strategies and Resources for Healthy Hospitalizations and Home.* Hay House (August 2003).

Dossey, Larry. *Reinventing Medicine: Beyond Mind-Body to a New Era of Healing.* HarperCollins; first edition (September 1999).

Dossey, Larry. *Healing Beyond the Body: Medicine and the Infinite Reach of the Mind.* Random House; first edition (October 16, 2001).

Edell, Dean. *Life, Liberty, and the Pursuit of Healthiness: Dr. Dean's Common-sense Guide for Anything That Ails You.* HarperCollins; first edition (December 23, 2003).

Fisher, Roger, Ury, William, and Patten, Bruce. *Getting to Yes: Negotiating Agreement Without Giving In.* Penguin USA; second edition (December 1991).

Groupman, Jerome. *The Anatomy of Hope: How People Prevail in the Face of Illness.* Random House (December 23, 2003).

Hyman, Mark, Liponis, Mark. *Ultraprevention: The 6-Week Plan That Will Make You Healthy for Life.* Scribner (September 16, 2003).

Kabat-Zinn, Jon. *Full Catastrophe Living: Using the Wisdom of Your Body and Mind to Face Stress, Pain, and Illness.* Delta; reprint edition (May 1, 1990).

Matthews, Dale A. *The Faith Factor: Proof of the Healing Power of Prayer.* Penguin USA (April 1999).

Santorelli, Santi. *Heal Thy Self: Lessons on Mindfulness in Medicine.* Harmony/Bell Tower (March 7, 2000).

Weil, Andrew T. *Natural Health, Natural Medicine.* Houghton Mifflin; revised edition (May 20, 1998).

REFERENCES

Chapter 1: Finding a Primary Care Provider

Backer LA. Strategies for better patient flow and cycle time. Fam Pract Manag 2002;9(6):45–50.

Chapter 2: The Pre-Hospital Emergency System

Cummins RO. ACLS Provider Manual. Dallas: American Heart Association; 2001.

Chapter 4: Coping in the Midst of Illness

Griffith JL, Griffith ME. Spirituality and coping with depression. Health and Spirituality Connection. 2002;5:3.

Matthews D. The Faith Factor. New York, NY: Penguin Books; 1999.

Pargament KL, Koenig HG, Nielson J. Religious coping and health status in medically ill hospitalized older adults. J Nerv Ment Dis. 1998;186(9):513–521.

Van Oyen WC, Ludwig TE, Vander LK, Granting forgiveness or harboring grudges: implications for emotion, physiology, and health. Psychol Sci. 2001; 12(2):117–123.

Chapter 6: Advance Care Planning

Gunter-Hunt G., Sieger MJ. A comparison of state advanced directive documents. *Gerontologist.* 2002;42(1):51–60.

Guyatte G, Cook DJ, Rocher G, Sjokvist P, et al. Cardiopulmonary resuscitation directives on admission to intensive-care unit: An international observational study. *Lancet.* 2001;358:1941–1945.

Perkins HS, Geppert GM, Gonzales A, Cortez JD, et al. Cross-cultural similarities and differences in attitudes about advanced care planning. *J Gen Int Med.* 2002;17:48–57.

Prendergrest TJ, Puntillo KP. Withdrawal of life support. Intensive care at the end of life. *JAMA.* 2002;288:2732–2744.

Snyder L. Advanced care planning. *American College of Physicians. PIER.* 2002. Available online at: http://pier.acponline.org/physicians/ethical_legal/ el143/background/el1 43_sl.html.

Chapter 8: Spirituality, Religion, and Health

Asser SM, Swan R. Child fatalities from religion-motivated medical neglect. *Pediatrics.* 1998;101(4):625–629.

Byrd RC. Positive therapeutic effects of intercessory prayer in a coronary care unit. *South Med J.* 1988;81:826–829.

Harris WS, Gowda M, Kolb JW, Strycacz CP, et al. A randomized controlled trial of the effects of remote, intercessory prayer on outcomes in patients admitted to the coronary care unit, *Arch Int Med.* 1999;159(19):2273–2278.

Kaczorowski JM. Spiritual well-being and anxiety in adults diagnosed with cancer. *Hospice J.* 1989;5:105–116.

Koeneg HG, George LK, Peterson BL, Religiosity and Remission of Depression in Medically Ill Older Patients. *Am J Psych.* 1998;155(4):536–542.

Koenig H., Cohen HJ, George LK, Hays JC, et al. Attendance at religious services, interleukin-6, and other biological parameters of immune function in older adults. *Int. J. Psych Med.* 1997;27(3):233–250.

Koenig HG, Hays JC, Larson DB, George LK, et al, Does religious attendance prolong survival? A six-year follow-up study of 3,968 older adults. *J Gerontol A Biol Sci Med Sci.* 1999;54(7):M370–376.

Koenig HG, Larson DB. Use of hospital services, religious attendance, and religious affiliation. *South Med J.* 1998;91(10):925–932.

Matthews D. The Faith Factor. New York, NY: Penguin Books; 1999.

Matthews DA, McCullough ME, Larson DB, Koenig HG, et al. Religious commitment and health status: a review of the research and implications for family medicine. *Arch Fam Med.* 1998;7(2):118–124.

McCullough ME, Hoyt WT, Larson DB, Koenig HG et al. Religious involvement and mortality: a meta-analytic review. *Health Psychology.* 2001;19(3):211–222.

Pettus, M. Developing a spirituality-medicine curriculum in a community teaching hospital. *Academic Medicine.* 2002;77(7):745.

Puchalski CM, Romer AL. Taking a spiritual history allows clinicians to understand patients more fully. *J Pall Med.*2000;3:129–137.

Yates JW, Chalmer BJ, St James P, Follansbee M, et al. Religion in patients with advanced cancer. *Med Pediatr Oncol.* 1981; 9(2):121–128.

Chapter 9: Making Difficult Medical Decisions

Fisher R, Fisher E. Patient decision making: in search of good decisions. *Effective Clinical Practices.* July/August 1999;2:189–190.

Chapter 11: Taking Medications

Newman JG. Did I take my medications today? Tips to help you remember. *Pharmacy Times.* 2002. August Insert.

U. S. Food and Drug Administration. Office of Generic Drugs. May 1998. Available online at: http://www.fda.gov/cder/ogd/.

Chapter 12: Contemplating Nursing Home Placement

Nursing Homes. An Overview. Article available online at: http://www.medicine.gov/nursing/overview.asp.

Chapter 13: Preparing for Surgery

Birkmeyer JD, Siewers AE, Marth NJ, Goodman DC.Regionalization of high-risk surgery and implications for patient travel times [abstract]. *JAMA*, November 26, 2003; 290(20):2703–2708.

Birkmeyer JD, Stukel TA, SIEWERS AE, Goodney PP.Surgeon volume and operative mortality in the United States. *New Engl J Med.* 2003; 349(22):2117–2127.

Chapter 14: Complementary and Alternative Medicine

De Smet PA, Herbal remedies. *New Engl J Med.* 2002;347:2046–2056.

Ernst E. The risk-benefit profile of commonly used herbal therapies: ginkgo, St. John's Wort, ginseng, Echinacea, saw palmetto, and kava. *Ann Int Med.* 2002;136:42–53.

Fleetwood J. Complementary and Alternative Health. May 2002. Available online at: http://pier.acponline.org/physicians/ethical_legal/el443/background/el443-sl .html.

Kronenberg F, Fugh-Berman A. Complementary and alternative medicine for menopausal symptoms: a review of randomized, controlled trials. *Ann Int Med.* 2002;137:805–814.

National Center for Complementary and Alternative Medicine. Information available online at: http://nccam.nih.gov.

Chapter 15: Health-Care Literacy

Baker L, Wagner T, Singer S, Bundorf MK. Use of the Internet and e-mail for health-care information. *JAMA.* 2003;289:2400–2401.

Chin T. Patients think if it's pretty, it must be smart. *American Medical News.* 2002;45:1.

Houts PS, Witmer JT, Egeth HE, Loscalzo MJ, Zabora JR. Using pictographs to enhance recall of spoken medical instructions. *Patient Education Couns.* 2001: 43(3):231–242.

Kurtzweil P. How to spot health fraud. *FDA Consumer Magazine*. Nov-Dec 1999. Available at: http://www.fda.gov/fdac/features/1999/699_fraud.html.

Schillinger D, Grumbach K, Piette J, Wang F, et al. Association of health literacy with diabetes outcomes. *JAMA*. 2002;288:475–482.

Williams MV, Baker DW, Honig EG, et al. Inadequate literacy is a barrier to asthma knowledge and self-care. *Chest*. 1998;114:1008–1015.

Williams MV, Parker RM, Baker DW. Recognizing and overcoming inadequate health literacy, a barrier to care. *Clev Clin J Med*. 2002;69:415–418.

Wilson J. The crucial link between literacy and health, Ann Int Med. 2003;139(10):875–878.

Chapter 16: Managing Conflict

Fisher R, Ury, W. *Getting to Yes*. New York, NY: Penguin Books; 1983.

Goleman D. *Emotional Intelligence*. New York, NY: Bantam Books;1995.

Marcus LJ, Kritek P, Dorn B, Miller V, Wyatt J. *Renegotiating Health Care: Resolving Conflict to Build Collaboration*. San Francisco: Jossey-Bass; 1995.

Stone, D, Patton B, Heen S. *Difficult Conversations*. New York, NY: Bantam Books; 1999.

Chapter 17: Health-Care Coverage

Krafchick S. How do health insurance companies cover pre-existing conditions? July 2002. Available online at: http://content.health.msn.com/content/dmk/dmk_article_5462871.

McCoy P. Claim denied! February 2000. Available online at: http://content.health.msn.com/question_and_answer/article/1691.50156.

McCoy P. Opting for long-term insurance. March 2000. Available online at: http://content.health.msn.com/question_and_answer/article/1691.50203.

McCoy P. Weighing insurance options. July 2002. Available online at: http://content.health.msn.com/question_and_answer/article/1691.50105.

McCoy, P. Supplementing Medicare. July 2002. Available online at: http://content.health.msn.com/question_and_answer/article/1691.50091.

Medicare information available online at: http://www.medicare.gov.

Shields J. How do I get the best coverage? Sept. 2000. Available online at: http://content.health.msn.com/question_and_answer/article/1691.50630.

Shields J. Insurance out of town. July 2000. Available online at: http://content.health.msn.com/question_and_answer/article/1691.50453.

Shields J. When health plans refuse to pay. August 2000. Available online at: http://content.health.msn.com/question_and_answer/article/1691.50532.

Wilson R. Choosing the right health plan. July 2002. Available online at: http://content.health.msn.com/question_and_answer/article/1691.50068.

Chapter 20: Parting Wisdom

Hu FB, Willett WC, Optimal diets for prevention of CHD. *JAMA.* 2002; 288:2569–2578.

Sox HC. Disease prevention guidelines from the U.S. Preventive Services Task Force. *Ann Int Med.* 2002;136(2):155–156.

Wart PJ. The type of fat affects diabetic risk. December 2002. Available online at: http://vanderbiltowc.wellsource.com/dh/content.asp?id=653.

Whooley MA, Avins AL, Miranda J, Browner WS. Case-finding instruments for depression. two questions are as good as many. *J Gen Intern Med.* 1997; 12(7):439–445.

INDEX

ABOUT THE AUTHOR

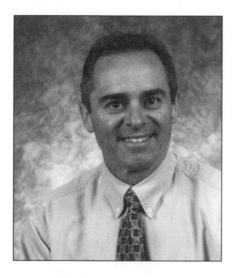

Mark C. Pettus, M.D. is the Chief of Staff and Associate Chairman of the Department of Medicine at Berkshire Medical Center in Western Massachusetts. He also serves as the Associate Program Director in Internal Medicine at Berkshire Medical Center. He is Board Certified in Internal Medicine and Nephrology and is a Clinical Associate Professor of Medicine at the University of Massachusetts Medical School. He is a diplomate of the Harvard School of Public Health's Advanced Program in Health Care Negotiations and Conflict Resolution. His areas of interest, in addition to patient care, are bedside skills, interpersonal skill development, medical education, the faith-health connection, conflict resolution, negotiation, and leadership in health care. He is a consultant and speaks regionally and nationally on a variety of health-related topics. Visit his website at www.savvypatient.com.